Language and Literacy Development

Language and Literacy Development

An Interdisciplinary Focus on English Learners with Communication Disorders

Linda I. Rosa-Lugo
Florin M. Mihai
Joyce W. Nutta

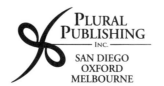

PLURAL
PUBLISHING
— INC. —

SAN DIEGO
OXFORD
MELBOURNE

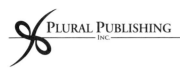

5521 Ruffin Road
San Diego, CA 92123

e-mail: info@pluralpublishing.com
Web site: http://www.pluralpublishing.com

49 Bath Street
Abingdon, Oxfordshire OX14 1EA
United Kingdom

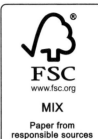

FSC
www.fsc.org
MIX
Paper from
responsible sources
FSC® C011935

Typeset in 11/13 Garamond Book by Flanagan's Publishing Services, Inc.
Printed in the United States of America by McNaughton & Gunn

Cover design by Omar D. Martinez. Cover images are of Matthew Cory
French and Tailin Jade Thompson. Copyright 2012 by Omar D. Martinez.

Library of Congress Cataloging-in-Publication Data

Rosa-Lugo, Linda I.
 Language and literacy development : an interdisciplinary focus on English
learners with communication disorders / Linda I. Rosa-Lugo, Florin Mihai,
Joyce W. Nutta. — 1st ed.
  p. ; cm.
 Includes bibliographical references and index.
 ISBN-13: 978-1-59756-332-1 (alk. paper)
 ISBN-10: 1-59756-332-3 (alk. paper)
 I. Mihai, Florin. II. Nutta, Joyce W. III. Title.
 [DNLM: 1. Communication Disorders. 2. Language Development. WL 340.2]

 616.85'5—dc23
          2012000428

Contents

Foreword

A significant challenge facing our nation is the cultivation of a literate citizenry. The well-being of our democracy depends on it. The work of educational institutions is largely focused on meeting this challenge that is complicated by many factors, including response to the needs of large and growing populations of English learners (ELs), as well as students with communication disorders in our schools. The current emphasis on preparation of children and adolescents to meet the high expectations of the Common Core State Standards, geared to postsecondary education and workforce readiness, further intensifies the challenge. When addressing the literacy needs of children and adolescents with communication disorders who are also learning English as another language, the challenge increases exponentially.

Educators from a variety of disciplines and with different job responsibilities need to know how to help these youth to become literate within the context of escalating curriculum demands. Although it is true that considerable attention has been paid in the literature to the education of ELs and to the problems of students with communication disorders, rarely has the work of both disciplines been integrated sufficiently to create a comprehensive context for addressing the literacy needs of ELs with communication disorders. Happily, this book helps to fill this void and makes a major contribution to education in general by doing so, not just to the disciplines of teaching English to speakers of other languages (TESOL) and speech-language pathology. It will be a great asset to a variety of professionals in schools, as well as to researchers formulating inquiries to elucidate effective practices.

However, English for speakers of other languages (ESOL) teachers and speech-language pathologists (SLPs) will be especially thankful for the detailed information that the book provides, because a shared information base is a springboard for collaboration. One can certainly argue that the complexity of facilitating literacy proficiency in ELs with communication disorders calls for approaches involving meaningful collaboration among all professionals working with these students, but special partnerships among ESOL professionals and SLPs are essential to this work. Background information about the populations and the disciplines themselves, catalog of relevant legal issues, clarification of terminology, practical application of important theories and practical assessment, and instruction/intervention suggestions will provide grist for the collaboration mill.

What I especially appreciate about this book is that the medium is the message; that is, Drs. Rosa-Lugo, Mihai, and Nutta have indeed engaged in meaningful collaboration themselves to bring together these professional worlds in order to guide professionals in meeting the complex needs of English learners with communication disorders. More of this kind of substantive interdisciplinary work is sorely needed to solve the complex problems educators face in helping youth prepare for a productive future. Kudos and thanks to these authors with the hope that their collaborative example will set the stage for partnerships among researchers and practitioners on behalf of children and adolescents with communication disorders in our schools who are struggling to meet high curriculum standards while learning the English language as another language.

Barbara J. Ehren, Ed.D., CCC-SLP, ASHA Fellow
Board Recognized Specialist in Child Language
Professor
Director of the Doctoral Program
Department of Communication Sciences and Disorders
University of Central Florida

Organization of the Text

The primary focus of this book is to provide the reader with information on language and literacy development for English learners (ELs) with communication disorders. Specifically, we discuss evidence-based practical strategies in the identification, assessment, and intervention of ELs with communication disorders. We also provide the reader with a description of the challenges surrounding the assessment and management of ELs with communication disorders. Written from the perspective of two disciplines, communication sciences and disorders (CSD) and ESOL (English for speakers of other languages) the authors merge their expertise to discuss the knowledge, skills, and competencies each professional must demonstrate in order to facilitate language and literacy development in ELs with communication disorders. The primary audience for this book is for school-based speech-language pathologists. The book is also intended for all professionals who are responsible for teaching language and literacy skills, such as the ESOL professional, general and special educators, bilingual teachers, reading coaches, and school administrators.

Chapter 1 presents the rationale for the content of this book. In each chapter, key terms are presented to provide the reader with core common terminology that is used to discuss ELs. The importance of evidence-based practice (EBP) and its use by speech-language pathologists (SLPs) and ESOL professionals in working with ELs are discussed. An illustrative case study is offered to highlight and examine some of the challenges and complexities faced in the identification, assessment, and management of ELs with communication disorders. Specifically, the challenge of differentiating that a child is in the process of acquiring a second language from a disability requires that professionals possess specific competencies and expertise. To successfully and effectively address the language and literacy development of ELs, both groups of professionals must understand each other's training, knowledge, and expertise—in other words, each professional must understand what they each "bring to the table" to work collaboratively to address the language and literacy development of ELs with communication disorders.

Chapter 2 presents some of the challenges faced by SLPs and ESOL professionals in working with ELs. SLPs and ESOL professionals providing services to ELs with communication disorders are required to work within their scope of practice, knowledge base, skills, competencies, and education. An overview of the specialized competencies necessary for SLPs and ESOL professionals to work with ELs with communication disorders in several service delivery models, as well as their new and expanded role in language and literacy, are discussed. The professional organizations of both disciplines, ASHA and TESOL, have official position statements on a broad range of issues related to ELs (e.g., identification of ELs with special educational needs; language and literacy development of ELs). These position statements provide both professionals with recommended competencies and preferred practices and are used to guide their practice within the standards set for each of the professions.

Chapter 3 provides an overview of the increasing EL population, their characteristics, and key legal mandates governing the assessment and intervention of ELs. This chapter also provides similar information for ELs with special needs in general, and ELs with communication disorders in particular.

Chapter 4 provides readers with basic background information on first and second language acquisition. In order for SLPs to conduct an accurate assessment of a communication disorder, they must be able to distinguish normal progression in a second language from those aspects of language that represents a communication disorder.

Chapter 5 offers a definition of literacy and provides the reader with an overview of literacy development in ELs. An emphasis is placed on L2 reading, L2 writing, and schema, and how these operations contribute to the literacy development of ELs and ELs with communication disorders.

Chapters 6 and 7 provide the reader with a definition of language proficiency and how this construct has been assessed. The importance of identification practices and protocols used by SLPs and ESOL professionals to determine language proficiency and how this information is used to conduct accurate assessments of ELs, and specifically ELs with communication disorders is discussed.

Chapter 8 explores classroom practices and strategies used to promote language and literacy development in ELs and ELs with communication disorders.

The last chapter focuses on the importance of collaboration and team work by SLPs and ESOL professionals in facilitating language and literacy development for ELs with communication disorders.

Acknowledgments

This was by far the most difficult page to write. We wanted to make sure to thank everyone who supported and contributed to this project. We also wanted to convey how it feels to finally complete this interdisciplinary work. This book required the partnership of two professions, speech-language pathology and English for speakers of other languages (ESOL). We could not have asked for better partners. We did not know each other well at the beginning of this project. Nonetheless, we spent countless hours sharing similar stories, experiences, and concerns about our work with English learner students and their families. These conversations led us to better understand what we each do to support language and literacy development in diverse school-age children. Despite our different yet complementary professional disciplines, these dialogues offered us the opportunity to explore how we could work together in a more meaningful way to provide optimal learning environments and effective interventions for English learners.

We thank the Plural Publishing family for allowing us to share the findings of those conversations in this book and specifically to Dr. Sadanand Singh, who saw value in this interdisciplinary project. He provided us with our book title.

The first author is indebted to the University of Central Florida for their support in the form of a one-year sabbatical leave and to the graduate students of the Department of Communication Sciences and Disorders, who provided feedback during the writing of this manuscript.

Specifically, we thank the USDOE, OSEP office for funding the personnel preparation grant "University of Central Florida Collaborative for Preparing School Speech-Language Pathologists to Serve English Language Learners with Communication Disorders (Project SLP~ELL)." This initiative allowed the three authors to partner across disciplines to work with the grant scholars. These experiences provided much of the focus for this book.

We express our gratitude to those who assisted in the review of the manuscript and offered suggestions that were helpful in the writing of this book. We thank the various authors and publishing companies who provided us with permission to reprint tables and figures to support the content in this book. In particular we are grateful for the graduate students enrolled in our respective programs who spent countless hours proofreading, editing, and giving us feedback on the manuscript (Valentin Alonso, Lauren Armstrong, Alexandra Arredondo, Deanna Lopez, Ivanna Ortiz, and Alison Youngblood).

We would like to thank Omar D. Martinez for the book cover, with a special thank you to the parents of Matthew Cory French and Tailin Jade Thompson for allowing them to appear on the book cover.

We dedicate this book to students who are English learners and to the professionals who work with passion to facilitate the language and literacy success of school-age students. We hope that our focus on collaboration will have a positive impact on English learners, and specifically English learners with communication disorders.

Finally, we could not have accomplished this work without the support of our friends and colleagues. Specifically, we thank our families for their unwavering support and words of confidence ("You can do this . . . "). Thank you for supporting us in our professional endeavors.

Linda I. Rosa-Lugo
Florin M. Mihai
Joyce W. Nutta

1

English Learners — The Merging of Two Disciplines

Introduction

English learners (ELs) represent the fastest growing segment of the school-age population in the United States (Matthews & Ewen, 2006; National Clearinghouse for English Language Acquisition [NCELA], 2006). Nearly one in five Americans speaks a language other than English at home and projections suggest that "language minority students" (those who speak a language other than English at home and who have varying levels of proficiency in English) will comprise over 40% of school-age children by 2030 (Padolsky, 2005; Thomas & Collier, 2001).

Although ELs can be found in all the states across the United States, they tend to be heavily concentrated in six states: California, Texas, Florida, New York, Illinois, and Arizona. In many states, the growth of the EL population is a direct result of steady immigration from North, Central, South America and Asia through the 1990s and into the beginning of the 21st century. The language background of ELs is very diverse and, according to the US Census Bureau data (http://www.census.gov), reflects approximately 350 native languages. However, almost 80% identify Spanish as their native language (Hopstock & Stephenson, 2003). Seventy-six percent of all ELs enrolled at the elementary level and 72% of all secondary education speak Spanish as their native language (Capps, Fix, Murray, Ost, Passel, & Herwantoro, 2005). The next most commonly reported native languages were Vietnamese (2.4%) and Hmong (1.8%). Table 1–1 lists the ten most common language groups of ELs in the US.

Almost 45% of US teachers have at least one student designated as an EL in their classrooms (Hopstock & Stephenson, 2003). These students represent a myriad of backgrounds and experiences. They are either newly arrived immigrants or refugees (learning the language and getting acquainted with US culture), US born in households where English is not the primary language of communication, or sojourners (people from other countries who are working or studying in the US for a finite period of time) (Capps, Fix, Murray, Ost, Passel, & Herwantoro, 2005). Overall, in 2000, from the total of over 3 million ELs, only 36% were first generation (foreign-born children of foreign-born parents), 42% were second generation (US-born children of foreign-born parents), and 22% were third generation (US-born

Table 1–1. *Ten Most Common Languages Spoken by ELs*

Language	Percentage of ELs
Spanish	76.9%
Vietnamese	2.4
Hmong	1.8
Korean	1.2
Arabic	1.2
Haitian Creole	1.1
Cantonese	1.0
Tagalog	0.9
Russian	0.9
Navajo	0.9

Source: Adapted from *Descriptive Study of Services to LEP Students with Disabilities Special Topic Report #2. Analysis of Office of Civil Rights Data Related to LEP Students,* by P. J. Hopstock and T. G Stephenson, 2003, Washington, DC: US Department of Education, OELA. Retrieved from http://www.ncela.gwu.edu

children of US-born parents). If we look at the percentages of ELs at the elementary and secondary level by generation, we notice that they are consistent with the overall percentages discussed previously, clearly showing that the majority of ELs are US born (Tables 1–2 and 1–3).

In the US, ELs are educated in a variety of instructional environments in the school setting. These can include: (1) all-English instruction with some support related to their limited English proficiency; (2) all-English instruction with no support related to their limited English proficiency; or (3) programs that make some use of their home language. If ELs have special needs, such as a communication disorder, then a number of well-delivered research based instruction, intervention and delivery models are considered and implemented to address their communication disorders (e.g., pull-out speech-language therapy in a small group; push-in therapy in the classroom; see Chapter 2 for more information on program options) (Moore-Brown & Montgomery, 2005). Despite the array of instructional environments, inter-

Table 1–2. *Elementary and Secondary School ELs by Generation*

School Level	1st Generation ELs	2nd Generation ELs	3rd Generation ELs	US-Born ELs
Elementary	24%	58%	18%	76%
Secondary	44%	27%	29%	56%

Source: Data from R. Capps, M. Fix, J. Murray, J. Ost, J. Passel, and S. Herwantoro, 2005, *The New Demography of America's Schools: Immigration and the No Child Left Behind Act.* Washington, DC: The Urban Institute.

Table 1–3. *Country of Birth of ELs*

Country	Percentage
United States	47.3%
Mexico	25.9
Colombia	2.1
China	2.0
Russia	1.4
Puerto Rico	1.3
Yemen	1.3
Iraq	1.0
India	0.8
Brazil	0.8
Other	16.1

Source: Data from R. Capps, M. Fix, J. Murray, J. Ost, J. Passel, and S. Herwantoro, 2005, *The New Demography of America's Schools: Immigration and the No Child Left Behind Act.* Washington, DC: The Urban Institute.

vention designs and delivery methods for ELs, there are critical questions educators should ask themselves. First, is the amount, quality, and design of the support and instruction ELs receive appropriate? Additionally, do the instructional practices and service delivery models that are being used in the public school setting facilitate student achievement, specifically for ELs with communication disorders (Goldenberg, 2008)?

In the absence of careful planning and implementation of effective instructional practices, ELs are at risk of becoming academic underachievers with limited vocational and economic opportunities. The level of academic achievement among ELs, measured as a subgroup, is lower than that of proficient English-speaking learners. This is not surprising given that they are learning a new language. Language learning is a complex, dynamic process that forms the foundation for academic skills. In fact, students classified as "limited English proficient (LEP)" are often deemed to have lower academic abilities and may be placed in lower ability groups than native English-speaker peers (President's Advisory Commission on Educational Excellence for Hispanic American, 2003). These students often do not meet state norms for reading in English according to education agency reports from 41 states (Kindler, 2002).

Beginning with basic communication skills, ELs face an uphill battle to acquire the sophisticated verbal skills needed for college entry or career success. Moreover, there is a wide range of educational policies and practices that either help or hinder this process. The challenge for school professionals is to determine how best to work together to provide appropriate and effective instruction for students who are ELs. The emphasis on shared responsibility for all students demands a foundation of shared knowledge from which school professionals can work.

In order to build this foundation, this book focuses on the knowledge, skills and competencies of two specific school professionals, the speech-language pathologist (SLPs) and the English for speakers of other languages (ESOL) professional who works with ELs in the public school setting. The role of these two professionals in the public school setting and how their disciplines interact in working with ELs in language and literacy is explored. Possible ways in which they may collaborate to work with school-age children who are developing English proficiency and literacy, and who exhibit communication disorders are also explored. The roles and responsibilities of each professional as defined by their respective national organizations (e.g., ASHA [American Speech-Language-Hearing Association] and TESOL [Teachers of English to Speakers of Other Languages]), and, the collaboration that is required of the SLP and the ESOL in the identification, assessment, and intervention of ELs is discussed as we consider the use of evidence-based approaches and practical strategies that can be used to facilitate language and literacy in ELs by the SLP and ESOL professional.

Are SLP and ESOL Professionals Prepared to Work with ELs?

A Changing Society

ELs present a specific challenge to school professionals due to the linguistic diversity and proficiency they possess in their first and second languages (Collier, 2000; Klingner, Artiles, Kozleski, Harry, Zion, & Tate et al., 2005; Roseberry-McKibbin, 2000). These students are required to grapple with the dual demands of learning to speak English and achieve academically. Yet they often do not enter school with similar English language skills and academic preparedness as their English speaking counterparts. ELs lag significantly behind their fluent English-speaking peers in language and literacy and are at risk for underachievement and subsequently dropping out of high school (August, 2003; Haskins & Rouse, 2005). To obtain an understanding of the challenges faced by ELs and the role of each professional (e.g., speech-language pathologist and English as a second language professional) in working with these children, and specifically ELs with communication disorders the following question is posed: *How well are SLPs and ESOL professionals prepared to work with ELs?*

EL-Focused Professional Preparation

In the absence of qualified ESL or bilingual education teachers, teaching English language skills and academic content to EL students has become the responsibility of *all* school staff. Research has shown that there has been limited availability of school professionals with adequate preparation in effective practices to work with ELs (Barron & Menken, 2002; Calderon, 2007) and more specifically to work with ELs with communication disorders (Edgar & Rosa-Lugo, 2007; Roninson, 2003; Rosa-Lugo, Rivera, & McKeown, 1998). Providing quality instruction to ELs requires professionals who are skilled in a variety of curricular and instructional strategies. Research on teacher training and preparedness suggests that educators who do not hold bilingual or ESL certification are not well prepared to meet the needs of these children (Ballantyne, Sanderman, & Levy. 2008; Karabenick & Clemens Noda, 2004; Menken & Atunez, 2001; Reeves, 2006; US Department of Education (NCES), 1997, 1999, 2001; Zehler et al., 2003). Consequently, it is essential that school-based SLPs and ESOL engage in professional development as well as self-inquiry that will lead to implementation of culturally responsive instructional practices.

School professionals do not necessarily come from the same cultural and linguistic backgrounds as their students. Because of this, it is essential that professionals make conscious and sustained efforts to learn about their students and to commit to becoming a culturally competent professional. There is growing evidence that professionals are not as well prepared as they should be for the changing demographics reflected in the classrooms across the United States. Despite the abundance of research and availability of professional development focusing on working with ELs, professionals note that they have not received adequate information on addressing the needs of ELs and feel inadequate and ill prepared to meet the needs of these students (Flynn & Hill, 2005; Lewis, Parsad, Carey, Bartfai, Smerdon, & Green, 1999).

Professional staff development has been one method that has been used to develop culturally competent professionals. Mainstream teachers in urban areas with large numbers of ELs report that they have participated in professional development focusing on the needs of ELs. However, they note that training has not been sufficient to prepare them to foster English language acquisition while also teaching the content knowledge and skills these students need to achieve academically (Cosentino de Cohen, Deterding, & Clewell, 2005). Lynch and Hanson (1998) suggest that effective staff development requires attention to participants' cultural self-awareness, attitudes/expectations, beliefs, knowledge, and skills as well as a foundation of shared knowledge from which professionals can work together. Twenty states currently require that new teachers have some EL preparation: however, states' requirements vary considerably, with some peripherally mentioning ELs in their standards for preservice teachers, and others (Arizona, California, Florida, and New York) requiring specific coursework or separate certification to address the educational needs of ELs (Ballantyne, Sanderman, & Levy, 2008). In a survey of postsecondary institutions offering EL teacher preparation, Menken and Atunez (2001) in conjunction with the American Association of Colleges for Teacher Education (2002) found that less than one-sixth of all postsecondary institutes required EL-oriented content in their preparation of mainstream teachers.

At the state and district levels, staff development opportunities for practicing teachers are similarly underrepresented. A 2001 National Center for Education Statistics (NCES) study of staff development reported that EL education was the least likely topic of focus (US Department of Education, NCES, 2001). Although 80% of those surveyed had participated in staff development that related to their state or district curriculum, only 26% had staff development relating to ELs. Zehler et al. (2003) found that of teachers who had at least three ELs in their classroom, 62% had reported attending training related to ELs within the past five years with the median amount of training being only four hours.

Surveys of attitudes and feelings of preparedness indicate that teachers are uneasy with their lack of knowledge in this area. In the 2001 NCES survey, only 27% of teachers felt that they were "very well prepared" to meet the needs of ELs, whereas 12% reported that they were "not at all prepared" (US Department of Education, NCES, 2001). In a separate survey of over 1,200 teachers, 57% indicated that they needed more information to work effectively with ELs (US Department of Education, 1999, p. 10). In research conducted with 279 teachers in a school district with a minimal number of ELs, Reeves (2006) found that 81.7% believed that they did not have adequate training to work effectively with ELs, and 53% wanted more preparation. Given the steady increase in the EL population it is safe to assume that a growing number of teachers see the need for—and feel the lack of—professional development.

Schools in rural communities enroll very few students for whom English is a second or new language. Although low numbers of ELs are characteristic of most schools situated in rural schools, their also exists a dramatic need for quality interventions for EL students. Professional staff is likely to be unprepared for the changing realities of having children of limited English proficiency in the classroom. Similar to the need expressed by teachers in urban areas, teachers in rural schools report a need for competence in EL methodology, multiculturalism, EL curriculum development, EL assessment, and second language acquisition theory (Berube, 2000, 2002).

Smaller-scale attitudinal surveys of teachers have often focused on teacher attitudes toward and knowledge about ELs as a proxy for preparedness, reasoning that if teachers do not have accurate information about the cultural, linguistic and learning characteristics of ELs then they are not well prepared to teach them. Teachers of ELs often hold beliefs of this population that have either been disproven or are seriously contested. For example, Reeves (2006) found that 71.1% of teachers surveyed believed that ELs should be able to learn English within 2 years. In a survey of 729 teachers in a school district in which almost one-third of students were ELs, Karabenick and Clemens Noda (2004) found that a majority (52%) believed that speaking one's first language at home inhibited English language development. Nearly one-third (32%) thought that if students are not able to produce fluent English, they are also unable to comprehend it. The authors also reported that many mainstream teachers do not "distinguish between oral communication proficiencies and cognitive academic language capabilities" (p. 63). Several researchers, including those above (see also Bartolomé, 2002; Lee & Oxelson, 2006; Phuntsog, 2001), have found that culturally sensitive and comprehensive training of educators leads to a shift in these attitudes toward ELs.

The need to prepare SLPs to work with ELs and to demonstrate cultural competence has also been addressed in the literature (ASHA, 1985, 2011a, 2011b; Battle, 2002; Kayser, 1996, 2008). Several researchers have examined the preparedness of SLPs to work with ELs (Artiles & Klingner, 2006; Campbell, Brennan, & Steckol, 1992; McConnell-Stephen, Weiler, Sandman, & Dell'aira, 1994; Nixon, McCardle, & Leos, 2007; Rosa-Lugo & Fradd, 2000; Roseberry-McKibbin, Brice, & O'Hanlon, 2005; Roseberry-McKibben & Eicholtz, 1994). Studies note that a significant percentage of SLPs are not proficient enough in a language other than English to provide services to ELs, do not feel competent or confident in conducting nonbiased assessment or using alternate assessments, and do not feel prepared to provide evidence-based culturally and linguistically appropriate treatment (Caesar & Kohler, 2007; Chabon & Lee-Wilkerson, 2007; Kohnert et al., 2003; Kriticos, 2003; Roseberry-McKibbin, 2008). On the other hand, ESOL professionals are adequately prepared to work with ELs but often do not have the preservice or in-service preparation to work with ELs with communication disorders.

To summarize, there is a pressing need for further professional preparation for teachers and SLPS at all stages in their careers. In studying the preparedness of educators and SLPs to work with ELs, several recommendations have been offered. Preservice and/or in-service initiatives such as inclusion of coursework and clinical practice with individuals from diverse backgrounds is one such recommendation as is an increased emphasis on research on communication disorders in diverse populations (Coleman, 2000; Horton-Ikard, Munoz, Thomas-Tate, & Keller-Bell, 2009; Stockman, Boult, & Robinson, 2004). Other researchers have recommended modifications of traditional assessment practices and the use of culturally appropriate intervention strategies and evidence-based practices in working with ELs.

A recommendation most offered for SLP and other key professionals is that they should develop "cultural competence" or become "culturally competent" to work with ELs (ASHA, 1985; Anderson, 1992; Campbell, Brenna, & Steckol, 1992). To better understand this recommendation and the competencies and skills set needed by SLPs and ESOL professionals to work with ELs, it is important to understand what is meant by "cultural competence."

Development of Culturally Competent Professionals

What Is a Culturally Competent Professional?

Cultural competence, as defined by Lynch and Hanson (1998), is described "as having respect for difference, eagerness to learn, and a willingness to accept that there are many ways of viewing the world" (p. 356). Although the term "cultural competence" has been used interchangeably with other terms (i.e., cultural sensitivity and/or cross-cultural competence) they all refer to ways of thinking and behaving that enable members of one cultural, ethnic, or linguistic group to work effectively with members of another. Cross, Bazron, Dennis, and Isaacs (1989) describe a path toward cultural competence that illustrates that cultural competence is a process with varied rules and facts to be learned. Cultural competence includes: (1) an awareness of one's own cultural limitations; (2) openness, appreciation, and respect for cultural differences; (3) a view of intercultural interactions as learning opportunities; (4) the ability to use cultural resources in interventions; and (5) an acknowledgment of the integrity and value of all cultures (Green, 1982, p. 356).

Attaining cultural competence is an ongoing process and requires systematic study of individuals including the impact that their cultural and linguistic background has had on academic achievement, and/or clinical service (Battle, 2002). Numerous books, chapters, and journal articles have been used to raise critical issues and offer solutions when working with ELs. For example, authors have written about: (a) the general characteristics of racial, ethnic, and cultural groups (Lynch & Hanson, 1998; Kayser, 2008; Roseberry-McKibben, 2008; Taylor, 1986); (b) the nature of linguistic differences among certain culturally and linguistically diverse groups and the implications for SLPs and other professionals (Battle, 2002; Centeno, Anderson, & Obler, 2007; Coleman, 2000; Goldstein, 2004; Goldstein & Washington, 2001; Kohnert, 2008; Rivers, Rosa-Lugo, & Hedrick, 2004; Seymour, Bland-Stewart, & Green, 1998), and (c) the impact cultural characteristics have on the language and literacy development of ELs (Brisk & Harrington, 2007; Calderon, 2007; Curtin, 2009; Diaz-Rico & Weed, 2006; Farrell, 2009; Freeman, Freeman, & Ramirez, 2008; Klingner, Hoover, & Baca, 2008; Peregoy & Boyle, 2005; Quiocho & Ulanoff, 2009; Roseberry-McKibben, 2008).

National organizations such as the American Speech-Language-Hearing Association (ASHA) and Teachers of English to Speakers of Other Languages (TESOL) have outlined the professional standards and the knowledge, skills, and competencies expected of professionals who work with ELs (see Appendix A for further information on ASHA and TESOL position papers). These resources serve as starting points for learning about different cultural groups, their linguistic characteristics, and the role of families and the community in the development of language and literacy in ELs, and specifically those with communication disorders. Although these resources provide valuable information, simply reading them will not lead one to become a culturally competent professional. They can, however, serve to facilitate discussion, generate questions, and propel us to reexamine our cultural competence.

Although it is impossible for an individual to be knowledgeable about all the cultural and linguistic characteristics of ELs, it is recommended that professionals strive for increased cultural sensitivity toward people whose cultural, linguistic, and social backgrounds are different from their own. Strategies such as obtaining information about a family's culture and language, working with people from the cultural community who can guide service providers in culturally appropriate interactions with clients and their families, examining similarities and differences in students and their families, and evaluating our own values and assumptions have proven helpful in developing cultural competency (Roseberry-McKibben, 2008). The practice of viewing individuals from a narrow lens can be dangerous. When people are viewed as "representative" of a specific cultural and/ or linguistic group without considering the great heterogeneity that exists within cultural groups, this can lead to subjective and erroneous stereotypes and/or generalizations. Simply put, a "culturally competent professional" recognizes that each person in any cultural group is first an individual and is willing to explore and question their biases and perceptions when working with individuals that are different from their own cultural and linguistic background.

Key Terms and Concepts

EL Terminology

As in other professions, working with students for whom English is not the primary language requires mastering a unique jargon. A culturally competent professional must be familiar with key terminology related to working with ELs. Often, the term EL specifically refers to students who are learning English and already have a native language, but other labels have been used to describe these students. For example, within the public schools in the United States, common terms include "language-minority," "limited English proficient," "second-language learners," and/or "bilingual." The terms "language-minority" and "limited English proficient" are both official designations under federal law. However, each of these labels is problematic because there is inconsistent uniformity in defining and describing ELs. To ensure some continuity a consistent definition of what constitutes an EL is necessary (Short & Fitzsimmons, 2006).

Description of English Learners

A number of terms are often used to *describe* ELs. For example, terms such as culture, race, and ethnicity have been cause for miscommunications or misunderstandings. **Culture** is the shared beliefs, traditions, and values of a group of people; learned patterns of thoughts and behavior (Payne, 1986); and the framework that guides and bounds life practices (Hanson, 1992). Culture is associated with or influenced by factors such as age, gender, religion, education, child rearing practices, geographic region, and socioeconomic status (SES). Presently, culture has taken on various shades of meaning in the social science literature and a number of definitions have been proposed (see Frisby, 1992; Garcia, 1982; Goldman & McDermott, 1987). Scholars note that the term "culture" has sometimes been erroneously used synonymously with race—however, the terms are not the same. Two people may be of the same race and yet identify with two very different cultural groups.

Race has traditionally been defined as a classification that distinguishes one group of people from another based on physical characteristics (e.g., skin color, facial features) (Kammey, Ritzer, & Yetman, 1990). Physical characteristics are one means of differentiating people; however the criteria used to distinguish one racial group from another varies from one society to another (Kammey et al., 1990). It appears that categorizing people by race has been discredited and is not useful in addressing the linguistic needs of ELs with communication disorders (Kendall, 1997).

Ethnicity is another term that has often been confused with culture and race. Ethnicity is the social definition of groups of people based on cultural similarities. Ethnicity includes race and also factors such as customs, nationality, language, and heritage (Coleman & McCabe, 2000). Sociologists suggest that ethnic groups share five main characteristics: (1) unique cultural traits (e.g., language, clothing, holidays); (2) a sense of community; (3) a feeling of ethnocentrism or a belief that one's own culture and way of life are superior to all others; (4) ascribed membership—a status conferred at birth; and (5) territoriality, defined as a tendency to occupy a distinct geographic area (such as Chinatown) by choice or for self-protection (Kammey et al., 1990).

Several other terms have been included in the *description* of ELs. Wei (2006) outlined approximately 35 terms that have been used to describe ELs. For example, terms have been used to describe: (a) their language proficiency (non-English speaking [NES]; Limited English speaking [LES]; Fluent English speaker [FES]; Bilingual); (b) their stage of language proficiency (preproduction, emergent production); (c) the conditions under which bilingualism occurs (simultaneous; sequential); (d) the types of bilingualism (semilingual, additive bilingualism, subtractive bilingualism, dual language); (e) the instructional environments (sheltered English; dual language instruction); (f) the way they organize, classify, and assimilate information in a language (learning style, field dependent, field independent); and (g) how they have transitioned into the mainstream culture (acculturation, assimilation). As Goldstein (2004) points out, scholars (see Abedi, 2003; Baker, 2001; de Houwer, 1990; Hakuta, 1986; Romaine, 1995; Valdes & Figueroa, 1994) have defined and described ELs in a variety of ways. These descriptions highlight the complexity of issues associated with this student population from the perspective of SLP and ESOL.

Recommended Competencies for SLPs and ESOL Professionals

What Competencies Are Critical in Working with ELs?

Professionals who work with ELs need to develop specific competencies and a skill set to help ELs achieve high academic standards. In 2004, the knowledge and skills needed by SLPs and audiologists to provide culturally and linguistically appropriate identification, assessment, and intervention services were outlined and described by the American Speech-Language-Hearing Association (ASHA, 2004) The knowledge and skills to acquire professional cultural competency focused on three fundamental knowledge domains: knowledge of self, knowledge of others, and knowledge of the theoretical and empirical literature on dual-language development, use and disorders (Kohnert et al. 2003; Rosa-Lugo & Champion, 2007). Specifically, ASHA (2004) suggests knowledge and skills that SLPs should develop in order to work with ELs. SLPs should:

A. Engage in self-scrutiny;
B. Demonstrate an understanding of cultural characteristics and the impact that these characteristics have on students' performance in the classroom learning environment;
C. Be able to distinguish between normal characteristics of second language acquisition, a communication difference, and/or a communication disorder using appropriate assessment measures; and
D. Provide appropriate, culturally responsive, and evidence-based practices (Battle, 2002; Kayser, 1995; Kohnert et al., 2003; Roseberry-McKibben, 2008).

Similarly, the knowledge and skills needed by ESOL professionals to effectively work with ELs werc outlined in several position papers by Teachers of English to Speakers of Other Languages (TESOL) (2003a, 2003b, 2005a, 2005b, 2007, 2008). Specifically, the position papers stressed the need for ESOL professionals to: (a) engage in lifelong learning, (b) understand the academic and linguistic needs of ELs with special needs, and (c) access and apply research based approaches from a variety of disciplines to improve the achievement and academic success of ELs.

To equip SLPs and ESOL professionals with explicit, research-based pedagogical knowledge and skills that they can use in the classroom, professional development related to diversity must go beyond cultural sensitivity and appreciation (Garcia & Guerra, 2004). Both professionals must be provided with opportunities to obtain knowledge and develop expertise in the basic constructs of language proficiency, bilingualism, and second language development; the role of the first language and culture in learning, the demands found in the general education curriculum for ELs placed in mainstream English-only classrooms (Clair & Adger, 1999), the academic and linguistic demands of ELs with special needs (Antunez, 2002), and evidence-based approaches and strategies. Thus, the primary goals of SLP and ESOL professionals are to address the language development, instructional, and literacy needs of ELs (ASHA, 2001; TESOL, 2001) and to use evidence-based approaches to facilitate the academic success of school-age ELs. These shared goals present opportunities to discuss the implementation of evidence-based approaches and strategies that can be used by SLPs and ESOL professionals to work with ELs with communication disorders.

Evidence-Based Practice

What Is the Significance of Evidence-Based Approaches and Strategies in Working With ELs?

The current climate of accountability, particularly in our nation's schools, emphasizes personal and institutional responsibility for actions and decisions concerning our nation's schoolchildren. This climate stems, in part, from the spiraling costs of special education services. The No Child Left Behind Act (NCLB) of 2001 (NCLB, 2002) placed a strong emphasis on accountability and emphasized the need for school-based professionals to deliver instruction and interventions that have demonstrated efficiency (the time taken to reach a desired outcome) and effectiveness (the likelihood that the desired outcome will be achieved). The NCLB Act also required that all school districts use instructional strategies that are rooted in scientifically based research. School-based SLPs and professionals in many other disciplines embody the 21st century's twofold emphasis on reform based on accountability and research. Together, these concepts contextualize discussions of evidence-based practice (EBP) as it applies to meeting the needs of school-age ELs, specifically those with communication disorders.

The term *evidence-based practice (EBP)* refers to an approach in which current, high-quality research evidence is integrated with practitioner expertise and client preferences and values in the process of making clinical decisions (ASHA, 2005a). Research refers to a spirited inquiry and systematic investigation that contributes to the knowledge base of a field. For example, research-based knowledge provides a principled basis for understanding language teaching and learning, and making decisions about policies, plans, and actions. Research has the potential to help English-language teaching professionals improve the processes, outcomes, and conditions for language teaching, learning, and assessment. It also can help the profession address urgent social and political issues around the world, improve the materials used for second language teaching in schools, as well as clarify debates and debunk myths regarding second language acquisition. A strong commitment to research as a means of improving professional knowledge is vital to the field of teaching of English to speakers of other languages (TESOL, 2005b) and the discipline of speech-language pathology.

The goal of evidence-based practice is to integrate clinical expertise and best current evidence (ASHA, 2005a). In response to the evidence-based practice movement, ASHA created a framework for ranking levels of evidence that is specific to the field of communication disorders and sciences (*ASHA Leader*, 2007; Justice & Fey, 2004). For example, currently, evidence-based systematic reviews have been completed for specific areas of intervention (see Gorman, 2007; Mullen 2007; Thomason, Gorman, & Summers, 2007). Similarly, summaries of studies that have been peer-reviewed and published in professional journals have provided school-based SLPs with evidence-based support for the use of specific interventions (Gillam & Gillam, 2006; Schraeder, 2008). General clinical strategies and techniques are available for use by SLPs across a variety of intervention programs regardless of the student's disability type (Schraeder, 2008). ASHA has published policy statements related to the designation of competencies associated with the various needs (disorders or conditions) of persons being served. Each policy statement, derived from the ASHA Code of Ethics (ASHA, 2010a), details the scope of practice, the necessary education and training, precautions, and knowledge and skills needed in the particular area of service delivery.

Application of EBP by the SLP involves more than simply making clinical decisions based on literature reviews. To date, a systematic review of what works with ELs with communication disorders, and specifically, across disability type is not readily available. What does exist are recommendations extracted from the professional literature of peer-reviewed and published studies specific to working with ELs (Justice & Fey, 2004; Restrepo & Towle-Harmon, 2008). Specifically, it is recommended that school-based SLPs should:

1. Be culturally competent (ASHA 2004, 2005b, 2010b; Battle, 2002; Schraeder, 2001);
2. Reflect on their cultural competence (ASHA, 2006; McCarthy, 2003); and
3. Collaborate with other school professionals to work with ELs (Blosser, 2006; Hegde & Davis, 1995; Rosa-Lugo & Fradd, 2000).

Serving English Learners — The Collaboration of Two Disciplines

How Can Two Disciplines Collaborate to Serve ELs in General, and Specifically with ELs with Communication Disorders?

The role of the school-based SLP has changed dramatically (ASHA, 1991, 1999, 2001, 2010b; Beck & Dennis, 1997; Ehren, 2000). Today's SLP faces challenges such as demands for greater accountability, lifelong learning, educational and health care reform, and a changing society (Taylor, 1992). The growing cultural heterogeneity of our society demands that students preparing to become SLPs be knowledgeable about persons from communication disorders backgrounds. They must have a solid foundation in order to execute all of the roles and responsibilities faced in the school setting and they must be able to apply this knowledge to their clinical practice. ASHA (1999, 2003) outlines the knowledge SLPs must have and the clinical competencies they must demonstrate (Kwiatkowski, Murray-Branch, & Schraeder, 2005). Over the years, the roles and responsibilities of the school-based SLP have been heavily influenced by local, state, and federal mandates. Wording in the Individual Disabilities Education Act (IDEA) (USDOE, 2009) and the No Child Left Behind Act (NCLB, 2002) called for the involvement of SLPs in the school setting in prevention, assessment, intervention, documentation, counseling, supervision, research, leadership, and advocacy. It also called for the forging of partnerships with general education and special education colleagues to address academic and curricular areas (Moore-Brown & Montgomery, 2005) for ELs.

The role of the ESOL professional has also evolved over the past several decades (TESOL, 2008). Under the NCLB Act of 2001 (USDOE, 2002), new guidelines for teacher preparedness have been established to ensure that teachers in every classroom in the US are highly qualified. With NCLB's primary emphasis on core subjects and content area mastery, ESOL providers are required to:

A. Construct learning environments that support students' language and literacy development, content-area achievement, and students' cultural identities;
B. Know, understand, and use standards-based practices and strategies related to planning, implementing, and managing second language and content instruction; and
C. Collaborate with their colleagues across disciplines and serve as a resource to all staff, to improve learning for all students (TESOL, 2003a, 2003b, 2005a).

The disproportionate representation of ELs in special education and the challenges in identifying ELs with special needs also requires that ESOL professionals understand the differences between disabilities and second language acquisition (Artiles & Ortiz, 2002; Collier, 2000; Klingner et al., 2005; Roseberry-McKibben, 2002; TESOL, 2007).

To ensure that appropriate assessment practices are not at odds with research-based understandings of language competency and accepted practices in educational testing, it is essential that the SLP and ESOL professional engage in *purposeful collabora-*

tion and develop and demonstrate expertise in the identification, assessment and management of ELs, to include ELs with communication disorders (ASHA, 1998). Expertise has been described as what experts know and can do. O'Sullivan and Doutis (1994) identified several traits and characteristics of experts across disciplines. These include an ability to be a confident, knowledgeable, involved communicator, integrative thinker, and a problem solver who simultaneously and effectively quantifies outcomes of treatment, while maintaining the flexibility to adjust to new situations (Guilford, Graham, & Scheuerle, 2007).

Developing expertise requires identifying and describing important skills and behaviors. The following case study is offered as an example of an opportunity for the SLP and the ESOL professional to merge their expertise and competencies in working with an EL referred for an assessment and possible special education services. This case study is included to stimulate discussion and provide practice in the application of key issues presented in this chapter.

Case Study

Rey is a 7-year-old male who was referred to the speech-language pathologist by his parent and teacher. The reason for the referral was to ascertain the reasons for his poor academic achievement and behavior. Rey was educated in Puerto Rico from kindergarten through the first grade and moved to Florida with his family. He was placed in the second grade in an English-only classroom setting. He is currently in the second grade and has been described as "demonstrating behavior problems, needing multiple cues to remain on task, and not following directions, preferring to talk with peers or draw rather than follow directions for assignments." His parents speak Spanish in the home but report that Rey prefers to speak English.

A bilingual speech-language pathologist conducted an assessment using a variety of assessment instruments and/or informal procedures to determine his language proficiency and linguistic strengths and weaknesses. Results of testing indicated that Rey's Spanish oral proficiency was characteristic of students with "very limited Spanish." Similarly, results of testing indicated his English oral proficiency to be characteristic of students with "very limited English." To assess his overall general language performance in Spanish and English, a global measure of language was administered. His scores in Spanish yielded scores that fell in the normal range for Spanish language skills. However, his scores in English fell below the average range. Additionally, a measure of vocabulary and pragmatics (i.e., the knowledge and use of the rules of language) in both languages was administered. Results of these assessments suggested that his receptive and expressive language skills in his first language (L1) are commensurate with his nonverbal cognitive level. Subsequent to obtaining a language sample, the SLP concluded that Rey was able to initiate conversation in English and Spanish and able to code-switch (i.e., use both languages competently). The bilingual SLP noted that Rey appears to be losing some proficiency in Spanish with an increase in English proficiency. The SLP concluded that Rey appeared to be experiencing some "arrested language development (Schiff-Myers, 1992).

To determine if Rey has a communication disorder that is having an impact on his academic achievement and behavior will require collaboration among key professionals. Given the complexity of language and its development, it is not surprising that the SLP will struggle to determine if this student has a language disorder or is experiencing difficulties that are normal for ELs. The ESOL professional will be required to consider Rey's language and literacy performance in light of test results, classroom performance, and in comparison to other school-age children of his age and background. Reflecting on this case study, the reader is asked to ponder the following question: What do the SLP and ESOL professionals have to consider in first and second language development to determine if Rey is experiencing a language disorder or if he is in the process of acquiring a second language? The following chapters provide essential information about first and second language development, bilingual phenomena, what constitutes a language disorder and/or a language difference, and what distinguishes one from the other.

References

Abedi, J. (2003). The No Child Left Behind Act and English language learners: Assessment and accountability issues. *Educational Researcher*, *33*(1), 4–14.

American Association of Colleges for Teacher Education. (2002). Educators' preparation for cultural and linguistic diversity: A call to action 2002. Retrieved from http://www.aacte.org/index.php?/Programs/Multicultural-/-Diversity/aacte-statements-on-multicultural-education.html

American Speech-Language-Hearing Association. (1985). *Clinical management of communicatively handicapped minority language populations* [Position statement]. Retrieved from www.asha.org/policy

American Speech-Language-Hearing Association. (1991). A model for collaborative service delivery for students with language-learning disorders in the public schools. *ASHA*, *33*(Suppl. 5), 44–50.

American Speech-Language-Hearing Association. (1998). *Provision of instruction in English as a second language by speech-language pathologists in school settings* [Technical report]. Retrieved from www.asha.org/policy

American Speech-Language-Hearing Association. (1999). *Guidelines for the roles and responsibilities of the school-based speech-language pathologist*. Retrieved from www.asha.org/policy

American Speech-Language-Hearing Association. (2001). *Roles and responsibilities of speech-language pathologists with respect to reading and writing in children and adolescents* [Position statement]. Retrieved from www.asha.org/policy

American Speech-Language-Hearing Association. (2003). *Implementation guide: A workload analysis approach to caseload standards in schools*. Rockville, MD: Author.

American Speech-Language-Hearing Association. (2004). *Knowledge and skills needed by speech-language pathologists and audiologists to provide culturally and linguistically appropriate services* [Knowledge and skills]. Retrieved from www.asha.org/policy

American Speech-Language-Hearing Association. (2005a). *Evidence-based practice in communication disorders* [Position statement]. Retrieved from www.asha.org/policy

American Speech-Language-Hearing Association. (2005b). *Cultural competence*. [Issues in ethics]. Retrieved from www.asha.org/policy

American Speech-Language-Hearing Association. (2006). *Professional performance review process for the school-based speech-language pathologist*. Retrieved from www.asha.org/policy

American Speech-Language-Hearing Association. (2010a). *Code of ethics* [Ethics]. Retrieved from www.asha.org/policy and http://www.asha.org/docs/html/ET2010-00309.html

American Speech-Language-Hearing Association. (2010b). *Roles and responsibilities of speech-language pathologists in schools* [Professional issues statement]. Retrieved from www.asha.org/policy

American Speech-Language-Hearing Association. (2011a). *Cultural competence in professional service delivery* [Position statement]. Retrieved from www.asha.org/policy

American Speech-Language-Hearing Association. (2011b). *Cultural competence in professional service delivery* [Professional issues statement]. Retrieved from www.asha.org/policy

Anderson, N. B. (1992). Understanding cultural diversity. *American Journal of Speech-Language Pathology, 1,* 11–12.

Antunez, B. (2002). The preparation and professional development of teachers of English language learners. *ERIC Digest.* Washington, DC: ERIC Clearinghouse on Teaching and Teacher Education (ERIC Document Reproduction Service No. ED 477 724). Retrieved April 10, 2009.

Artiles, A. J., & Klingner, J. K. (Eds.). (2006). Forging a knowledge base on English language learners with special needs: Theoretical, population, and technical issues. *Teachers College Record, 108,* 2187–2438.

Artiles, A. J., & Ortiz, A. A. (Eds.). (2002). *English language learners with special education needs: Identification, assessment, and instruction.* Washington, DC, and McHenry, IL: Center for Applied Linguistics and Delta Systems.

ASHA Leader. (2007). The state of the evidence: ASHA develops levels of evidence for communication sciences and disorders. *ASHA Leader, 12*(3), 8–9, 24–25.

August, D. (2003). Supporting the development of English literacy in English language learners: Key issues and promising practices. Report no. 61, Baltimore, MD: CRESPAR/Johns Hopkins University. Retrieved from http://www.csos.jhu.edu/crespar/techReports/Report61.pdf

Baker, C. (2001). *Foundations of bilingual education and bilingualism* (3rd ed.). Clevedon, UK: Multilingual Matters.

Ballantyne, K. G., Sanderman, A. R., Levy, J. (2008). *Educating English language learners: Building teacher capacity.* Washington, DC: National Clearinghouse for English Language Acquisition. Retrieved from http://www.ncela.gwu.edu/practice/mainstream_teachers.htm

Barron, V., & Menken, K. (2002, August). What are the characteristics of the shortage of teachers qualified to teach English language learners? *AskNCELA, 14.* Retrieved from http://www.ncela.gwu.edu/expert/faq/14shortage.htm

Bartolomé, L. (2002). Creating an equal playing field: Teachers as advocates, border crossers, and cultural brokers. In Z. F. Beykont (Ed.), *The power of culture: Teaching across language difference* (pp. 167–191). Cambridge, MA: Harvard Education Publishing Group.

Battle, E. E. (Ed.). (2002). *Communication disorders in multicultural populations* (2nd ed.). Newton, MA: Butterworth-Heinemann.

Beck, A., & Dennis, M. (1997). Speech-language pathologists' and teachers' perceptions of classroom-based interventions. *Language, Speech, and Hearing Services in Schools, 28*, 146–153.

Berube, B. (2000). *Managing ESL programs in rural and small urban schools.* Arlington, VA: TESOL.

Berube, B. (2002). The three R's for ESL instruction in U.S. rural schools: A test of commitment. *TESOL Matters, 12*(4). Retrieved from http://www.tesol.org/s_tesol/sec_document.asp?CID=193&DID=955

Blosser, J. (2006). Partnering with teachers for speech-language service deliver. Retrieved from http://www.speechpathology.com/

Brisk, M. E., & Harrington, M. (2007). *Literacy and bilingualism: A handbook for all teachers.* Mahwah, NJ: Lawrence Erlbaum.

Caeser, L., & Kohler, P. (2007). The state of school-based bilingual assessment: Actual practice versus recommended guidelines. *Language, Speech, and Hearing Services in School, 38*, 190–200.

Calderón, M. (2007). *Teaching reading to English language learners grades 6–12: A framework for improving achievement in the content areas.* Thousand Oaks, CA: Corwin Press.

Campbell, L. R., Brennan, D. G., & Steckol, K. F. (1992). Preservice training to meet the needs of people from diverse cultural backgrounds. *ASHA, 34*, 27–32.

Capps, R., Fix, M., Murray, J., Ost, J., Passel, J., & Herwantoro, S. (2005). *The new demography of America's schools: Immigration and the No Child Left Behind Act.* Washington, DC: The Urban Institute. Retrieved from http://www.urban.org/publications/311230.html

Centeno, J. G., Anderson, R. T., & Obler, L. K. (2007). *Communication disorders in Spanish speakers: Theoretical, research and clinical aspects. Communication disorders across languages.* Clevedon, UK: Multilingual Matters.

Chabon, S., & Lee-Wilkerson, D. (2007). Dialogues on diversity in speech-language pathology: Not for the faint of heart. In J. Branche, J. Mullennix, & E. Cohen (Eds.), *Diversity across the curriculum: A guide for faculty in higher education.* Bolton, MA: Anker.

Clair, N., & Adger, C. T. (1999). Professional development for teachers in culturally diverse schools. *ERIC Digest.* ERIC Document Reproduction Service No. ED 435 185.

Coleman, T. (2000). *Clinical management of communication disorders in culturally diverse children.* Boston, MA: Allyn & Bacon.

Coleman, T., & McCabe-Smith, L. (2000). Key terms and concepts. In T. Coleman (Ed.), *Clinical management of communication disorders in culturally diverse children* (pp. 3–12). Boston, MA: Allyn & Bacon.

Collier, C. (2000). *Separating difference and disability: Strategies for identification and instruction.* Ferndale, WA: CrossCultural Developmental Education Services.

Cosentino de Cohen, C., Deterding, N., & Clewell, B.C. (2005). *Who's left behind? Immigrant children in high and low LEP schools.* Washington, DC: The Urban Institute.

Cross, T., Bazrn, B., Dennis, K., & Isaacs, M. (1989). *Toward a culturally competent system of care* (Vol. 1). Washington, DC: CAASP Technical Assistance Center, Georgetown University Child Development Center.

Curtin, E. M. (2009). *Practical strategies for teaching English language learners.* Upper Saddle River, NJ: Pearson.

De Houwer, A. (1990). *The acquisition of two languages from birth: A case study.* Cambridge, UK: Cambridge University Press.

Diaz-Rico, L. T., & Weed, K. Z. (2006). *The crosscultural, language, and academic development handbook: A complete K–12 reference guide* (3rd ed.). Boston, MA: Pearson.

Edgar, D., & Rosa-Lugo, L. I. (2007). The critical shortage of speech-language pathologists in the public school setting: Features of the work environment that affects recruitment and retention. *Language, Speech, and Hearing Services in Schools, 38,* 1–16.

Ehren, B. (2000). Maintaining a therapeutic focus and sharing responsibility for student success: Keys to in classroom speech-language services. *Language, Speech, and Hearing Services in Schools, 31,* 219–229.

Farrell, G. (2009). *Teaching reading to English language learners.* Thousand Oaks, CA: Corwin Press.

Flynn, K., & Hill, J. (2005). *English language learners: A growing population.* Denver, CO: Mid-continent Research for Education and Learning.

Freeman, Y. S., Freeman, D. E., & Ramirez, R. (2008). *Diverse learners in the mainstream classroom: Strategies for supporting all students across content areas, English language learners, students with disabilities, gifted/talented students.* Portsmouth, NH: Heinemann.

Frisby, C. L. (1992). Issues and problems in the influence of culture on the psychoeducational needs of African-American children. *School Psychology Review, 21*(4), 532–551.

Garcia, R. (1982). *Teaching in a pluralistic society: Concept, models, strategies.* New York, NY: Harper and Row.

Garcia, S. B., & Guerra, P.L. (2004). Deconstructing deficit thinking: Working with educators to create more equitable learning environments. *Education and Urban Society, 36*(2), 150–168.

Gillam, S. L., & Gillam, R. B. (2006). Making evidence based decisions about child language intervention in schools. *Language, Speech, and Hearing Services in Schools, 37,* 304–315.

Goldenberg, C. (2008). Teaching English language learners. What the research says and does not say. *American Educator, 32*(2), 8–44. Retrieved from http://homepages.ucalgary.ca/~hroessin/documents/Goldenberg,_2008,_America_Ed_Summary_of_research.pdf

Goldman, S., & McDermott, R. (1987). The culture of competition in American schools. In G. Spindler (Ed.), *Education and cultural process* (2nd ed.) (pp. 282–299). Prospect Heights, IL: Waveland Press.

Goldstein, B. A. (Ed.). (2004). *Bilingual language development and disorders in Spanish-English speakers.* Baltimore, MD: Brookes.

Goldstein, B., & Washington, P. (2001). An initial investigation of phonological patterns in 4-year-old typically developing Spanish-English bilingual children. *Language, Speech, and Hearing Services in Schools, 32,* 153–164.

Gorman, C. (2007). Are doctors just playing hunches? *Time, 169*(9), 52–54.

Green, J. (1982). *Cultural awareness in the human services.* Englewood Cliffs, NJ: Prentice-Hall.

Guilford, A., Graham, S., & Scheuerle, J. (2007). (Eds.). *The speech-language pathologist. From novice to expert.* Upper Saddle River, NJ: Pearson.

Hakuta, K. (1986). *Mirror of language. The debate on bilingualism.* New York, NY: Basic Books.

Hanson, M. J. (1992). Ethnic, cultural, and language diversity in intervention settings. In M. J. Hanson & E. W. Lynch (Eds.), *Developing cross-cultural competence: A guide for working with young children and their families* (pp. 3–18). Baltimore, MD: Brookes.

Haskins, R., & Rouse, C. (2005). *Closing achievement gaps. The future of children policy brief.* Washington, DC: The Future of Children.

Hegde, M. N., & Davis, D. (1995). *Clinical methods and practicum in speech-language pathology.* San Diego, CA: Singular.

Hopstock, P. J., & Stephenson, T. G. (2003). *Descriptive study of services to LEP students and LEP students with disabilities. Special*

Topic Report #2. Analysis of Office of Civil Rights Data related to LEP students. Washington DC: US Department of Education, OELA. Retrieved from http://www.ncela.gwu.edu

Horton-Ikard, R., Munoz, M., Thomas-Tate, S., & Keller-Bell, Y. (2009). Establishing a pedagogical framework for the multicultural course in communication sciences and disorders. *American Journal of Speech-Language Pathology, 18,* 192–206.

Justice, L. M., & Fey, M. E. (2004), September 21). Evidence-based practice in schools: Integrating craft and theory with science and data. *ASHA Leader,* 4–5, 30–32.

Kammey, K. C. W., Ritzer, G., & Yetman, N. R. (1990). *Sociology: Experiences changing society.* Boston, MA: Allyn & Bacon.

Karabenick, S. A. & Clemens Noda, P. A. (2004). Professional development implications of teachers' beliefs and attitudes toward English language learners. *Bilingual Research Journal, 28*(1), 55–75.

Kayser, H. (1995). Assessment of speech and language impairments in bilingual children. In H. Kayser (Ed.), *Bilingual speech-language pathology: An Hispanic focus* (pp. 243–264). San Diego, CA: Singular.

Kayser, H. (1996). Cultural/linguistic variation in the United States and its implications for assessment and intervention in speech-language pathology: An epilogue. *Language, Speech, and Hearing Services in the Schools, 27*(4), 385–387

Kayser, H. (2008). *Educating Latino preschool children.* San Diego, CA: Plural.

Kendall, D. (1997). *Race, class, and gender in a diverse society: A text-reader.* Upper Saddle River, NJ: Pearson.

Kindler, A. L. (2002). *Survey of the states' limited English proficient students and available educational program and services: 2000–2001 summary report.* Washington, DC: National Clearinghouse for English Language Acquisition and Language Instruction Educational Programs.

Klingner, J. K., Artiles, A. J., Kozleski, E., Harry, B., Zion, S., Tate, W., . . . Riley, D. (2005). Addressing the disproportionate representation of culturally and linguistically diverse students in special education through culturally responsive educational systems. *Education Policy Analysis Archives, 13*(38).

Klingner, J., Hoover, J., & Baca, L. (Eds). (2008). *Why do English language learners struggle with reading?* Thousand Oaks, CA: Corwin Press.

Kohnert, K. (2008). *Language disorders in bilingual children and adults.* San Diego, CA: Plural.

Kohnert, K., Kennedy, M. R. T., Glaze, L., Kan, P. F., & Carney, E. (2003). Breadth and depth of diversity in Minnesota: Challenges to clinical competency. *American Journal of Speech-Language Pathology, 12,* 259–272.

Kritikos, E. (2003). Speech-language pathologists' beliefs about language assessment of bilingual/bicultural individuals. *American Journal of Speech-Language Pathology, 12*, 73–91.

Kwiatkowski, J., Murray-Branch, J., & Schraeder, T. (2005). *Clinical skills learner outcomes tracking system.* Unpublished assessment tool, University of Wisconsin at Madison, Madison, WI.

Lee, J. S., & Oxelson, E. (2006). "It's not my job": K–12 teacher attitudes toward students' heritage language maintenance. *Bilingual Research Journal, 30*(2), 453–477.

Lewis, L., Parsad, B., Carey, N., Bartfai, N., Smerdon, B., & Green, B. (1999). *Teacher quality: A report on the preparation and qualifications of public school teachers (NCES 199-080).* Washington, DC: National Center for Education Statistics.

Lynch, E. W., & Hanson, M. J. (Eds.). (1998). *Developing cross-cultural competence: A guide for working with young children and their families.* Baltimore, MD: Brookes.

Matthews, H., & Ewen, D. (2006). *Reaching all children? Understanding early care and education participation among immigrant families.* Washington, DC: Center for Law and Social Policy. Retrieved from http://eric.ed.gov/ERICDocs/data/ericdocs2sql/content_storage_01/0000019b/80/29/dc/dc.pdf

McCarthy, M. P. (2003, October). Promoting problem-solving and self-evaluation in clinical education through a collaborative approach to supervision. *Perspectives on Administration and Supervision, 20*–26.

McConnell-Stephen, P. L., Weiler, E. M., Sandman, D. E., & Dell'aira, A. (1994). Survey of speech-language psychologists regarding training in dialects. *Hearsay, 9*, 15–19.

Menken, K., & Atunez, B. (2001). *An overview of the preparation and certification of teachers working with limited English proficient students.* Washington, DC: National Clearinghouse of Bilingual Education. Retrieved from http://www.ericsp.org/pages/digests/ncbe.pdf

Moore-Brown, B., & Montgomery, J. K. (2005). *Making a difference for America's children. Speech-language pathologists in public schools.* Eau Claire, WI: Thinking Publications.

Mullen, R. (2007, March 06). The state of the evidence: ASHA develops levels of evidence for communication sciences and disorders. *ASHA Leader.*

National Clearinghouse for English Language Acquisition. (2006). *The growing number of limited English proficient students.* Retrieved from www.ncela.gwu.edu/files/uploads/4/GrowingLEP_0506.pdf

Nixon, S., McCardle, P., & Leos, K. (2007). Epilogue: Implications of research on English language learners for classroom and clinical practice. *Language, Speech, and Hearing Services in Schools, 38,* 272–277.

No Child Left Behind Act of 2001. (2002). Pub. L. No. 107-110, 115 Stat. 1446.

O'Sullivan, M., & Doutis, P. (1994). Research on expertise. Guideposts for expertise and teacher education in physical education. *QUEST, 46,* 176–185.

Padolsky, D. (2005). How many school-aged English language learners (ELLs) are there in the U.S.? *AskNCELA, 1.* Retrieved from http://www.ncela.gwu.edu/expert/faq/01leps.htm

Payne, K. (1986). Cultural and linguistic groups in the United States. In O. Taylor (Ed.), *Nature of communication disorders in culturally and linguistically diverse populations.* San Diego, CA: College-Hill Press.

Peregoy, S. F., & Boyle, O. F. (2005). *Reading, writing, and learning in ESL: A resource book for K–12 teachers.* New York, NY: Pearson Education.

Phuntsog, N. (2001). Culturally responsive teaching: What do selected United States elementary school teachers think? *Intercultural Education, 12*(1), 51–64.

President's Advisory Commission on Educational Excellence for Hispanic Americans. (2003). *From risk to opportunity: Fulfilling the educational needs of Hispanic Americans in the 21st century.* Washington, DC: Author.

Quiocho, A. L., & Ulanoff, S. H., (2009). *Differentiated literacy instruction for English language learners.* Boston, MA: Allyn & Bacon.

Reeves, J. (2006). Secondary teacher attitudes toward including English-language learners in mainstream classrooms. *Journal of Educational Research, 99*(3), 131–143.

Restrepo, M. A., & Towle-Harmon, M. (2008, September 23). Addressing emergent literacy skills in English-Language Learners. *ASHA Leader.*

Rivers, K., Rosa-Lugo, L. I., & Hedrick, D. (2004). Performance of African-American adolescents on a measure of language proficiency. *Negro Educational Review, 55*(2–3), 117–127.

Romaine, S. (1995). *Bilingualism.* Boston, MA: Blackwell.

Roninson, O. Z. (2003). "But they don't speak English!" Bilingual students and speech-language services in public schools. *Newsletter of the ASHA Special Interest Division 16: Perspectives on School-Based Issues, 4*(1), 42–46.

Rosa-Lugo, L. I., & Champion, T. (2007). The influence of knowledge and experience on responding to diversity in speech-language pathology. In A. Guilford, S. Graham, & J. Scheuerle (Eds), *The speech-*

language pathologist. From novice to expert (pp. 89–104). Upper Saddle River, NJ: Pearson.

Rosa-Lugo, L. I., & Fradd, S. (2000). Preparing professionals to serve English language learners with communication disorders. *Communication Disorders Quarterly, 22*(1), 29–42.

Rosa-Lugo, L. I., Rivera, E. A., & McKeown, S. W. (1998). Meeting the critical shortage of speech-language pathologists to serve the public schools: Collaborative rewards. *Language, Speech, and Hearing Services in Schools, 29*, 232–242.

Roseberry-McKibbin, C. (2000). Distinguishing language differences from language disorders in linguistically and culturally diverse students. In K. Fieiberg (Ed.), *Educating exceptional children* (pp. 78–81). Guilford, CT: Dushkin/McGraw-Hill.

Roseberry-McKibbin, C. (2002). *Multicultural students with special language needs* (2nd ed.). Oceanside, CA: Academic Communication Associates.

Roseberry-McKibbin, C. (2008). *Increasing language skills of students from low income backgrounds.* San Diego, CA: Plural.

Roseberry-McKibbin, C., Brice, A., & O'Hanlon, L. (2005). Serving English language learners in public schools: A national survey. *Language, Speech, and Hearing Services in Schools, 36*, 48–61.

Roseberry-McKibben, C. A., & Eicholtz, G. E. (1994). Serving LEP children in schools: A national survey. *Language, Speech, and Hearing Services in Schools, 25*(3), 156–164.

Schiff-Myers, N. (1992). Considering arrested language development and language loss in the assessment of second language learners. *Language, Speech, and Hearing Services in Schools, 23*, 28–33.

Schraeder, T. (2001, October). Three current hot issues related to professional ethics. *School-Based Issues, 2*(1), 28.

Schraeder, T. (2006). *School services in speech-language pathology.* Madison, WI: Pigwick Papers.

Schraeder, T. (2008). *A guide to school services in speech-language pathology.* San Diego, CA: Plural.

Seymour, H. N., Bland-Stewart, L., & Green, L. J. (1998). Difference versus deficit in child African American English. *Language, Speech, and Hearing Services in Schools, 29*, 96–108.

Short, D. J., & Fitzsimmons, S. (2006, January). *Literacy development of bilingual adolescents: Issues and recommendations.* Paper presented at the meeting of National Association of Bilingual Education, Phoenix, AZ.

Stockman, I. J., Boult, J., & Robinson, G. (2004, July 20). Multicultural issues in academic and clinical education: A cultural mosaic. *ASHA Leader*, 6–7, 20.

Taylor, J. (1992). *Speech-language pathology services in schools* (2nd ed.). Boston, MA: Allyn & Bacon.

Taylor, O. (1986). *Treatment of communication disorders in culturally and linguistically diverse populations*. Austin, TX: Pro-Ed.

Teachers of English to Speakers of Other Languages. (2001). *Position statement on language and literacy development for young English language learners*. Retrieved from http://www.tesol.org/s_tesol/bin .asp?CID=32&DID=371&DOC=FILE.PDF

Teachers of English to Speakers of Other Languages. (2003a). *TESOL position statement on teacher quality in the field of teaching English to speakers of other languages*. Retrieved from http://www.tesol .org/s_tesol/bin.asp?CID=32&DID=374&DOC=FILE.PDF

Teachers of English to Speakers of Other Languages. (2003b). *TESOL position statement on Preparation of pre-k–12 educators for cultural and linguistic diversity in the United States*. Retrieved from http://www.tesol.org/s_tesol/bin.asp?CID=32&DID=1301&DOC= FILE.PDF

Teachers of English to Speakers of Other Languages. (2005a). *TESOL position statement on highly qualified teachers under No Child Left Behind*. Retrieved from http://www.tesol.org/s_tesol/bin.asp?CID =32&DID=3400&DOC=FILE.PDF

Teachers of English to Speakers of Other Languages. (2005b). *TESOL position statement on research and policy*. Retrieved from http:// www.tesol.org/s_tesol/bin.asp?CID=32&DID=3401&DOC=FILE.PDF

Teachers of English to Speakers of Other Languages. (2007). *TESOL position statement on the identification of English language learners with special educational needs*. Retrieved from http://www.tesol .org/s_tesol/bin.asp?CID=32&DID=8283&DOC=FILE.PDF

Teachers of English to Speakers of Other Languages. (2008). *Position statement on teacher preparation for content-based instruction (CBI)*. Retrieved from http://www.tesol.org/s_tesol/bin.asp?CID=32 &DID=10882&DOC=FILE.PDF

Thomas, W. P., & Collier, V. (2001). *School effectiveness for language minority students*. Washington, DC: National Center for Bilingual Education.

Thomason, K. M., Gorman, B. K., & Summers, C. (2007). English literacy development for English language learners: Does Spanish instruction promote or hinder? *EBP Briefs, 2*(2), 1–15.

US Department of Education. (1997). *1993–94 schools and staffing survey: A profile of policies and practices for limited English proficient students: Screening methods, program support, and teacher training (NCES 97–472)*. Washington, DC: Author. Retrieved from http://nces .ed.gov/pubs97/97472.pdf

US Department of Education. (1999). *Status of education reform in public elementary and secondary schools: Teachers' perspectives (NCES, 1999-045)*. Washington, DC: Author. Retrieved from http://www.eric.ed.gov/ERICDocs/data/ericdocs2sql/content_storage_01/0000019b/80/29/c0/d8.pdf

US Department of Education. (2001). *Teacher preparation and professional development: 2000 (NCES 2001-088)*. Washington, DC: Author.

US Department of Education. (2002). *Executive summary: The No Child Left Behind Act of 2001*. Washington, DC: Author.

US Department of Education. (2009). *Office of Special Education and Rehabilitative Services, Office of Special Education Programs, 28th annual report to Congress on the implementation of the Individuals with Disabilities Education Act, 2006* (Vol. 2). Washington, DC: Author.

Valdés, G., & Figueroa, R. A. (1994). *Bilingualism and testing: A special case of bias*. Norwood, NJ: Ablex.

Wei, L. (2006). *The bilingualism reader* (2nd ed.). New York, NY: Routledge.

Zehler, A., Fleischman, H., Hopstock, P., Stephenson, T., Pendzick, M., & Sapru, S. (2003). *Policy report: Summary of findings related to LEP and SPED-LEP students* (Report submitted to US Department of Education, Office of English Language Acquisition, Language Enhancement, and Academic Achievement of Limited English Proficient Students). Arlington, VA: Development Associates.

2

English Learners — Perspective from Two Disciplines

Key Terms

ASHA — American Speech-Language-Hearing Association

CAA — Council on Academic Accreditation in Audiology and Speech-Language Pathology

CCC — Certificate of Clinical Competence

CD EL — English Learner with a Communication Disorder

CLD — Culturally and Linguistically Diverse

CSD — Communication Sciences and Disorders

EBP — Evidence-Based Practice

EL — English Learner

ELL — English Language Learner

ESOL — English for Speakers of Other Languages

IDEA — Individuals with Disabilities Education Act

IDEIA — Individuals with Disabilities Education Improvement Act

KASA — Knowledge and Skills Acquisition

LEP — Limited English Proficient

NCATE — National Council for Accreditation of Teacher Education

continues

NCLB—No Child Left Behind

RtI—Response to Intervention

SLA—Second Language Acquisition

SLP—Speech-Language Pathologist

SLPCF—Speech-Language Pathology Clinical Fellowship

TESOL—Teachers of English to Speakers of Other Languages

Introduction

The discipline of communication sciences and disorders (CSD) includes the study of the human communication process, the science of human communication, breakdowns in the processes of human communication (referred to as communication differences or disorders), and the efficacy of the applied disciplinary practices (Guilford, Graham, & Scheuerle, 2007). Three primary professions are represented under the umbrella term "communication sciences and disorders." These include speech, language, and hearing sciences; audiology; and speech-language pathology. Other disciplines, such as deafness and deaf education, are often included as related areas of practice because many of these professionals develop and apply educational and rehabilitative techniques for individuals with severe and profound hearing impairments (Guilford, 2003).

What Is the Profession of
Communication Sciences and Disorders?

The term speech-language pathology has primarily been used to describe the role of professionals primarily concerned with individuals who could not communicate. Early efforts in establishing the professional discipline of speech-language pathology came from psychology, education, medical science, and linguistics. Currently, this professional field focuses on the prevention, etiology, diagnosis, prognosis, and treatment of communication delays, disorders, or differences across the scope of practice (ASHA, 2007). The term "communication sciences and disorders" has consistently been used since the 1980s. It is offered as a program of study in approximately 250 US graduate programs in the discipline; however, not all of these programs offer both speech-language pathology and audiology degrees (ASHA, 2011).

Speech-language pathology is a dynamic and continuously developing profession. The goal of the profession of speech-language pathology and its members is provision of the highest quality treatment and other services consistent with the fundamental right of those served to participate in decisions that affect their lives (Lubinski & Fratteli, 2001). Over the past 25 years, the client populations, work settings, and assessment and treatment methods have changed dramatically. Passage of educational legislation (i.e., Individuals with Disabilities Education Act [IDEA] and No Child Left Behind [NCLB]) focusing on the rights of school-age children has had a strong impact on the profession. Additionally, legislation focusing on individuals with disabilities and their communicative needs has resulted in the establishment of comprehensive diagnostic and treatment procedures for individuals across the life span.

An important characteristic of the practice of speech-language pathology is that, to the extent possible, clinical decisions are based on the best available evidence. ASHA has defined evidence-based practice in speech-language pathology as an approach in which current, high-quality research evidence is integrated with practitioner expertise and the individual's preferences and values into the process of clinical decision making (ASHA, 2005a). A high-quality basic, applied, and efficacy research base in communication sciences and disorders and related fields of study is essential to providing evidence-based clinical practice and quality clinical services. Currently, SLPs provide services in settings that are deemed appropriate, including but not limited to health care, educational, community, vocational, home settings, and private practices (ASHA, 2010a).

Professional Association — American Speech-Language-Hearing Association (ASHA)

The American Speech-Language-Hearing Association (ASHA) is the professional, credentialing, and scientific organization for SLPs, audiologists, and speech/language/hearing scientists in the United States and internationally. Founded in 1925, it currently provides an array of membership services, has numerous scholarly journals and publications, special-interest divisions, and educational activities that support lifelong learning to its current 145,481 members (ASHA, 2010 b). The purpose, nature, and scope of ASHA can be found in its bylaws (ASHA, 2008) and governance structure (Figure 2–1).

The competencies needed by SLPs and audiologists are essential if patients and clients are to receive appropriate and quality care. Competencies are based on the professional body of knowledge and application of this knowledge to the assessment and treatment of individuals with communication disorders (Ehren, Lefkowitz, & Roth, 1997). SLPs must have the requisite knowledge, specialized skills, and techniques to work with a diverse population across the life span and settings. Graham and Guilford (2000) offer a model of clinical expertise that outlines five factors and associated indicators often cited as critical to the development of expertise within the profession. These five factors include interpersonal skills, professional skills, problem-solving skills, technical skills, and knowledge and experience. Although expertise in speech-language pathology is a broad concept, Graham (1998) notes that the factors and associated indicators represented in their model provide an overview of the competencies necessary for all SLPs in the development of expertise in the profession of speech-language pathology. One important role served by ASHA is the assurance that SLPs have the professional skills and knowledge to provide optimum services to individuals with communication disorders. ASHA provides standards for professional education, certification, and licensure necessary for entry into the professions of speech-language pathology and audiology. Specifically, the Council on Academic Accreditation in Audiology and Speech-Language Pathology (CAA) of the American Speech-Language-Hearing Association

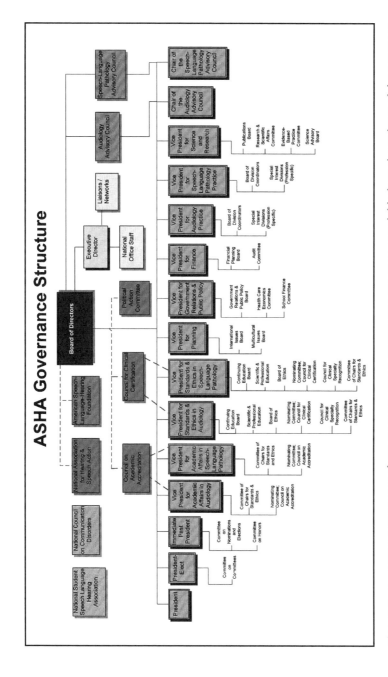

Figure 2–1. *ASHA governance chart. Source: ASHA governance structure. Available from the website of the American Speech–Language–Hearing Association: http://www.asha.org/uploadedFiles/about/governance/ASHAGovStructure.pdf. Copyright 2009 by American Speech–Language–Hearing Association. All rights reserved. Reprinted with permission.*

37

is the accrediting agency for audiology and speech-language pathology education programs. The CAA formulates standards for the accreditation of graduate education programs that provide entry-level professional preparation in audiology and/or speech-language pathology.

Graduates of an accredited program in speech-language pathology require academic and clinical education that reflects current knowledge, skills, technology, and scope of practice. These standards, specified by ASHA in 2005 (ASHA, 2005b) and often referred to as the "KASA Standards," requires students to demonstrate that they have acquired a specific set of knowledge and skills standards through participation in their graduate program (see Appendix B). KASA is an acronym standing for Knowledge and Skills Acquisition. There is a "Knowledge" portion of KASA and a "Skills" portion. The Skills portion relates to clinical competencies across nine specific clinical areas, referred to as "the Big Nine" (see Table 2–1). Every academic program accredited by the CAA is impacted by KASA; however, programs differ in determining how students will demonstrate their competency in achieving these skills.

Graduates must pass the national examination adopted by ASHA (i.e., PRAXIS) for purposes of certification in speech-language pathology and after completion of academic course work and practica, the student must successfully complete a 36-week Speech-Language Pathology Clinical Fellowship (SLPCF). Upon successful completion of the SLPCF the clinical fellow is awarded the Certificate of Clinical Competence (CCC) in Speech-Language Pathology by the Council on Clinical Certification (ASHA, 2005b).

Although the credential issued by ASHA is the CCC professional certification, licenses issued by governmental agencies are usually required for SLPs who work in settings such as schools or health care agencies. The credentials issued by governmental agencies are either the professional license or teacher certification. The specific content of the licensure laws varies from state to state. Maintenance of the CCC requires that the licensee participate in continuing education to maintain currency and continues to uphold the standards of practice acceptable to the profession. To facilitate continuing professional development, ASHA publishes a number of scholarly journals and newsletters, offers continuing education opportunities (e.g., annual conven-

Table 2–1. ASHA Standards for Speech-Language Pathology, Standard III-C (2005)

"Big Nine" Clinical Areas	
Clinical Area	Descriptor
Articulation	Articulation and phonology
Fluency	Fluency, stuttering
Voice	Voice and resonance, including respiration and phonation
Language	Receptive and expressive language (phonology, morphology, syntax, semantics, and pragmatics) in speaking, listening, reading, writing, and manual modalities
Hearing	Hearing, including the impact on speech and language
Swallowing	Swallowing (oral, pharyngeal, esophageal, and related functions, including oral function for feeding; orofacial myofunction)
Cognitive Aspects	Cognitive aspects of communication (attention, memory, sequencing, problem-solving, executive functioning)
Social Aspects	Social aspects of communication (including challenging behavior, ineffective social skills, lack of communication opportunities)
Communicative Modalities	Communication modalities (including oral, manual, augmentative, and alternative communication techniques and assistive technologies)

Source: 2005 Standards and Implementation Procedures for the Certificate of Clinical Competence in Speech-Language Pathology (revised March 2009). Retrieved from the website of the American Speech-Language-Hearing Association: http://www.asha.org/Certification/slp_standards/. All rights reserved. Adapted with permission.

tion; seminars; self-study), has 16 special interest divisions representing specific areas of practice, maintains a website (http://www.asha.org), and offers an award for continuing education (ACE).

To ensure that the standards for practice are followed, ASHA requires that every individual who is: (a) a member of the American Speech-Language-Hearing Association, whether certified or not, (b) a nonmember holding the Certificate of Clinical Competence from ASHA, (c) an applicant for membership or certification, or (d) a clinical fellow seeking to fulfill standards for certification abide by the Code of Ethics (ASHA, 2010c). Adherence to the standards assures the public that no harm will occur from improper evaluation or treatment. Ultimately, SLPs must be knowledgeable about the Code of Ethics and scope of practice, as these are essential for professional development and practice. ASHA's Practice Policy Documents, along with other important documents of the association, provide SLPs with direction on best practices and standards in the profession (Davidson & Denton, 2010).

ASHA Practice Policy Documents

ASHA has published a multitude of documents and policy statements that outline the competencies associated with the various needs (disorders or conditions) of persons being served (see Appendix A). These documents detail the scope of practice, the necessary precautions (educational and training), and the knowledge and skills needed to meet the unique needs of individuals with communication disorders across settings and the life span (ASHA, n.d.).

Appendices A and B include many of the policy statements and standards that provide the SLP with guidelines for practice across populations and settings. For example, with the ever-increasing diversity in schools, SLPs are required to work with other professionals to ensure that all students receive quality, culturally competent services. In the ASHA 2010 professional issues statement on the role and responsibility of SLPs in the schools, SLPs are required to "develop competencies to distinguish a language disorder from a language difference, consider socioeconomic factors and/or a lack of adequate prior instruction, and the process of acquiring the dialect of English used in the schools to promote efficient and effective outcomes for students" (ASHA, 2010d, 2010e).

The advent of groundbreaking research on culturally and linguistically diverse (CLD) populations in the early 1980s marked the beginning of the distinction between communication differences and disorders (Saad & Polovoy, 2009). As the difference versus disorders research increased, a series of ASHA position papers, guidelines, and technical reports specific to providing culturally and linguistically appropriate services were developed (e.g., *Social Dialects Position Paper* [ASHA, 1983]; *Clinical Management of Communicatively Handicapped Minority Language Populations* [ASHA, 1985]; *Bilingual SLPs and Audiologists: Definition* [ASHA, 1989]; *Knowledge and Skills Needed by Speech-Language Pathologists and Audiologists to Provide Culturally and Linguistically Appropriate Services* [ASHA, 2004]). Additionally, ASHA's Office of Multicultural Affairs (OMA) became responsible for: (a) addressing cultural and linguistic diversity issues related to professionals and persons with communication disorders and differences, and (b) providing the profession with information and resources that are important to the service and delivery to culturally and linguistically diverse populations, and specifically ELs.

Competencies for SLPS Who Work with ELs

The growing population of ELs in US schools has been well documented. Nearly one in five Americans speak a language other than English at home, and almost 45% of US teachers have at least one student designated as an EL in their classrooms. There is a critical shortage of trained school SLPs to meet the specialized needs of ELs with disabilities. Students learning English are disadvantaged by lack of personnel trained to conduct linguistically and culturally relevant educational assessments (Bedore, Peña, Garcia, & Cortez, 2005; Klingner et al., 2005; Mattes & Saldana-Illingworth, 2009; National Association for Bilingual Education & ILIAD Project, 2002; Solórzano, 2008) and to address their language- and disability-related needs simultaneously (Battle, 2002; Caesar & Kohler, 2007; Kohnert, 2008; Rosa-Lugo & Fradd, 2000; Rosa-Lugo, Rivera, & McKeown, 1998).

Approximately 20 years ago, ASHA adopted a resolution that "encouraged undergraduate, graduate and continuing education programs to include specific information, course content and/or clinical practica that address the communication needs of individuals within socially, culturally, economically and linguistically diverse populations" (ASHA, 1987). In response to the need to serve an increasingly diverse population, ASHA mandated that, as of January 1, 1993, accredited graduate programs in communication sciences and disorders must offer course content pertaining to culturally diverse groups (ASHA, 1992). The goal was to ensure that SLPs develop the knowledge and competencies to serve ELs with communication disorders and clients who speak nonstandard dialects (ASHA, 1983, 2003a), as well as to continue to increase the percentage of ASHA professionals from CLD groups, which to date has remained low.

The roles and responsibilities of school-based SLPs have changed over the years in response to legislative, regulatory, societal, and professional influences. Schools are striving to meet the mandate of leaving no child behind, despite the challenges associated with teaching students from multiple cultural, linguistic, and experiential backgrounds, including those who are new to the English language. The responsibility of determining whether a student's academic difficulties stem from learning a second language or from the presence of a disability, or from both, requires that SLPs have the skills and competencies to facilitate the necessary changes that would move the profession "from past practice patterns to those that reflect current legislation, research, and practice guidelines" with respect to practice in the school setting, specifically with underrepresented populations (ASHA, 2010d; Caesar & Kohler, 2007; Rosa-Lugo & Champion, 2007). SLPs must be knowledgeable about general curricular goals and benchmarks and skilled in more educationally relevant approaches that support and reflect content area learning for ELs (ASHA, 2001; Mihai, 2010; Nutta, Bautista, & Butler, 2010).

In 1998 ASHA issued a position statement and technical report entitled *Provision of Instruction in English as a Second Language by SLPs in School Settings* (1998a, 1998b). This position paper noted that, increasingly, SLPs are being requested to work in a role traditionally assigned to instructors of ESOL. Due to the growing population of students who are ELs and the increasing requests for SLPs to function in this role, SLPs requested clarification on their role in working with ELs in the school setting. ASHA's position statement clearly indicates that

ESOL instruction should be provided *only* by professionals with appropriate training and experience. ESOL instruction requires academic preparation and experience in such areas as second language acquisition theory, comparative linguistics, ESOL methodologies, assessment, and practica. ASHA recognized that the required knowledge, skills, and competencies for providing such service may extend beyond those provided in CSD preservice educational training program; thus, they recommended that SLP and ESOL professionals work collaboratively in the preassessment, assessment, and intervention stage of service in the language and academic development of ELs with communication disorders.

Interestingly, in 2007 Teachers of English to Speakers of Other Languages (TESOL) issued a position statement on *The Identification of English Language Learners with Special Educational Needs*. This position paper acknowledged that identifying ELs with special needs is a complex and difficult process and requires culturally responsive expertise and purposeful collaboration (TESOL, 2007). In this age of changing demographics, SLPs are not exempt from the possibility of being asked to provide services to ELs. As a result, SLPs and ESOL professionals are being tapped to respond to the call for new collaborative roles and responsibilities in identifying and serving ELs with disabilities (Rosa-Lugo & Champion, 2007; Rosa-Lugo & Fradd, 2000; Roseberry-McKibben, 2003, 2008a).

Who Are English Learners with a Communication Disorder (CD ELs)?

Determining the population of children and adults with speech and language disorders has been challenging because there are several populations that may have communication disorders secondary to another disability. Furthermore, when ELs struggle academically professionals must determine all the variables to ascertain if the child's learning problems results from a language disorder or if the student is progressing through the stages of learning a second language. Researchers have indicated that (Goldstein, 2004; Harry & Klingner, 2006; Kayser, 2002; Kohnert,

2008; Roseberry-McKibbin, 2007, 2008a, 2008b) students with communication disorders often exhibit specific characteristics such as difficulty learning language at a normal rate, even with support and assistance in both languages; gaps in vocabulary and decreased mean lengths of utterances; difficulties communicating with peers as well as in the home; difficulty across literacy events; lack of organization in the use of language to convey thoughts; and poor academic achievement despite having adequate academic proficiency in English. Researchers concur that typical language abilities serve as the focal point for determining a language disorder. The literature consistently suggests that if a student has a language disorder he/she will usually demonstrate problems not only in English but in English and the primary language, or the acquisition of any language (Goldstein, 2004; Kohnert, 2008; Roseberry-McKibben, 2008a).

Service Delivery Models for CD ELs

The choice of effective service delivery is a major challenge for school-based SLPs. In general, one of the greatest challenges of school-based SLPs is how to deliver speech-language services in a way that results in the most change in students within the daily schedule and logistics of the school environment (Flynn, 2010). A service delivery model is often conceptualized as an organized configuration of resources to achieve a particular educational outcome. It must address questions such as: Where will the service be delivered? Who will deliver the service? How frequently will the service be provided? And for how long?

Service delivery in the schools (Blosser & Kratcoski, 1997; Moore & Montgomery, 2008; Paul, Blosser, & Jakubowitz, 2006; Peters-Johnson, 1998; Throneburg, Calvert, Strum, Paramboukas, & Paul, 2000; Whitmire, 2002) has evolved over the years and dramatically influenced the role of school-based SLPs. Blosser and Kratcoski (1997) chronicled speech-language delivery models over three decades and posed a framework for decision making and service delivery that would take into consideration the provider, the activities, and the context (PACs) necessary to meet the needs of individuals with a communication disorder (Figure 2–2). They encouraged SLPs to expand and incorporate ser-

	1970s	1980s	1990s	2000
Focus for Treatment	Mechanistic view of language	Pragmatics	Functional, interactive communication Preparation for learning, living, and working	Outcomes
Speech-language pathologist's role	Specialist model	Expert model	Collaborative-consultative model	Facilitator of the service delivery
Emerging issues	Language use is important	Language and learning are linked	Inclusion, transition, efficacy, account-ability, outcomes	To be decided
	syntax semantics phonology	content form use	communication learning collaboration	context providers activities

Figure 2–2. *The evolution of speech-language pathologist service delivery models.* Source: *"A Framework for Determining Appropriate Service Delivery Options," by J. L. Blosser and A. Kratcoski, 1997,* Language, Speech, and Hearing Services in Schools, 28, *p. 100. Copyright 2007 by American Speech-Language-Hearing Association. All rights reserved. Reprinted with permission.*

vice delivery options that would serve all children in the least restrictive environment (LRE), as outlined in the Individuals with Disabilities Education Improvement Act (IDEIA) of 2004.

New service delivery models have been recommended that range from the traditional pull-out model to the family-centered model, self-contained classrooms, the resource room model, consultative/collaborative service delivery models, and several types of classroom-based approaches (Table 2–2; Brandel & Loeb, 2011; Cirrin et al., 2010; Flynn, 2010; Friend & Cook, 2010; Katz, Maag, Fallon, Blenkarn, & Smith, 2010; Moore & Montgomery, 2008; Schooling, Venediktov, & Leech, 2010).

Table 2–2. Service Delivery Model for Speech-Language Pathologists

	Cases Served	Services Provided	Group Size	Time	Rationale for Caseload Size	Caseload Maximum
Itinerant Program (Direct Service)	All communicative disorders All ranges	Program development, management, coordination, and evaluation Direct services Provision of speech-language services in coordination with classroom teachers and/or other special educators	Individual/ small group, up to 3 students/ session	½ hr. (mild) to 2 hrs./day 2 to 5 times a week	Moderate-severe cases require more service Increased clinical time required to produce change Amount and type of service needed is considered in determining caseload numbers	Up to 25 severe; up to 22–25 maximum
Resource Room Program (Direct Service)	All communicative disorders Moderate to severe	Program development, management, coordination, and evaluation Direct services and/or self-study	Individual/ small group, up to 5 students/ session	1 to 3 hrs./ day 4 to 5 times a week	Moderate-severe case may require more intensive service Consistent with some state regulations for classes of special ed.	Up to 15–25 students

continued

	Cases Served	Services Provided	Group Size	Time	Rationale for Caseload Size	Caseload Maximum
Resource Room Program (Direct Service) *continued*		Provision of speech-language services in coordination with classroom teachers and/or other special educators				
		Classroom teacher is primarily responsible for academic instruction				
Self-Contained Program (Direct Service)	Severe and/or multiple communicative disorders	Program development, management, coordination, and evaluation	Up to 10 students per SLP	Full school day	Consistent with some state regulations for classes of special education	Up to 10 students without aide
	Primary handicapping condition is communication	Direct speech-language services plus academic instruction provided by SLP with SEA guidelines	Up to 15 students per SLP and aide	Full-time placement	Provides for intensive services	Up to 15 students with aide

47

Table 2-2. *continued*

	Cases Served	Services Provided	Group Size	Time	Rationale for Caseload Size	Caseload Maximum
Consultation Program (Indirect Service)	All communicative disorders All ranges	Program development, management, coordination, and evaluation Indirect services: Develops clinical programs carried out by others	Individual/small group (through indirect service)	½ hr. to 3–4 hrs./day (variable)	Amount of time needed in relation to organizational and structural variety of personnel or agencies involved Variability of student needs and the needs of those being trained	10–15 severe 15–55 mild to moderate

Source: From *Making a Difference for America's Children: Speech–Language Pathologists in Public Schools, Second Edition* (p. 180), by B. J. Moore and J. K. Montgomery, 2008, Austin, TX: PRO-ED. Copyright 2008 by PRO-ED, Inc. Reprinted with permission.

To specifically serve CD ELs, service delivery models will have to incorporate culturally responsive approaches that are evidence-based. Speech-language pathologists will have to consider the use of nonbiased assessment, the role of the native language, the use of interpreters in intervention, accents and dialects spoken by ELs, evidenced-based interventions, and ways to successfully collaborate with professionals and families who are culturally and linguistically diverse (Moore & Montgomery, 2008; Ortiz & Yates, 2001).

Given the many activities that school-based SLPs are required to accomplish (Figure 2–3), the issue of caseload and

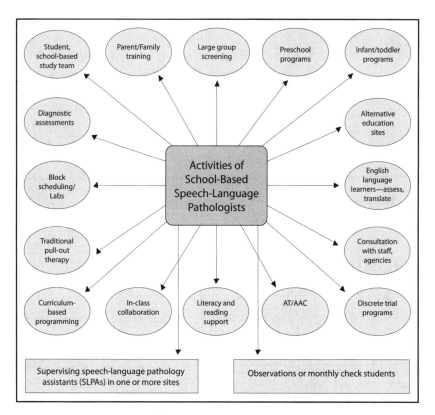

Figure 2−3. *Activities of the SLP.* Source: *From* Making a Difference for America's Children: Speech-Language Pathologists in Public Schools, Second Edition *(p. 185), by B. J. Moore and J. K. Montgomery, 2008, Austin, TX: PRO-ED. Copyright 2008 by PRO-ED, Inc. Reprinted with permission.*

workload has also been considered. The term caseload typically refers to the number of students with Individualized Education Programs (IEPs) or Individualized Family Service Plans (IFSPs) that school SLPs serve through direct and/or indirect service delivery options. Workload refers to all activities required and performed by school-based SLPs (ASHA, 2002). Several methods and strategies have been recommended for developing a workload approach to service delivery to ensure that SLPs can engage in the required workload activities and implement best practices in school speech-language pathology to meet the individual needs of students (ASHA, 2002, 2003b; Giess, 2010).

The Individuals with Disabilities Education Improvement Act of 2004 also allows services for students who are having academic difficulties but are not identified as having a disability. This initiative, known as Response to Intervention (RtI), is an alternative to the use of a discrepancy model to assess underachievement. This model, also known in the literature as a prevention model (Schraeder, 2008), uses a multitiered approach to provide a seamless system of instruction and interventions to struggling learners at increasing levels of intensity guided by child outcome data. Esparza-Brown and Doolittle (2008) proposed an RtI model for use with ELs that calls for collaboration among professionals and increased opportunities for professional dialogue. They outlined a three-tiered framework that considers students' ecologies and cultural and linguistic needs in addition to the skills that professionals must possess when working with an EL student. Rinaldi and Samson (2008) support the use of a three-tiered RtI model with ELs and suggest that professionals use a data-driven decision-making process to inform assessment and implementation of evidence-based interventions and to determine disability in ELs.

Ultimately, SLPs play an important role in using RtI to identify ELs with disabilities and to provide instruction to students who are struggling in the general education setting. These roles have required some fundamental changes in the way SLPs engage in assessment and intervention activities (Ehren, Montgomery, Rudebusch, & Whitmore, 2006).

The current climate of accountability requires SLPs to apply evidence-based practice (EBP) when making assessment and intervention decisions. Specific to ELs, SLPs must identify and execute the most ethical and appropriate services. However, making clinical decisions for ELs and their families can be challenging. Selecting the language of instruction (Gutierrez-Clellan, 1999; Nixon, McCardle, & Leos, 2007; Schiff-Myers, 1992); using interpreters (Langdon & Cheng, 2002); acknowledging accents and dialects (ASHA, 2003a; Langdon, 1999; Wilkinson & Payne, 2005); and working with families are all factors that influence service provision to ELs (Caesar & Kohler, 2007; Moore & Montgomery, 2008; Roseberry-McKibben, 2008b). A decision-making framework to assist the SLP select and implement a culturally and linguistically appropriate service delivery model has been recommended by Chabon, Esparza-Brown, and Gildersleeve-Neumann (2010). This systematic approach proposes that SLPs should: (a) examine relevant evidence and clinical expertise, (b) consider the perspectives, values, and beliefs of the individuals involved, and (c) evaluate all data in relation to the ASHA Code of Ethics (ASHA, 2010c) in order to identify and implement the most ethical and appropriate services. Although a number of recommendations have been provided within the discipline of communication sciences and disorders, Cirrin et al. (2010) concluded that clinicians have little research evidence on which to base decisions about service delivery options for ELs with CDs.

In the absence of conclusive data on providing services to ELs with CDs, it is imperative that we look to other disciplines such as general and special education, linguistics, and bilingual education or English as a second language (ESL) to provide us with additional data and resources. Specifically, the 1998 ASHA position paper on the role of SLPs working with ESL professionals in school settings lays the beginning groundwork for a collaborative process for both professionals to merge their skills and knowledge to facilitate learning outcomes and language proficiency in ELs (ASHA, 1998a, 1998b). Therefore, it is critical that SLPs understand this discipline and the skills and competencies of the ESOL professional.

English Learners — Perspectives of the ESOL Professionals

The field of English for Speakers of Other Languages (ESOL) is grounded in the discipline of second language acquisition (SLA). This area of study combines research and theory in a variety of fields to address how languages other than the native (first) language are learned. Linguistics has historically been the foundation of SLA research and theory. This is fitting as SLA examines language, specifically language acquired after acquisition of the native tongue. Scholars in the areas of applied linguistics, psycholinguistics, and sociolinguistics have been the primary developers of SLA theory, but disciplines such as cognitive psychology, literacy studies, and critical pedagogy, among others, have also influenced the direction of SLA. Second language acquisition encompasses not only ESOL but also any other language learned after the first. In other words, researching how an American exchange student learns Spanish in Colombia or a German high school student learns French in Berlin is also the focus of SLA. However, there are specific issues that pertain to the context of teaching ESOL. Like any other subject matter, ESOL has an abundance of jargon and acronyms. Just as ELs must learn new vocabulary to communicate in English, professionals need to know the language of ESOL. The term ESOL refers to both a subject and an instructional approach. ESOL as a subject is a sequence of increasingly complex linguistic competencies, involving both comprehension and expression. The aim of the subject of study is to become fully proficient in listening, speaking, reading, and writing the language. In other words, the target is to be nativelike in proficiency. For example, being able to understand the question, "What is your name?" and being able to state an appropriate response would be a typical early competency. Furthermore, being able to correctly use comparative and superlative adjectives such as "more advantageous than" and "the most advantageous" would be a more advanced competency in an ESOL course. School districts also treat ESOL as an instructional approach or intervention, meaning that common types of accommodations and modifications of instruction for English learners may fall under the terms ESOL services or ESOL strategies.

ESOL is not the only accepted acronym for this field. Other common terms include English as a second language (ESL), English as an additional language (EAL), and English as a new language (ENL). The term ESOL is most frequently used in K–12 school settings, whereas ESL is used more in postsecondary environments, although this is not always the case. English as a new language and English as an additional language are less frequently used and were developed to more precisely describe the field. In other words, nonnative speakers who are learning English may already know two or three languages, so calling English a second language is inaccurate for many students. English for speakers of other languages does not necessarily convey that these speakers are not proficient in English (they could have been brought up bilingually or English could be their first of two or more languages acquired). As evidenced by the variety of terms to refer to the field, no term has been coined that is perfectly descriptive of the diverse conditions that comprise ESOL.

Professional Association — TESOL

The professional organization that represents ESOL specialists is Teachers of English to Speakers of Other Languages, or TESOL (http://www.tesol.org). Although ESOL is part of the acronym TESOL, it is interesting to note that the preposition that is bounded by the E and S differs between the two acronyms. The subject area or field is English *for* Speakers of Other Languages, but the profession is Teachers of English *to* Speakers of Other Languages.

TESOL began in 1966, supported by five existing professional organizations in related fields: (1) the Center for Applied Linguistics, (2) the Modern Language Association, (3) the National Association for Foreign Student Affairs, (4) the National Council of Teachers of English, and (5) the Speech Association of America (TESOL, n.d.a). The mission of this organization is to "develop and maintain professional expertise in English language teaching and learning for speakers of other languages worldwide" (TESOL, n.d.b). Its values include: "professionalism in language education, individual language rights, accessible, high quality education, collaboration in a global community, interaction of research and reflective practice for educational improvement, and respect for diversity and multiculturalism" (TESOL, n.d.c).

As of November 2011, there were approximately 12,000 members (TESOL, n.d.d) representing 52 countries. The top five countries were as follows: 74% of TESOL members are from the United States, 4% from Japan, 3.5% from China, 3% from

Canada, and 1% from Mexico. In the United States, the state with the most members is California, followed by New York, Texas, Illinois, and Pennsylvania. In terms of grade level, 27% of members teach at the postsecondary level, 18% in adult education, 10% in secondary education, 10% in elementary education, and 6% in community colleges. The remaining members are in "other" or "undeclared" categories. The largest special interest groups, comprising 8, 7, and 7% of membership respectively, address English as a foreign language (EFL), meaning English taught in countries where it is not the native language (e.g., not in the United States, England, or Australia), teacher education, and adult education.

Although ASHA began promulgating position statements on issues affecting children in K–12 in the 1980s, TESOL did not issue position papers on these topics until the 1990s. As of winter 2011, TESOL has approximately 57 position statements, ranging from recognition of all varieties of English, including dialects, creoles, and World Englishes, to governance of intensive English programs at universities, to recommendations for the reauthorization of the Elementary and Secondary Education Act in the US.

TESOL Position Statements

A number of TESOL's position statements address issues pertaining to teaching ELs in the K–12 setting (see Appendix A). In addition, there are position statements that are specific to students with special needs. For example, in July 2009, TESOL issued a position statement on deaf students, asserting that they have the right to become proficient in sign language or written or spoken languages, such as English (TESOL, 2009). In March 2007, TESOL took a stance on the identification of ELs with special needs, maintaining that there is a disproportionate number of CLD students in special education, while arguing that in some cases ELs with special needs are not identified as such due to confusion over language development versus language disorders or learning disabilities (TESOL, 2007). The statement cites IDEIA (2004), which specifies provisions for assessing linguistically and culturally diverse students for special education services. TESOL believes that multiple means of assessment must be used for identifying learning disabilities in ELs. Moreover, they state that assessment should be conducted in the EL's dominant language, and the student's level of proficiency in English and the native language should be taken into account. Professionals working with students identified as ELs with special needs will be required to attain knowledge and competencies in bilingualism, second language acquisition, and sociocultural issues.

Competencies for Teachers of ELs — Specialists and Generalists

TESOL and the National Council for the Accreditation of Teacher Education (NCATE) have clearly defined the knowledge base and skill set for ESOL professionals who focus entirely on teaching ELs. These performance-based standards, used in the preparation and licensing of ESOL professionals, are often referred to as the TESOL/NCATE Standards for P–12 Teacher Education Programs (TESOL, 2010). The standards were originally approved in 2001 for P–12 ESL teacher education programs and revised in 2009. They focus on five domains: *language, culture, instruction, assessment,* and *professionalism.*

The first domain, *language,* includes the ability to describe language and the process of acquiring it. The second domain, *culture,* focuses on its nature and role as well as cultural groups and identity. The third domain, *instruction,* is divided into three sections and focuses primarily on planning, managing, and implementing instruction through the effective use of resources and technology. The fourth domain, *assessment,* includes general assessment issues, assessing language proficiency, and classroom-based assessment. In addition, recommendations for collaboration with other professionals, to include the SLP, are noted to specifically determine "differences among normal language development, language difference, and learning problems." (TESOL, 2010, pp. 57–58). The final domain, *professionalism,* encompasses research and history of the field, partnerships and advocacy, and professional development and collaboration.

Under each of the five domains are specialized standards. For example, in language, the first standard is describing language, and its first indicator is *Apply knowledge of phonology to help ESOL students develop oral, reading, and writing skills in English.* The criterion for meeting the standard requires that teachers use contrastive phonology of students' first language to analyze students' pronunciation in English, develop activities to help students acquire the English sound system, and use techniques to promote phonemic awareness.

In contrast to the TESOL/NCATE standards, the report *Educating English Language Learners: Building Teacher Capacity* (Ballantyne, Sanderman, & Levy, 2008) focuses on general information and skills that mainstream teachers who have one or more ELs in their regular classrooms should possess. They divide essential competencies into language acquisition and communicative competence, curriculum and instruction, content assessment, culture and education, and school and home communities. Assuming that the SLP or other professionals (e.g., regular classroom teacher; special education teacher; bilingual education teacher) will collaborate with an ESOL specialist as necessary, they maintain that mainstream teachers and/or other professionals require a less specialized and in-depth skill set and knowledge base to accommodate one or more ELs in the regular classroom.

Many states have set requirements for professionals that work with ELs. For example, in Florida, the Consent Decree (also known as the META or ESOL Consent Decree) of 1990 is the framework for compliance with federal and state laws and jurisprudence regarding the education of ELs (FLDOE, n.d.). The Consent Decree outlines specific requirements and competencies for personnel who instruct and interact with ELs and monitors compliance to ensure that ELs have equal access to comprehensible instruction. The Florida Department of Education (FLDOE), Bureau of Student Achievement through Language Acquisition, has set requirements for state certification, and competencies and skills for professionals who work with ELs (FLDOE, 2010). The SLP who is working with ELs with communication disorders is one of the professionals that are required to complete prescribed in-service staff development to ensure that they are able to provide essential services to ELs.

Who Are ESOL Students?

Even more intricate than the terms for the field of ESOL are the terms that describe the students. At one time, students were described by the subject they were taught — ESOL students. However, not all students who are not proficient in English are ESOL students. Some may be in bilingual programs, whereas others may be mainstreamed with in-class support, etc. Therefore, a term was needed that reflected the nature of the students rather than the subject. The federal term that became prevalent in the 1980s was limited English proficient, or LEP. This term troubled many in the field because it emphasized the students' limitations. Equally troubling was the unspoken assumption that having a native language other than English and developing as a bilingual was a limitation. On the contrary, developing fluency in more than one language is an asset that most native speakers of English would like to attain.

As federal terms are difficult to change, some states referred to the acronym of LEP as "language-enriched pupil," but over time that acronym has fallen into disfavor. Subsequently, the term English language learner (ELL) has become the most common descriptor, with the term now being shortened to English learner (EL). Some take issue with this term because its precision in describing these students is lacking. One could make the case that an EL is any student in an English-speaking environment, even native speakers of English, as they are learning to read and write in English. Although the term EL has this shortcoming, it is currently the preferred term to describe students who are identified as needing ESOL support services or ESOL instruction. Another term for EL students, language minority student, encompasses English language learner but goes beyond that term, including those students whose English proficiency is sufficient to no longer need support services or ESOL instruction. These former ELs require monitoring for a specific period after being moved from the EL category. Because current and former ELs speak a language other than English as their native language, they are termed language minority students.

The field of ESOL is unique in its varied emphases in different parts of the world. In Europe, ESOL is currently termed

English language teaching, with origins that reach back to the 15th century (Howatt & Widdowson, 2004). Because of British colonialism, English language instruction spread throughout the British Empire as a language of trade or lingua franca. In the United States, however, ESOL focused on the instruction of immigrants. The Naturalization Act of 1906 required English proficiency to become a naturalized citizen. Citizenship and "Americanization" classes emerged in response to the immigrant influx at the turn of the 20th century. Job sites and community organizations began to teach English along with citizenship classes. After World War I, immigration rates declined, with the lowest period of immigration during the 1930s. In subsequent decades, immigration continued to increase. During the US civil rights movement, language minority issues were raised by Latino populations in Arizona, California, and Texas (Roos, 1978). In 1964, the Civil Rights Act established a basis for equal access to educational programming and freedom from segregation and discrimination for ELs. The Bilingual Education Act of 1968 followed, opening the door to instruction in the native languages of ELs. In 1974, the Supreme Court ruling *Lau v. Nichols* declared that to abide by civil rights laws, public schools were required to accommodate the linguistic needs of ELs. To meet the spirit of the *Lau v. Nichols* ruling, schools have a variety of options for service delivery (Collier, 1998; Garcia, 1991; Gibbons, 2002; Montone, 1995; Rennie, 1993). In the next section, we will survey the most common service delivery options for ELs in the United States.

Instructional Program Models for English Learners

ESOL programs differ in multiple ways. Typically, ELs in ESOL programs are taught by specialists who hold certification or endorsement in ESOL. By having access to professionals with a depth of knowledge and skills in promoting second language acquisition, ELs in ESOL programs can receive more individualized and targeted instructional support.

One common service delivery model for ELs is the *pull-out ESOL model*. Pull-out ESOL programs remove ELs from one or more class periods per day to gather with other ELs for language development and subject matter support. Often, pull-out ESOL sessions replace one or more hours of English language arts instruction. ESOL teachers may use a special language arts curriculum for ELs, or they may work with the classroom teacher to identify vocabulary and grammar related to the content taught in the mainstream class.

Another model of service delivery for ELs is the *push-in ESOL model*. In contrast to the pull-out ESOL model, the push-in ESOL model involves coteaching with the classroom teacher and ESOL specialist. The ESOL specialist and classroom teacher collaborate in planning, delivering, and evaluating lessons for ELs who are integrated in the regular classroom. When the classroom teacher is leading a lesson, the ESOL specialist may sit in the back of the room with the ELs, using supplemental materials and targeted language to reach the ELs at their levels of English proficiency. Sometimes a bilingual aide may be the push-in specialist, working with ELs in both English and their native language to improve comprehension and performance.

Another model of service delivery is the *self-contained ESOL class*. Self-contained ESOL classes are offered where and when there is a critical mass of ELs at the same grade level. English learners are grouped with other ELs and are taught using "sheltered" instruction. Sheltered instruction has a long history in teaching ELs, and most recently it has come to mean teaching regular academic content at the level and pace appropriate for ELs (Echevarria, Vogt, & Short, 2008). Teachers of self-contained classes are ESOL specialists as well as certified in the subjects and/or grade levels they teach. Variations on self-contained classrooms are newcomer schools. Newcomer schools typically are provided at the secondary level for ELs who are at beginning to intermediate levels of proficiency. By grouping ELs together at a high school dedicated entirely to these students, teachers can provide intensive English instruction while teaching academic content at the students' level of English proficiency or even in the native language. Typically, students remain a year in newcomer schools before transitioning into a mainstream environment.

In many areas, there are not enough ELs to warrant hiring specialists who provide ESOL services and classes. This situation often leads to another option in the schooling of ELs, *mainstreamed education (inclusion)*. If mainstream (meaning regular classroom) teachers have appropriate training, ELs can be successful. In general, the smaller the gap between the EL's level of English proficiency and the language demands of the grade level/subject, the better chance of the EL's success in the mainstream. When the mainstream teacher has also learned about second language acquisition and instructional and assessment accommodations and modifications for ELs, successfully bridging the English proficiency/language demands gap is more likely. For example, an intermediate-level EL in a kindergarten class, where the language demands are simple and supported by a great deal of extralinguistic context, has a smaller gap to navigate than an intermediate EL in a 10th-grade social studies class, where students are expected to read the textbook and discuss and write about abstract concepts. As a rule of thumb, in the upper grades ELs need much more content comprehension support and English language development instruction than ELs in lower grades.

In the past, mainstreamed instruction for ELs has also meant a "sink or swim" approach to learning (Ovando, 2003). Children with low levels of English proficiency were placed in regular classrooms and were expected to catch up on their own. However, current research has indicated that mainstreamed ELs will achieve greater gains if their teachers use appropriate strategies for their comprehension of content and English language development.

Bilingual/Dual-Language Instruction

Another option to serve ELs in the school setting is *bilingual/ dual-language instruction* (Cloud, Genesee, & Hamayan, 2000; Collier & Thomas, 2004; Calderon, Slavin, & Sanchez, 2011). Often an area of controversy and misunderstanding, bilingual education has been part of the American educational system since the 1800s. Interestingly, German was the first language other than English used as a medium of instruction in the United

States, but with the dawn of World War I, an anti–bilingual education movement ended the practice. The current national debate on the merits of bilingual education ignores a great deal of empirical evidence that supports its effectiveness. We will look at the evidence in the following section; before we examine the research, it is important to define the many types of options for bilingual education.

According to the Center for Applied Linguistics (Rennie, 1993), there are three main categories of bilingual education programs: early exit, late exit, and two-way. Early exit programs typically conclude by the end of the second grade. Their purpose is to support reading skills in both languages through reading instruction in the first language (L1) and to phase out L1 instruction quickly. Late exit programs typically transition students into full English instruction over a longer period of time, usually lasting throughout the elementary school years. For either program, the transition period usually involves reducing the percentage of instruction in the native language and increasing the amount of instruction in English. Late exit programs typically progress to 60% English instruction prior to mainstreaming the students in instruction conducted entirely in English.

Two-way bilingual programs have a very different purpose —they are designed to develop full proficiency in two languages in English-speaking and EL students. Typically, two-way bilingual programs involve combining English speakers with English learners of one native language and offering instruction in the two languages. The definitive split is half of instruction in each language, but this ratio can vary according to community and school needs and resources. A more recent term for two-way bilingual programs is dual language, which offers a range of options for dividing instruction in two languages.

Although school districts choose different service delivery options based on multiple factors, including parental preference, the philosophical perspectives of administrators and board members, access to qualified teachers and other personnel, and cost, research on the impact of the program model on EL achievement is clear. In *A National Study of School Effectiveness for Language Minority Students' Long-Term Academic Achievement*, Thomas and Collier (2002) found compelling differences among program models. Results from this study showed differences in English and Spanish achievement, and achievement in different subject matters such as math based on the type of program ELs completed. ELs who received no ESOL and bilingual education services had substantial decreases in reading and math scores by the fifth grade compared to ELs who received the services. In addition, the greatest number of dropouts came from this category. Spanish-speaking students in bilingual programs scored higher in reading in their native language than English-speaking students did in English in grades 1 through 5, 7, and 8. They also scored higher than English-speaking students when tested on math in their native languages. In general, this study documents the academic achievement of ELs over the long-term (4–12 years) and across content areas. It offers a much-needed overview of programmatic successes in the education of ELs for policy makers.

Summary

This chapter detailed the roles and professional preparation characteristics of the SLP and ESOL professional. When both professionals serve the same students, ELs, it is critical to understand the professional preparation and competencies of each, their respective roles and responsibilities, and how they influence educational decisions and student language and learning outcomes. This chapter also discussed EL students from the perspective of each of the disciplines. For the ESOL professional, the EL student is in various stages of second language acquisition and needs support to develop oral, reading, and writing skills in English. For the SLP, the EL student has been referred due to a possible speech-language delay or disorder and might also be in the process of second language acquisition. It is the role of the SLP to provide appropriate intervention (e.g., prereferral activities or Response to Intervention strategies or intervention) assessments to make that determination. Both professionals must be familiar with the service delivery models used by the SLP and the instructional models used by ESOL professionals in educating ELs in order to facilitate intervention planning and implementation. The next chapter provides an overview of the increasing EL population, their characteristics, and key legal mandates governing the assessment and intervention of ELs.

References

American Speech-Language-Hearing Association. (n.d.). *ASHA practice policy*. Retrieved from http://www.asha.org/policy/type.htm

American Speech-Language-Hearing Association. (1983). Position paper: Social dialects and implications of the position on social dialects. *ASHA, 25*(9), 23–27.

American Speech-Language-Hearing Association. (1985). Clinical management of communicatively handicapped minority language populations. *ASHA, 27*(6), 29–32.

American Speech-Language-Hearing Association. (1987). *Multicultural professional education in communication disorders: Curriculum approaches*. Rockville, MD: Author.

American Speech-Language-Hearing Association. (1989). *Bilingual speech-language pathologists and audiologists: Definition* [Relevant paper]. Retrieved from http://www.asha.org/policy

American Speech-Language-Hearing Association. (1992). *Professional certification standards*. Rockville, MD: Author.

American Speech-Language-Hearing Association. (1998a). *Provision of instruction in English as a second language by speech-language pathologists in school settings* [Position statement]. Retrieved from http://www.asha.org/policy

American Speech-Language-Hearing Association. (1998b). *Provision of instruction in English as a second language by speech-language pathologists in school settings* [Technical report]. Retrieved from http://www.asha.org/policy

American Speech-Language-Hearing Association. (2001). *Roles and responsibilities of speech-language pathologists with respect to reading and writing in children and adolescents* [Guidelines]. Retrieved from http://www.asha.org/policy

American Speech-Language-Hearing Association. (2002). *A workload analysis approach for establishing speech-language caseload standards in the schools* [Guidelines, position statement, and technical report]. Retrieved from http://www.asha.org/policy

American Speech-Language-Hearing Association. (2003a). *American English dialects* [Technical report]. Retrieved from http://www.asha.org/policy

American Speech-Language-Hearing Association. (2003b). *Implementation guide: A workload analysis approach for establishing speech-language caseload standards in the schools.* Rockville, MD: Author.

American Speech-Language-Hearing Association. (2004). *Knowledge and skills needed by speech-language pathologists and audiologists to provide culturally and linguistically appropriate services* [Knowledge and skills]. Retrieved from http://www.asha.org/policy

American Speech-Language-Hearing Association. (2005a). *Evidence-based practice in communication disorders* [Position statement]. Retrieved from http://www.asha.org/policy

American Speech-Language-Hearing Association. (2005b). *Standards and implementation procedures for the certificate of clinical competence in speech-language pathology.* Retrieved from http://www.asha.org/certification/2005SLPStdRevisions.htm

American Speech-Language-Hearing Association. (2007). *Scope of practice in speech-language pathology* [Scope of practice]. Retrieved from http://www.asha.org/policy

American Speech-Language-Hearing Association. (2008). *Bylaws of the American Speech-Language-Hearing Association* [Bylaws]. Retrieved from http://www.asha.org/policy

American Speech-Language-Hearing Association. (2010a). *Employment settings.* Retrieved from http://www.asha.org/careers/professions/EmploymentSettings.htm

American Speech-Language-Hearing Association. (2010b). *Highlights and trends: ASHA counts for year end 2010.* Retrieved from http://www.asha.org/uploadedFiles/2010-Member-Counts.pdf

American Speech-Language-Hearing Association. (2010c). *Code of ethics* [Ethics]. Retrieved from http://www.asha.org/policy

American Speech-Language-Hearing Association. (2010d). *Roles and responsibilities of speech-language pathologists in schools* [Position statement]. Retrieved from http://www.asha.org/docs/html/PI2010-00317.html

American Speech-Language-Hearing Association. (2010e). *Roles and responsibilities of speech-language pathologists in schools* [Professional issues statement]. Retrieved from http://www.asha.org/policy

American Speech-Language-Hearing Association. (2011). *CAA-Accredited academic program statistics.* Retrieved from http://www.asha.org/academic/accreditation/CAA_Program_Stats.htm

Ballantyne, K. G., Sanderman, A. R., & Levy, J. (2008). *Educating English language learners: Building teacher capacity.* Washington, DC: National Clearinghouse for English Language Acquisition. Retrieved from http://www.ncela.gwu.edu/practice/mainstream_teachers.htm

Battle, D. (2002). *Communication disorders in multicultural populations* (3rd ed.). Woburn, MA: Butterworth-Heinemann.

Bedore, L. M., Peña, E. D., Garcia, M., & Cortez, C. (2005). Conceptual versus monolingual scoring: When does it make a difference? *Language, Speech, and Hearing Services in Schools, 36*, 188–200.

Blosser, J. L. & Kratcoski, A. (1997). PACs: A framework for determining appropriate service delivery option. *Language, Speech and Hearing Services in Schools, 28*, 99–107.

Brandel, J., & Loeb, D. F. (May 26, 2011). Program intensity and service delivery models in the schools: SLP survey results. *Language, Speech, and Hearing Services in Schools.*

Caesar, L. G., & Kohler, P. D. (2007). The state of school-based bilingual assessment: Actual practice versus recommended guidelines. *Language, Speech, and Hearing Services in Schools, 38,* 190–200.

Calderon, M., Slavin, R., Sanchez, M. (2011). Effective instruction for English learners. *Immigrant Children, 21*(1). Retrieved from http://www.futureofchildren.org/futureofchildren/publications/journals/article/index.xml?journalid=74&articleid=542

Chabon, S., Esparza-Brown, J. E., & Gildersleeve-Neumann, C. (2010, August 03). Ethics, equity, and English-language learners: A decision-making framework. *ASHA Leader.*

Cirrin, F. M., Schooling, T. L., Nelson, N. W., Diehl, S. F., Flynn, P. F. Staskowski, M., . . . Adamczyk, D. (2010). Evidence-based systematic review: Effects of different service delivery models on communication outcomes for elementary school-age children. *Language, Speech, and Hearing Services in Schools, 41,* 233–264.

Cloud, N., Genesee, F., & Hamayan, E. (2000). *Dual language instruction: A handbook for enriched education.* Boston, MA: Heinle and Heinle.

Collier, V. (1998). *Promoting academic success for E.S.L. students: Understanding second language acquisition for school.* Woodside, NY: Bastos.

Collier, V., & Thomas, W. P. (2004). The astounding effectiveness of dual language education for all. *NABE Journal of Research and Practice, 2*, 1–20.

Davidson, S., & Denton, D. (2010). Ethics compliance: Enforcing ASHA's Code of Ethics. *Perspectives on Fluency and Fluency Disorders, 20*(3), 71–75.

Echevarria, J., Vogt, M. E., & Short, D. (2008). *Making content comprehensible for English Learners: The SIOP model* (3rd ed.). Boston, MA: Allyn & Bacon.

Ehren, B. J., Montgomery, J., Rudebusch, J., & Whitmore, K. (2006). Responsiveness to intervention: New roles for speech-language pathologists. *ASHA Leader.*

Ehren, T., Lefkowitz, N., & Roth, C. (October, 1997). Developing, evaluating, and managing competencies across work settings. *ASHA Special Interest Division 11 Newsletter, 7*(3), 3–4.

Esparza-Brown, J., & Doolittle, J. (2008). A cultural, linguistic, and ecological framework for response to intervention with English language learners. National Center for Culturally Responsive Educational Systems (NCCRESt) Practitioner Briefs. Retrieved from http://www.nccrest.org/publications/briefs.html

Florida Department of Education (FLDOE). (n.d.). *League of United Latin American Citizens (LULAC) et al. v. State Board of Education Consent Decree.* United States District Court for the Southern District of Florida, August 14, 1990. Retrieved from http://www.fldoe.org/aala/rules.asp

Florida Department of Education (FLDOE). (2010). Approved Florida teacher standards for teacher endorsement. Retrieved from http://www.fldoe.org/aala

Flynn, P. (2010, August 31). New service delivery models: Connecting SLPs with teachers and curriculum. *ASHA Leader.*

Friend, M., & Cook, L. (2010). *Interactions: Collaboration skills for school professionals* (6th ed.). Boston, MA: Pearson.

ProGarcia, E. E. (1991). *The education of linguistically and culturally diverse students: Effective instructional practices.* NCRCDSLL Educational Practice Reports. Paper EPR01. Santa Cruz, CA: Center for Research on Education, Diversity & Excellence. Retrieved from http://repositories.cdlib.org/crede/ncrcdslleducational/EPR01

Gibbons, P. (2002). *Scaffolding language, scaffolding learning: Teaching second language learners in the mainstream classroom.* Portsmouth, NH: Heinemann.

Giess, S. (2010). *Implementing a workload approach to caseload: Methods and strategies.* Rockville, MD: American Speech-Language-Hearing Association.

Goldstein, B. (Ed.). (2004). *Bilingual language development and disorders in Spanish-English speakers.* Baltimore, MD: Brookes.

Graham, S. V. (1998). *Quality treatment indicators: A model for clinical expertise in speech-language pathology.* Doctoral dissertation, University of South Florida, Tampa.

Graham, S. V., & Guilford, A. M. (2000, November). *Beyond competence: Development of a model of clinical expertise.* American Speech-Language-Hearing Association annual conference, Washington, DC.

Guilford, A. (2003). Communication sciences and disorders. In M. A. Richard & W. G. Emener (Eds.), *I'm a people person: A guide to human services professions.* Springfield, IL: Charles C. Thomas.

Guilford, A. M., Graham, S. J., & Scheuerle, J. (Eds.). (2007). *The speech-language pathologist: From novice to expert.* Upper Saddle River, NJ: Pearson.

Gutierrez-Clellan, V. (1999). Language choice in intervention with bilingual children. *American Journal of Speech-Language Pathology, 8,* 291–302.

Harry, B., & Klingner, J. (2006). *Why are so many minority students in special education?* New York, NY: Teachers College Press.

Howatt, A. P. R., & Widdowson, H. G. (2004). *A history of English language teaching* (2nd ed.). Oxford, UK: Oxford University Press.

Individuals with Disabilities Education Improvement Act (IDEIA). (2004). PL 108-446, 20 U.S.C. §§ 1400 et seq.

Katz, L. A., Maag, A., Fallon, K. A., Blenkarn, K., & Smith, M. K. (2010). What makes a caseload (un)manageable? School-based speech-language pathologists speak. *Language, Speech, and Hearing Services in Schools, 41,* 139–151.

Kayser, H. (2002). Bilingual language development and language disorders. In D. E. Battle (Ed.), *Communication disorders in multicultural populations* (3rd ed.) (pp. 205–232). Woburn, MA: Butterworth-Heinemann.

Klingner, J. K., Artiles, A. J., Kozleski, E., Harry, B., Zion, S., Tate, W., . . . Riley, D. (2005). Addressing the disproportionate representation of culturally and linguistically diverse students in special education through culturally responsive educational systems. *Education Policy Analysis Archives, 13*(38). Retrieved from http://epaa.asu.edu/epaa/v13n38/

Kohnert, K. (2008). *Language disorders in bilingual children and adults.* San Diego, CA: Plural.

Langdon, H. W. (1999). Foreign accent: Implications for delivery of speech and language services. *Topics in Language Disorders, 19*(4), 49–65.

Langdon, H., & Cheng, L. L. (2002). *Collaborating with interpreters and translators: A guide for communication disorders professionals.* Austin, TX: Pro-Ed.

Lubinski, R., & Fratelli, C. (Eds.). (2001). *Professional issues in speech-language pathology and audiology.* San Diego, CA: Singular.

Mattes, L., & Saldana-Illingworth, C. (2009). *Bilingual communication assessment resource.* Oceanside, CA: Academic Communication Associates.

Mihai, F. (2010). *Assessing English language learners in the content areas.* Ann Arbor: University of Michigan Press.

Montone, C. L. (1995). *Piecing linguistically and culturally diverse learners: Effective programs and practices.* Paper presented at National Center for Research on Cultural Diversity and Second Language Learning, Santa Cruz, CA. Retrieved from ERIC database. (ED381036)

Moore, B. J, & Montgomery, J. K. (2008). *Making a difference for America's culture. Speech-language pathologist in public schools* (2nd ed.). Austin, TX: PRO-ED.

National Association for Bilingual Education (NABE) & ILIEAD Project. (2002). *Determining appropriate referrals of English Language Learners to special education: A self-assessment guide for principals.* Arlington, VA: Council for Exceptional Children.

Nixon, S. M., McCardle, P., & Leos, K. (2007). Epilogue: Implications of research on English language learners for classroom and clinical practice. *Language, Speech, and Hearing Services in Schools, 38*(3), 272–277.

Nutta, J., Bautista, N., & Butler, M., (2010). *Teaching sciences to English language learners.* New York, NY: Routledge.

Ortiz, A. A., & Yates, J. R. (2001). A framework for serving English language learners with disabilities. *Journal of Special Education Leadership, 14*(2):72–80.

Ovando, C. J. (2003). Bilingual education in the United States: Historical development and current issues. *Bilingual Research Journal, 27,* 1–24.

Paul, D., Blosser, J., & Jakubowitz, M. (2006). Principles and challenges for forming successful literacy partnerships. *Topics in Language Disorders, 26*(1), 5–23.

Peters-Johnson, C. (1998). Action: School services, survey of speech-language pathology services in school-based settings national study report. *Language, Speech, and Hearing Services in Schools, 29,* 120–126.

Rennie, J. (1993). ESL and bilingual program models. *ERIC Digest.* ERIC Clearinghouse on Languages and Linguistics. Digest based on an article in *Streamlined Seminar, 12*(1). National Association of Elementary School Principals. Retrieved from http://www.cal.org/resources/digest/rennie01.html

Rinaldi, C. & Samson, J. (2008). English language learners and response to intervention. *Teaching Exceptional Children, 40*(5), 6–14.

Roos, P. (1978). Bilingual education: The Hispanic response to unequal educational opportunity. *Law and Contemporary Problems, 42*(4), 111–140.

Rosa-Lugo, L., & Champion, T. (2007). The influence of knowledge and experience on responding to diversity in speech-language pathology. In A. M. Guilford, S. Graham, & J. Scheuerle, (Eds.), *The speech-language pathologist: From novice to expert* (pp. 80–104). Upper Saddle River, NJ: Pearson.

Rosa-Lugo, L. I., & Fradd, S. H. (2000). Preparing professionals to serve English-language learners with communication disorders. *Communication Disorders Quarterly, 22*(1), 29–42.

Rosa-Lugo, L. I., Rivera, E. A., & McKeown, S. W. (1998). Meeting the critical shortage of speech-language pathologists to serve the public schools — collaborative rewards. *Language, Speech, and Hearing Services in Schools, 29,* 232–242.

Roseberry-McKibbin, C. (2003). *Assessment of bilingual learners: Language difference or disorder? Video and workbook.* Rockville, MD: American Speech-Language-Hearing Association.

Roseberry-McKibben, C. (2007). *Language disorders in children. A multicultural and case perspective.* Boston, MA: Pearson Educational.

Roseberry-McKibbin, C. (2008a). *Multicultural students with special language needs: Practical strategies for assessment and intervention* (3rd ed.). Oceanside, CA: Academic Communication Associates.

Roseberry-McKibbin, C. (2008b). *Increasing the language and academic skills of children in poverty: Practical strategies for professionals.* San Diego, CA: Plural.

Saad, C., & Polovoy, C. (2009, May 05). Differences or disorders? In the 1980s, research focused on culturally and linguistically diverse populations. *ASHA Leader.*

Schiff-Myers, N. (1992). Considering arrested language development and language loss in the assessment of second language learner. *Language, Speech, and Hearing Services in Schools, 23,* 28–33.

Schooling, T., Venediktov, R., & Leech, H. (2010). *Evidence-based systematic review: Effects of service delivery on the speech and language skills of children from birth to 5 years of age.* Rockville, MD: American Speech-Language-Hearing Association, National Center for Evidence-Based Practice in Communication Disorders.

Schraeder, P. (2008). *A guide to school services in speech-language pathology.* San Diego, CA: Plural.

Solorzano, R. W. (2008). High stakes testing: Issues, implication, and remedies for English language learners. *Review of Educational Research, 78*(2), 260–329.

Teachers of English to Speakers of Other Languages (TESOL). (n.d.a). *The early history of TESOL.* Retrieved from http://www.tesol.org/s_tesol/bin.asp?CID=32&DID=8283&DOC=FILE.PDF

Teachers of English to Speakers of Other Languages (TESOL). (n.d.b). *Bylaws and standing rules. SR II. Mission.* Retrieved from http://www.tesol.org/s_tesol/seccss.asp?CID=413&DID=2038

Teachers of English to Speakers of Other Languages (TESOL). (n.d.c). *TESOL's mission and values.* Retrieved from http://www.tesol.org/s_tesol/sec_document.asp?CID=3&DID=220

Teachers of English to Speakers of Other Languages (TESOL). (n.d.d). *Membership statistics.* Retrieved from http://www.tesol.org/s_tesol/seccss.asp?CID=130&DID=1600

Teachers of English to Speakers of Other Languages (TESOL). (2007). *The identification of English language learners with special educational needs.* Retrieved from http://www.tesol.org/s_tesol/bin.asp ?CID=32&DID=8283&DOC=FILE.PDF

Teachers of English to Speakers of Other Languages (TESOL). (2009). *Position statement on the rights of deaf learners to acquire full proficiency in a native signed language.* Retrieved from http://www .tesol.org/s_tesol/seccss.asp?CID=32&DID=37

Teachers of English to Speakers of Other Languages (TESOL). (2010). *TESOL/NCATE standards for the recognition of initial TESOL programs in P–12 ESL teacher education.* Retrieved from http://www .tesol.org/s_tesol/seccss.asp?CID=219&DID=1689

Thomas, W., & Collier, V. (2002). *A national study of school effectiveness for language minority students' long-term academic achievement.* Santa Cruz, CA, and Washington, DC: Center for Research on Education, Diversity & Excellence. Retrieved from http://repositories. cdlib.org/crede/finalrpts/1_1_final/ and http://crede.berkeley.edu/ research/llaa/1.1_final.html

Throneburg, R. N., Calvert, L. K., Strum, J. J., Paramboukas, A. A., & Paul, P. J. (2000). A comparison of service delivery models: Effects on curricular vocabulary skills in the school setting. *American Journal of Speech-Language Pathology, 9*(1), 10–20.

Wilkinson, B. R., & Payne, K. T. (2005). Effect of clinician's accent on verbal performance of preschool children. *ECHO: E-Journal for Black and Other Ethnic Group Research and Practices in Communication Sciences and Disorders, 1*(2), 11–28.

Whitmire, K. (2002). The evolution of school-based speech-language services: A half century of change and a new century of practice. *Communication Disorders Quarterly, 23*(2), 68–76.

3

English Learners in the United States — Preschool Through Grade 12

Introduction

In an effort to understand the growing population of ELs and ELs with communication disorders in US schools, it is essential to first analyze and define terms associated with ELs. This chapter provides critical data related to their enrollment in US public schools, as well as their country of origin and language background. Finally, this chapter examines several key legislation initiatives that have influenced the education of ELs in the US in very important ways.

English Learners: In Search of Common Terminology

Children who are classified as ELs are the fastest growing segment of the school population in the United States. Over the past decade, ELs have increased by more than 15 million students (Flynn & Hill, 2005; Mathews & Ewen, 2006). Today ELs represent more than 10% of the total school population in prekindergarten through the 12th grade. This very significant percentage of public school students who are learning English is heterogeneous. Therefore, a list of characteristics that apply to all ELs in the United States is complex. One obvious example of this student population's diversity is represented by the language background of the US public school ELs, students who speak more than 350 languages (Hopstock & Stephenson, 2003).

There are various terms and definitions associated with ELs. However, these terms lack uniformity in defining and describing ELs. The terms EL and LEP (limited English proficient) have been used quite extensively in the educational literature to describe students who are not yet proficient in English and who require instructional support in order to fully access academic content in their classes. The term most commonly used in the literature is EL although the No Child Left Behind Act (NCLB) (2001a) continues to use the term LEP. Students referred to as LEP are often seen as a subset of ELs who have not yet attained English language proficiency (as measured by the particular assessment procedures of their state). However, both groups of students often continue to need support in acquiring and using language in the classroom, particularly with the complex academic language that leads to successful high school graduation and higher education opportunities (Francis, Rivera, Lesaux, Kieffer, & Rivera, 2006).

Florida has followed a national trend to use the term EL instead of LEP. The term LEP was changed from limited English proficiency to language-enriched pupils in an attempt to deemphasize the language deficit of EL and emphasize language accomplishment (Florida Department of Education, 2005). Additional terms commonly used by educators to describe nonnative English speakers are ELL (English language learner), ESL (English as a second language), ESOL (English for speakers of other languages), and/or culturally and linguistically diverse (CLD). Due to the variety of terms used to describe this specific group of students, researchers have argued that it would be advantageous to have standardized EL definitions and terms that could be used nationally. For example, Short and Fitzsimmons (2006) argue that a common definition of an EL is necessary to have clear and consistent national standards that will define this student population and allow valid and reliable cross-state comparisons vis-à-vis EL academic achievement and English language proficiency. Definitions associated with ELs at the federal and state level are reviewed here in order to facilitate the building of a common definition of ELs.

Federal

At the federal level, Public Law 107-110, also known as the No Child Left Bchind Act (NCLB, 2001a), defines an EL as a limited English proficient (LEP) student. The definition provided by this act states that an LEP student is:

> an individual: (1) who is aged 3 through 21; (2) who is enrolled or preparing to enroll in an elementary school or secondary

school; (3) (i) who was not born in the United States or whose native language is a language other than English; (ii) (I) who is a Native American or Alaska Native, or a native resident of the outlying areas; and (II) who comes from an environment where a language other than English has had a significant impact on the individual's level of English language proficiency; or (iii) who is migratory, whose native language is a language other than English, and who comes from an environment where a language other than English is dominant; and (4) whose difficulties in speaking, reading, writing, or understanding the English language may be sufficient to deny the individual (i) the ability to meet the State's proficient level of achievement on State assessments; (ii) the ability to successfully achieve in classrooms where the language of instructions is English; or(iii) the opportunity to participate fully in society. (NCLB, 2001a)

State

At the state level, there is no consistent definition of the EL student population. States and school districts use a wide range of standards and language proficiency tests to determine eligibility for programs for ELs. This often results in a wide variation in the definition of who is considered to be limited English proficient and who is qualified to receive appropriate services. Thus the definition varies from state to state. For example, states, such as Alabama, Nevada, New Hampshire, New Jersey, and Virginia define ELs as children who meet the definition of a limited English proficient child under the Elementary and Secondary Education Act (ESEA) of 1968. However, the Elementary and Secondary Education Act was reauthorized by the NCLB legislation; therefore, the NCLB and ESEA definitions of an LEP student are identical. Other states use modified versions of a definition of limited English proficiency, found in Title VII of the Improving America's Schools Act of 1994 (US Congress, 1994). One example of this is the definition of an EL in the state of Florida, as defined in the *League of United Latin American Citizens et al. v. Florida Board of Education*. ELs are:

(a) individuals who were not born in the United States and whose native language is a language other than English; or (b) individuals who come from home environments where a language other than English is spoken in the home; or (c) individuals who are American Indian or Alaskan natives and who come from environments where a language other than English has had a significant impact on their level of English language proficiency; and (d) individuals who, by reason thereof, have sufficient difficulty speaking, reading, writing, or listening to the English language to deny such individuals the opportunity to learn successfully in classrooms where the language of instruction is English. (Florida Department of Education, n.d.)

Finally, other states have adopted the definition (or a slightly modified version) recommended by the Council of Chief State School Officers (CCSSO). California is such an example: English learner students are those students for whom there is a report of a primary language other than English on the state-approved Home Language Survey *and* who, on the basis of the state approved oral language (grades kindergarten through grade twelve) assessment procedures and literacy (grades three through twelve only), have been determined to lack the clearly defined English language skills of listening comprehension, speaking, reading, and writing necessary to succeed in the school's regular instructional programs (California Department of Education, n.d.). The implication of the lack of a uniform system to define ELs becomes evident as we look at EL categories used by various states to describe student status (i.e., current placement or exited). In Florida, for example, ELs fall under specific categories (Table 3–1). However, if an EL moves from Florida to Virginia, placement in an EL category will be difficult because Virginia uses a different classification system based on their adoption of the World-Class Instructional Design and Assessment (WIDA) English Language Proficiency (ELP) levels (Table 3–2). Should the same student move to Alaska, placement in an EL category will be equally difficult, because Alaska uses categories quite different from those used in Florida or in Virginia (Table 3–3).

Table 3–1. *Classification System Used in the State of Florida*

Codes	Description
LY	The student is an English learner and is enrolled in classes specifically designed for English learners.
LF	The student is being followed up for a 2-year period after having exited from the ESOL program
LP	The student is in grades 3–12, tested fully English proficient on an aural/oral test and is an English learner pending the reading and writing assessment, or the student is in grades K–12, answered "yes" on the Home Language Survey question "Is a language other than English spoken in the home?" and is pending aural/oral assessment
LZ	The student is one for whom a 2-year follow-up period has been completed after the student has exited the ESOL program. Once a student completes the 2-year postreclassification monitoring period, they are recoded LZ and remain so for the remainder of their school career.
ZZ	Not applicable. (Students who responded in the negative to all three required Home Language Survey questions, that is, non-ELs, or who answered yes to one or more questions on the Home Language Survey but after assessment were not eligible for ESOL services).

Source: Data from *2010–2011 English Language Learners (ELL) Data Base and Program Handbook: English for Speakers of Other Languages (ESOL).* Florida Department of Education, 2011. Retrieved from www.fldoe.org/aala/pdf/edph1011.pdf

Building the Context for Understanding ELs

Demographics

There are approximately 5 million ELs enrolled in the pre-K–12 schools in the US. This number represents over 10% of the entire US public school population, which is approximately 49 million students (Ballantyne, Sanderman, & Levy, 2008). The statistics for the academic year 2005–2006 indicates that the number of

Table 3–2. *Classification System Used in the State of Virginia*

Codes	Description
WIDA ELP Level 1	Entering
WIDA ELP Level 2	Beginning
WIDA ELP Level 3	Developing
WIDA ELP Level 4	Expanding
WIDA ELP Level 5	Bridging (students no longer receive direct ESL services but are monitored for two years)
WIDA ELP Level 6	Reaching (formerly LEP; monitored for two additional years)

Source: Data from *Handbook for Educators for Students Who Are English Language Learners with Suspected Learning Disabilities.* Virginia Department of Education, 2009. Retrieved from http://www.doe .virginia.gov/instruction/esl/standards_resources/index.shtml; *Limited English Proficient Students: Guidelines for Participation in the Virginia Assessment Program.* Virginia Department of Education, 2011. Retrieved from http://www.doe.virginia.gov/testing/participation/ index.shtml

ELs represented over 10% of the entire US public school population, which is approximately 49 million students (Office of English Language Acquisition [OELA], 2008). The incredible rate of growth is reflected in Table 3–4. The total pre-K–12 population shows a 3.6% increase for the past decade, whereas the EL population has a 57% expansion for the same period of time. This growth is also reflected in the proportion of ELs. More and more ELs are part of schools today, from 6% in 1995–1996 to over 10% in the 2005–2006 academic year (National Clearinghouse for English Language Acquisition [NCELA], 2006). Perhaps this amazing rate of growth will stabilize in the future, but for now, the EL population growth will most likely continue.

Table 3–3. *Classification System Used in the State of Alaska*

Categories	
Codes	**Descriptors**
N	Potential LEP student who was assessed for identification, but not identified as LEP because he or she scored at the proficient level in all domains of speaking, listening, reading and writing
L1	1st year of identification as an LEP student. Student meets definition of LEP and has scored at some point below the proficient level on a state-approved assessment of English language proficiency
LP	Student has been identified as LEP in a previous school year and has not yet scored proficient on the state-approved assessment of English language proficiency.
LT	LEP student who has scored at the proficient level on the state-approved assessment of English language proficiency.
M1	First year of monitoring for former LEP student. The student should have had a code of LT the previous school year.
M2	Second year of monitoring for a former LEP student. Student should have had a code of M1 the previous school year.

Source: Data from *Guidance for Limited English Proficient (LEP) Student Identification Assessment and Data Reports.* Alaska Department of Education, 2010. Retrieved from http://www.eed.state.ak.us/

Although ELs can be found in all the states across the United States, they tend to be heavily concentrated in six states: California, Texas, Florida, New York, Illinois, and Arizona. For the academic year 2005–2006, approximately 60% of the EL population resided in these six states (Table 3–5). However, if we look at growth in the past decade, and not at density, these six states are not the ones that have experienced amazing rates of growth in their EL population. California's EL student population grew 18% in 2005–2006 compared with 1995–1996. However, other states such as Arkansas recorded a 300% or higher growth of their EL population (Table 3–6). Springdale Public School District, located in northwest Arkansas, is a relevant example of

Table 3–4. EL Enrollment Between 1995–1996 and 2005–2006

School Year	Pre-K–12 Enrollment	EL Enrollment	EL Proportion
1995–1996	47,582,665	3,228,799	6.79%
1996–1997	46,714,980	3,452,073	7.39%
1997–1998	46,023,969	3,470,268	7.54%
1998–1999	46,153,266	3,540,673	7.67%
1999–2000	47,356,089	4,416,580	9.33%
2000–2001	47,665,483	4,584,947	9.62%
2001–2002	48,296,777	4,750,820	9.84%
2002–2003	49,478,583	5,044,361	10.20%
2003–2004	49,618,529	5,013,539	10.10%
2004–2005	48,982,898	5,119,561	10.45%
2005–2006	49,324,849	5,074,572	10.29%

Source: Data from *The Growing Numbers of Limited English Proficient Students 1995/1996–2005/2006*, by National Clearinghouse for English Language Acquisition (NCELA), 2006. Retrieved from http://www.ncela.gwu.edu/files/uploads/4/GrowingLEP_0506.pdf

Table 3–5. The Six States with the Highest EL Population, 2005–2006

State	Total Enrollment	EL Population	Percentage of ELs
California	6,259,972	1,571,463	25.10
Texas	4,525,394	640,749	14.16
Florida	2,675,024	253,165	9.46
New York	2,708,570	234,578	8.66
Illinois	2,111,245	204,803	9.70
Arizona	1,094,260	152,962	13.98

Source: Data from *NCELA State Title III Information System*, by National Clearinghouse for English Language Acquisition (NCELA), n.d. Retrieved from http://www.ncela.gwu.edu/t3sis/

Table 3–6. *Five States with the Highest Rate of Growth Between 1995–1996 and 2005–2006*

State	ELL Growth from 1995–1996	Total Enrollment 2005–2006	ELL Enrollment 2005–2006
South Carolina	688%	701,544	20,013
Arkansas	361%	473,460	20,320
North Carolina	346%	1,416,576	83,627
Tennessee	296%	939,571	20,901
Kentucky	266%	674,583	10,171

Source: Data from *NCELA State Title III Information System,* by National Clearinghouse for English Language Acquisition (NCELA), n.d. Retrieved from http://www.ncela.gwu.edu/t3sis/

a place that experienced a dramatic EL population increase. It had virtually no ELs in the 1990s. However, in 2008 there were 7,000 ELs, or around 40% of the total enrollment in the district (Maxwell, 2009). The reason for this almost unbelievable growth has been a very successful economy around the area, driven by job growth at Tyson Foods and Wal-Mart, which attracted thousands of families from Mexico and the Marshall Islands in the South Pacific.

An analysis of the data collected in 2004–2005 (and compared with the 1994–1995 school year) reveals some interesting facts. First, for 2004–2005, the top five EL growth states were South Carolina, Kentucky, Indiana, North Carolina, and Tennessee (Payan & Nettles, 2008). Nevertheless, in the 2005–2006 academic year, Arkansas jumped to second place from ninth place the year before, displacing Indiana in the rankings. South Carolina, Tennessee, North Carolina, and Kentucky stayed in the top five states with the highest EL growth, but their places shifted significantly, with the exception of South Carolina. Additionally, the rates of growth were very different from what was reported a year later, as seen in the following list: South Carolina (714%), Kentucky (417%), Indiana (407%), North Carolina (317%), and Tennessee (369%).

Clearly, the EL student population is fluid and quite difficult to predict in terms of growth. It is possible that, as a result of declining economic opportunities and tougher law enforcement of illegal immigration, states might experience a slowdown in immigration rates, and, consequently, in the number of ELs enrolled in public schools. Although the immigration surge might be slowing temporarily, the fact that so many immigrants have chosen states which were not traditional immigration magnets makes it essential for decision makers at the state level to monitor the population statistics very carefully in order to ensure that there are sufficient resources allocated toward providing quality education for ELs.

Country of Birth and Language Background of ELs

In many states, the growth of the EL population was a direct result of steady immigration through the 1990s and into the beginning of the 21st century. According to the US Census Bureau data (2011), the number of foreign-born people living in the US stood at 35.7 million, a 45% increase from 10 years ago. Therefore, it is very natural to assume that all or almost all ELs are recent arrivals in the United States, having been born abroad. Nonetheless, the statistical data provided by the US Census Bureau (2011) refute this claim. Overall, in 2000, from the total of over 3 million ELs, only 36% were first generation (foreign-born children of foreign-born parents). 42% were second generation (US-born children of foreign-born parents), and 22% were third generation (US-born children of US-born parents). If we look at the percentages of ELs at the elementary and secondary level by generation, we notice that they are consistent with the overall percentages discussed previously, clearly showing that the majority of ELs arc US born (see Tables 1–2 and 1–3).

The language background of ELs is very diverse, with an evident dominance of Spanish speakers. Although EL students speak over 350 native languages, almost 80% percent identify Spanish as their native language. The next most commonly reported native languages are Vietnamese (2.4%) and Hmong (1.6 %) (see Table 1–1). Additionally, based on district EL services surveys, Spanish is the most common language of ELs in over 80% of the schools in the US (Hopstock & Stephenson, 2003). The other languages most common in schools are as follows: Russian (2.3%), Hmong (1.9%), Arabic (1.3%), and Korean (1.3%).

Looking at school levels, 76% of all ELs enrolled at the elementary level and 72% of all secondary education ELs speak Spanish (Capps, Fix, Murray, Ost, Passel, & Herwantoro, 2006). At the elementary level, the five most spoken languages after Spanish were Chinese (2.6%), Vietnamese (2.5%), Korean (1.4%), Hmong or Miao (1.3%), and French (1.1%). At the secondary level, after Spanish, French was the most common language spoken by ELs (3%), followed by Vietnamese (3%), Chinese (2.7%), Korean (1.6%), and Haitian Creole (1.4%).

Legislation Affecting ELs

Federal Legislation

There are several laws affecting the education of ELs, but two of them stand out: the Bilingual Education Act (BEA, 1968) and the No Child Left Behind Act (NCLB, 2001a). The Bilingual Education Act (BEA), also known as Title VII of the Elementary and Secondary Education Act, was passed by the US Congress in 1968. It was the first time the needs of low-income students whose dominant language was not English were recognized at the federal level. The act was reauthorized several times, each reauthorization bringing forth important changes. The 1974 and 1978 reauthorizations specifically focused on the inclusion of ELs to be served. The 1984 reauthorization included not only the EL students, but also their families by providing funding for family English literacy programs. Additionally, it funded the development of two-way bilingual programs. These two-way bilingual programs focused on the development of dual-language proficiency. In this model students receive instruction in English and another language in classrooms that are usually composed of half native speakers of English and half native speakers of another language. The 1994 and final reauthorization of the BEA strongly endorsed the idea that ELs should not just be transitioned to full language proficiency in English, but should have dual-language proficiency.

The second important piece of legislation, NCLB (NCLB, 2001a), was a reauthorization of the Elementary and Secondary Education Act (ESEA) and was passed by the US Congress in 2001. Two goals of NCLB were very important for ELs. The first goal required that by the year 2014, all children, ELs included, reach grade-level proficiency in English language arts and mathematics. The second goal referred specifically to ELs and required that all LEP students become proficient in English and reach high academic standards, at a minimum attaining proficiency or better in reading/language arts and mathematics. Titles I and III of the law contained most of the important provisions affecting ELs.

Under Title I (Improving the Academic Achievement of the Disadvantaged) of the NCLB Act (NCLB, 2001a), schools face a federal mandate to properly meet the educational needs of ELs. Language instruction curricula that are research based must be used to determine the academic progress of ELs (Flynn & Hill, 2005). Title I wanted "to ensure that all children have a fair, equal, and significant opportunity to obtain a high-quality education and reach, at a minimum, proficiency on challenging state academic achievement standards and state academic assessments" (NCLB, 2001a). To achieve this purpose, the following steps were recommended:

- Align curriculum, teaching, and assessment to state standards.
- Meet the educational needs of low-achieving children from the following categories: low-income, ELs, migratory, special education, Indian, etc.
- Strive to close the achievement gap between minority and nonminority children, with a focus on low-income students.
- Hold schools accountable for not improving the academic achievement of their students.
- Focus on improving teaching, learning, and assessment by using statewide assessment instruments aligned to state achievement and content standards.
- Promote effective scientifically based instructional strategies and challenging academic content.

- Provide ample opportunities to teachers and administrators for professional development.
- Encourage parental participation in the education of their children.

Beginning in third grade, Title I requires schools to improve the performance of their ELs in reading and math as measured by state assessments. Although the outcomes of instruction are measured in third grade improvement, activities begin long before then. These improvement activities are in response to the reauthorization of the Individuals with Disabilities Education Act (IDEA) of 2004 that requires early intervening services and response to intervention approaches (RtI) to support struggling learner. If schools constantly fail to improve the performance of their students, they are subject to various types of interventions, ranging from allowing parents to send their children to other schools and offering additional services, (e.g., from after-school programs to more extreme measures such as restructuring or closing).

Title III, Language Instruction for Limited English Proficient and Immigrant Students, had three parts: Part A, English Language Acquisition, Language Enhancement, and Academic Achievement Act; Part B, Improving Language Instructional Programs for Academic Achievement Act; and Part C, General Provisions (NCLB, 2001b).

Part A, English Language Acquisition, Language Enhancement, and Academic Achievement Act, had several goals. First, it aimed to make sure that ELs develop high levels of academic achievement in English and content areas, as measured by state standards. It also focused on developing, establishing, implementing, and sustaining language instructional programs and programs of English language development for ELs.

Part B, Improving Language Instructional Programs for Academic Achievement Act, intended to "help ensure that limited English proficient children master English and meet the same rigorous academic standards for academic achievement as all children are expected to meet, including meeting challenging State academic content and student academic achievement standards" (NCLB, 2001b). This purpose was to be fulfilled by developing and promoting accountability systems for educational programs serving ELs, developing language skills and multicultural understanding, and focusing on the development of English proficiency of ELs and, to the extent possible, the native language proficiency of ELs.

Part C, General Provisions, contained a listing of definitions used in Part A and B; outlined procedures for parental notification; and established a national clearinghouse to disseminate information about ELs.

It is very clear that the law places English proficiency, as well as the ability to fully function in an all-English environment, among its top priorities. As a result, dual-language programs that promote proficiency in both languages might be replaced by English immersion or transitional programs (which have the primary purpose of building English proficiency). The emphasis of these types of programs at the expense of bilingual programs has recently come under scrutiny. For example, in 2002, Boston, Massachusetts, voters approved a law requiring ELs to be taught all subjects in English rather than in their native language. Subsequently, the school dropout rate for ELs nearly doubled in the Boston area (Tung et al., 2009).

Court Rulings

Two Supreme Court cases and one federal court case had a significant impact on the education of ELs: *Lau v. Nichols*, *Plyer v. Doe*, and *Castañeda v. Pickard* (Table 3–7). *Lau v. Nichols* (1974) examined whether or not same education was fair education for ELs. Plaintiffs representing 1,800 students of Chinese descent sued the San Francisco school district for not providing access to education by not implementing language accommodations for ELs. The Supreme Court ruled in favor of the plaintiffs and stated that the San Francisco school district did not comply with Title VI of the Civil Rights Act (1964). According to the Supreme Court, the school district in question denied non-English speaking students of Chinese origin a meaningful opportunity to participate in the public school system. Providing students with equal access to desks, books, teachers, and curricula did not mean an equal educational opportunity if the students had limited English skills. The decision of the Supreme Court in the

Table 3–7. ELs and the Courts

Case	Description	Ruling
Lau v. Nichols (1974)	Supreme Court case started as a class action suit filed on behalf of Chinese-speaking children attending San Francisco schools	Identical education (same materials, teachers, curriculum, etc.) does not add up to equal education under Title VI of the 1964 Civil Rights Act.
Plyer v. Doe (1982)	Supreme Court Case considering revisions of Texas laws withholding state funds for educating children who had not been legally admitted to the United States and authorizing local school districts to deny enrollment to such students.	US public schools are prohibited to deny free public education to undocumented immigrant children.
Castañeda v. Pickard (1981)	A federal court case against ethnicity-based discriminatory practices that took place in the school district in Raymondville, Texas.	Creation of the Castañeda Test (theory, practice, results) to determine the quality of programs for EL students.

1974 *Lau v. Nichols* case had significant and immediate effects in the US. It directly led to the establishment of standards for identifying ELs, for assessing their language proficiency, and for meeting their instructional needs. Additionally, even though the decision did not require any specific solution to address the limited English proficiency of ELs, it favored the establishment of bilingual programs in states like Texas or California as a way of avoiding violations of Title VI of the Civil Rights Act.

The second Supreme Court case, *Plyer v. Doe* (1982), ruled on a Texas statute that denied access to education to children of illegal immigrants. The Texas statute was a 1975 revision of education laws that allowed the withholding of state funds for educating children who had not been legally admitted to the United States. Additionally, the revision authorized school districts to deny enrollment to students who could not produce documentation of their legal status in the United States. The Supreme Court struck down the statute and ensured that all immigrant school-age children, whether here illegally or legally, who live in the United States have the right to attend public schools. Therefore, public schools in the US are not allowed to deny admission to schools to any student based on immigration status, to require students or parents to produce evidence of their immigration status, or require social security numbers of students.

The third case, *Castañeda v. Pickard* (1981), was a federal court case against the school district in Raymondville, Texas. The plaintiff claimed his Mexican American children were discriminated by the school district because of their ethnicity. Reversing an initial ruling in the federal district court, the United States Court of Appeals for the Fifth District agreed with the plaintiff and created a set of specific criteria for quality programming and for determining whether or not a school district is in compliance with the Equal Educational Opportunity Act. This compliance test has been known as the Castañeda Test and requires the satisfaction of three criteria for ensuring quality programming for ELs. The first criterion is theory: the school programs must be based on sound educational theory or legitimate experimental strategy. The second criterion is practice: the school programs must be implemented with adequate instructional practices, resources, and staff. The last criterion is results: the school program must demonstrate its effectiveness through evaluation, not only in the teaching of English, but also in the broad access to the content areas of the curriculum (Alexander, Alexander, & Alexander, 2000).

Building the Context for Understanding English Language Learners with Special Needs

Definitions and Terminology Related to ELs with Special Needs

So far, this chapter has examined several important characteristics of ELs in an effort to understand this growing student population. After an analysis of the definition of and terms associated with ELs, this chapter looked at critical data related to their enrollment in US public schools, as well as their country of origin and language background. Finally, it examined several key legislation initiatives that have influenced the education of ELs in the US in very important ways. To understand the category of ELs who are enrolled in special education programs, it is helpful to review important definition and terms that are relevant for ELs with special needs.

Definitions

School-age children who are diagnosed with a special need are often served in special education settings or receive special education services. These settings are dictated by the mandates set forth by the NCLB Act (2001a). Legislation notes that services for children with special needs must be offered in the least restrictive environment (LRE).

According to the federal definition, special education is specially designed instruction that is provided to children with disabilities to meet their unique needs at no cost to the parents (NCLB, 2001b). This includes instruction conducted in the classroom, in the home, in hospitals and institutions, and in other settings, as well as instruction in physical education. Special education may include a related service, if the service is considered special education rather than a related service under state standards (i.e., speech-language pathology services). The content, methodology, or delivery of instruction is often adapted to meet the needs of the child with special needs and to address the unique needs of the child that result from the child's disability. This ensures that the child has access to the general curriculum, so that the child can meet educational standards. In general, special education refers to a range of educational and social services provided by various educational entities to individuals with disabilities between the ages of 3 and 21 years of age (Table 3–8).

ELs with Special Needs: Terminology

The 1975 Education for All Handicapped Children Act (EAHCA) and the Individuals with Disabilities Education Act (IDEA) of 1997,

Table 3–8. *List of Disabilities as Defined by Federal Legislation*

Term	Definition
Autism	Having a developmental disability significantly affecting verbal and nonverbal communication and social interaction, generally evident before age 3 that adversely affects a child's educational performance. Other characteristics often associated with autism are engagement in repetitive activities and stereotyped movements, resistance to environmental change or change in daily routines, and unusual responses to sensory experiences.
Deaf	Having a hearing impairment so severe that the child cannot understand what is being said even with a hearing aid.
Deaf-Blind	Having concomitant hearing and visual impairments causing such severe communication, developmental, and educational problems that the child cannot be accommodated in programs exclusively designed for the deaf or for the blind.
Hearing Impairment	Having a hearing impairment, whether permanent or fluctuating, that is not included under the definition of deafness.
Mental Retardation	Having significantly subaverage general intellectual functioning existing concurrently with deficits in adaptive behavior and manifested during the developmental period.
Multiple Disabilities	Having a combination of impairments (with the exception of deaf-blindness) causing such severe educational problems that the child cannot be accommodated in a special education program designed only for one of the impairments.
Orthopedic Impairment	Having a severe orthopedic impairment (amputation, absence of a limb, cerebral palsy, poliomyelitis, bone tuberculosis, etc.).
Other Health Impairment	Having limited strength, vitality, or alertness due to chronic or acute health problems (heart condition, rheumatic fever, asthma, hemophilia, leukemia, etc.).

continues

Table 3–8. continued

Term	Definition
Serious Emotional Disturbance	Having a condition exhibiting one or more of the following characteristics, displayed over a long period of time and to a marked degree: • An inability to learn that cannot be explained by intellectual, sensory, or health factors • An inability to build or maintain satisfactory interpersonal relationships with peers or teachers • Inappropriate types of behavior or feelings under normal circumstances • A general pervasive mood of unhappiness or depression • A tendency to develop physical symptoms or fears associated with personal or school problems.
Specific Learning Disability	Having a disorder in one or more of the basic psychological processes involved in understanding or in using language, spoken or written, that may manifest itself in an imperfect ability to listen, think, speak, read, write, spell, or do mathematical calculations. The term includes such conditions as perceptual disabilities, brain injury, minimal brain dysfunction, dyslexia, and developmental aphasia. It does not include children who have learning problems that are primarily the result of visual, hearing, or motor disabilities; mental retardation; or environmental, cultural, or economic disadvantage.
Speech or Language Impairment	Having a communication disorder such as stuttering, impaired articulation, language impairment, or voice impairment.
Traumatic Brain Injury	Having an acquired injury to the brain caused by an external physical force, resulting in total or partial functional disability or psychosocial impairment, or both. The term applies to open or closed head injuries resulting in impairments in one or more areas, such as cognition; language; memory; attention; reasoning; abstract thinking; judgment; problem solving; sensory, perceptual and motor abilities; psychosocial behavior; physical functions; information processing; and speech.

Table 3–8. *continued*

Term	Definition
Visual Impairment	Having impairment in vision (including blindness) that, even with correction, adversely affects a child's educational performance. The term includes both partial sight and blindness.

Source: Data from "Categories of Disability Under IDEA," by National Dissemination Center for Children with Disabilities (NICHCY), 2009. Retrieved from http://nichcy.org/disability/categories

which came into being when the EAHCA was renamed IDEA in 1997, are two important pieces of legislation governing the identification, assessment, and instruction of students with special needs in general and ELs with special needs in particular. They contain key terminology used to describe children with special needs. These laws do not specifically address ELs with special needs; however, they provide an exclusionary statement that cautions professionals against misidentification of ELs. Multidisciplinary teams must provide assurances that students' problems are not the result of limited English proficiency, cultural or environmental disadvantage, or lack of educational opportunity or experiences. The exclusionary clause is one of the most important safeguards for ELs being considered for special education placement.

ELs with Special Needs: Demographics

Survey data provided by school districts show that ELs with special needs represent 9% of all ELs in US public schools (Zehler, Fleischman, Hopstock, Pendzick, & Stephenson, 2003). This percentage is smaller compared with the percentage of all non-EL students who are in special education, which is 13.5%. There are several possible explanations for this discrepancy. One explanation could be that the survey does not capture the number of ELs already in special education programs. Another possible explanation is that ELs with special needs are under-identified due to inadequate identification and referral procedures. Finally, they may have a primary diagnosis (e.g., autism) with a secondary diagnosis of a speech and/or language disorder and may not be captured statistically as an EL or a child who has a communication disorder.

EL students with special needs are enrolled in over 33,000 schools in the United States. Although these students are present in a large number of schools and districts, most of them are concentrated in a small number of schools. For example, 62.2% of schools with at least one EL with special needs have fewer than 10 EL students with special needs, and only 5.8% have more than 40 ELs with special needs. At the district level, the situation is comparatively similar, emphasizing the fact that ELs with special needs are in areas with high EL concentration. 54.6% of districts have fewer than 10 ELs with special needs and enroll a mere 2.6% of the total EL special needs population. Only 3.4% of districts have more than 500 ELs with special needs, but they enroll more than 57% of the EL special needs population nationwide.

In terms of special education classification, the percentage of ELs with special needs is smaller than the percentage of the total population, as seen in Table 3–9. Important differences in the percentages between the two student populations are in three categories: specific learning disability, emotional disturbance, and other health impairment.

As previously noted when discussing the national data comparing the representation of ELs with the representation of non-ELs in special education programs, ELs are clearly underrepresented in these education programs. Consequently, a smaller percentage of ELs receive services than would be expected given the proportion of the overall population they represent. However, underrepresentation is not the only characteristic of the demographical statistics describing ELs with special needs. EL students are likely to be overrepresented in certain special education categories, such as speech-language impairment or emotional disturbance (McCardle, Mele-McCarthy, Cutting, Leos, & D'Emilio, 2005). Additionally, the percentage of ELs who are on special education rosters in urban schools is significantly higher than the national non-EL special education percentage (Donovan & Cross, 2002). The overrepresentation of ELs in special education classes (Yates & Ortiz, 1998) suggests that professionals

Table 3–9. *Percentage of General Population Students and EL Special Needs Students*

Disability	General Population Percentage	SpEd EL Percentage
Specific Learning Disabilities	6.64%	5.16%
Speech-Language Impairments	2.72	2.17
Mental Retardation	1.20	0.72
Emotional Disturbance	1.00	0.23
Other Health Impairments	0.73	0.20
Developmental Delay	0.32	0.15
Autism	0.26	0.12
Multiple Disabilities	0.25	0.10
Hearing Disabilities	0.18	0.16
Orthopedic Impairments	0.16	0.14
Visual Impairments	0.06	0.05
Traumatic Brain Injury	0.04	0.02
Deaf/Blind	0.01	0.005

Source: Data from *Descriptive Study of Services to LEP Students and LEP Students with Disabilities. Special Topic Report No. 4: Findings on Special Education LEP Students*, by A. M. Zehler, H. L. Fleischman, P. J. Hopstock, M. L. Pendzick, & T. G. Stephenson, 2003, Arlington, VA: Development Associates.

continue to have difficulty distinguishing students who truly have communication disorders from students who are failing for other reasons, such as limited English. The underrepresentation of ELs with special needs at the national level and overrepresentation in certain school settings emphasizes once more the need to develop better tools for accurate identification of ELs with special needs and professionals with the skills and competencies to conduct linguistically and culturally relevant educational assessments (Valdéz & Figueroa, 1996).

Country of Birth and Language Background of ELs with Special Needs

Just like general education ELs, most ELs with special needs were born in the United States; in fact, even more ELs with special needs than general education ELs are born in the United States (68.6% of ELs with special needs compared with 47.3% of general education ELs) (Zehler, Fleischman, Hopstock, Stephenson, & Sapru, 2003). Table 3–10 lists the countries of birth for all ELs with special needs.

There are also similarities between ELs with special needs and general education ELs when we compare the language back-

Table 3–10. Country of Birth of ELs with Special Needs

Country	Percentage
United States	68.6%
Mexico	19.6
Iraq	1.6
Russia	0.9
Poland	0.9
El Salvador	0.8
Saudi Arabia	0.7
Peru	0.7
Puerto Rico	0.6
Ecuador	0.5
Other	5.1

Source: Data from *Descriptive Study of Services to LEP Students and LEP Students with Disabilities. Special Topic Report No. 4: Findings on Special Education LEP Students,* by A. M. Zehler, H. L. Fleischman, P. J. Hopstock, M. L. Pendzick, & T. G. Stephenson, 2003, Arlington, VA: Development Associates.

grounds of the two groups. From the entire ELs with special needs population, 80.4% are speakers of Spanish. Spanish speakers represent 76.9% of the US EL population (Hopstock & Stephenson, 2003). This similarity in percentages could be explained by the fact that there might be more bilingual staff available and more appropriate identification instruments. Other languages that display this contrast between the representation in special education and the general EL representation are Navajo, with 1.9 % of the ELs with special needs population speaking Navajo compared to 0.9% of general education ELs, and Lao, with 0.7% of ELs with special needs speaking Lao compared to 0.4% one of general education ELs. The top ten languages spoken by ELs with special needs are presented in Table 3–11.

Table 3–11. *Ten Most Commonly Spoken Languages by ELs with Special Needs*

Language	Percentage
Spanish	80.4%
Navajo	1.9
Hmong	1.7
Vietnamese	1.6
Cantonese	1.0
American Indian	1.0
Haitian Creole	0.8
English	0.8
Laotian	0.7
Arabic	0.6

Source: Data from *Descriptive Study of Services to LEP Students and LEP Students with Disabilities. Special Topic Report No. 1: Native Language of LEP Students,* by P. J. Hopstock and T. G. Stephenson. Submitted to US Department of Education, OELA. Arlington, VA: Development Associates.

Legislation Affecting ELs with Special Needs

Federal Legislation

There have been several efforts to ensure that special education students in general and ELs with special needs in particular have equitable access to education and receive appropriate service tailored to their needs. This chapter focuses on one crucial piece of legislation: the 1975 Education for All Handicapped Children Act (EAHCA), now known as the Individuals with Disabilities Education Act (IDEA). The 1975 law was a basic bill of rights for children with disabilities; these children had to demonstrate at least one disability to qualify for special services. This legislation was developed with the purpose of providing access to educational services to students.

The 1975 law had several important provisions (EAHCA, 1975). The first provision was *Zero Reject*. This provision implied that all children, regardless of disability and severity, were provided access to free and appropriate public education (FAPE). The second provision of the law was *Nondiscriminatory Assessment*, which stipulated that students must be diagnosed using nondiscriminatory standardized evaluation to be administered in the student's native language by properly trained administrators. It is important to note that the law clearly prohibited any test to be administered in any language other than the primary language spoken by the student.

Procedural Due Process and *Parental Participation* are two more important components of the Education for All Handicapped Children Act; they guaranteed parents' participation in educational decisions affecting their children, as well as parents' protection if they disagreed with school decisions. Parents were responsible for giving permission for testing and evaluation of their children for special services, participated in the decision whether or not their child should receive special education services, and advocated for their child (Birnbaum, 2008).

Another component of the law was the *Least Restrictive Environment (LRE)*, which states that the best placement for a child with special needs was in the regular classroom. Only when the nature or the severity of the disability prevented the student from being educated in a regular classroom should the student be placed in a more restricted setting or in an environment outside the public school classroom.

Perhaps the most important part of the EAHCA was the call for an *Individualized Education Program (IEP),* a legal document expressly written for a student requiring special services. When students were eligible for special education services, the school was required to convene an IEP team and develop an appropriate educational plan for the child. The IEP team included the student's parents or guardians, a special education teacher, at least one general education teacher, a school or district representative with knowledge regarding the availability of school resources, a professional qualified to interpret the instructional implications of the child's evaluation results (for example, the school psychologist), and a translator for parents with limited English proficiency. The 2004 reauthorization of IDEA required the IEP to be written to meet the needs of the student and to include the following:

◆ The student's current level of academic and functional performance
◆ A statement of annual goals, including academic and functional goals
◆ Procedures for evaluation of goals
◆ A list of special education services, related services, and supplementary aids to be provided to the student, as well as program modifications or supports provided to school personnel on behalf of the child
◆ The dates for the beginning of services, the frequency, duration, and location for the provision of services, and the extent to which the student is able to participate in the general curriculum
◆ List of accommodations to be provided during assessments that measure the student's academic and functional performance

The reauthorization of IDEA in 2004 reflected a number of amendments added between the original authorization of the Education for All Handicapped Children Act in 1975 and the current legislation. A 1986 reauthorization expanded the original legislation to cover children between ages 3 and 5, and a 1990 reauthorization encouraged the use of "person-first" language when describing disabilities. Additionally, through its 1990 amendments, for the first time IDEA specifically addressed the needs of students who are ELs and disabled:

> Studies have documented apparent discrepancies in the levels of referral and placement of limited English proficient children in special education. The Department of Education has found that services provided to limited English proficient student often do not respond primarily to the pupil's academic needs. These trends pose special challenges for special education in the referral, assessment, and services for our nation's student from non English language backgrounds. (IDEA, 1997)

In 1991, IDEA was again reauthorized and now required the development of an *Individualized Family Service Plan (IFSP)* for children and their families between birth and age 3. This plan required information about the child's status, family information, outcomes, early intervention services, dates and duration of services, and service coordinator. The IDEA changes of 1996 served to address and protect the educational rights of students who were disabled but challenges continued in meeting the needs of school-age ELs, especially children with communication disorders (Murdick, Gartin, & Crabtree, 2002).

Court Rulings

Although the course rulings of *Lau v. Nichols*, *Plyer v. Doe*, and *Castañeda v. Pickard* did not specifically address ELs with disabilities, the rulings made it more likely that students who were ELs would not be referred to special education because of a lack of educational opportunity or appropriate instruction. An important case that specifically dealt with the identification and placement of ELs in special education programs was *Diana v. State Board of Education* (1970). Plaintiffs, on behalf of Mexican American children in Monterey County, California, complained that the school system was wrongly identifying Spanish-speaking students as mentally challenged based on IQ tests administered in English. The judge ordered that an IQ test for Mexican American children be developed and all Mexican American children who had been placed in special education be reassessed in their first language and in English, or by using nonverbal IQ tests.

Fernandez (1992) identified two other important court cases that involved ELs with special needs (Table 3–12). The first one was *Jose P. v. Ambach* (1983), which was a class action suit on behalf of students who claimed they were denied access to adequate education because of the school's failure to evaluate

Table 3–12. ELs with Special Needs and the Courts

Case	Description	Ruling
Diana v. State Board of Education (1970)	A California District Court case in which the plaintiffs, on behalf of Mexican American children, complained that IQ tests in English were unfair.	The judge ordered IQ tests to be developed in students' native language, plus students who were misplaced were reassessed.
Jose P. v. Ambach (1979)	Federal District Court class action suit where plaintiffs claimed they were denied access to educational programs due to the inability of schools to evaluate and place them in special programs.	The schools were required to use bilingual resources to identify SpEd ELs, provide bilingual nondiscriminatory evaluations, provide bilingual alternatives at each stage of special education placement process, protect the rights of parents and students, and hire community workers to help with the involvement of parents in the assessment process and development of their IEPs.
Y. S. v. School District of Philadelphia (1986)	A federal class action suit where plaintiffs claimed educational decisions were incorrect because they were based on tests developed for English speakers.	The settlement included drastic changes in evaluation, curriculum, planning, and counseling of ELs and SpEd ELs.

and place them in special programs. The judge ordered several measures to provide language-appropriate services. The school board was required to complete a survey of all students with disabilities, recording by language the number of those who were ELs. The judge also required the school board to put together a description of each program for students with disabilities, including bilingual programs for ELs. An outreach office was created with the purpose of distributing information in English and other languages about special education programs. Procedures were to be developed for the provision of competent interpreters for EL parents, for evaluations of EL students, and for identifying appropriate bilingual tests.

The second case, *Y. S. v. School District of Philadelphia* (1986) was a federal class action suit. Y., a Cambodian refugee, was one of the students named in the case; Y. was enrolled in ESOL courses but received no other bilingual services. Three years after enrolling in school, Y. was placed in a class for students who were mentally challenged. Plaintiffs claimed that the decision to classify Y. was incorrect, because the decision was made based on a test developed for English-speaking students. The settlement reached between plaintiffs and school district officials required the district to implement several changes. First, the placement of all EL Asian students in general and special education was reviewed. Then, a remedial plan to address the needs of such students was developed. It included evaluation and counseling in their native language, a revised curriculum for the district's ESOL program, and a special education component of the remedial plan. The district agreed to hire and train bilingual staff and to improve communication with the students. It also agreed that all oral and written communication to parents would be provided in the parents' native language.

Building the Context for Understanding ELs with Communication Disorders

Terminology and Demographics

Communication disorders are among the most common disabilities in the United States. According to the 24th Annual Report to Congress on the Implementation of Individuals with Disabilities Education Act, "speech or language impairment" was the most prevalent disability category in schools, accounting for 55.2% of all preschoolers served in 2000–2001 (US Department of Education, 2001). In addition, the majority (56.3%) of the preschoolers who were served for speech or language impairment in the United States were Hispanic. For students ages 6 through 12 who were served under IDEA, "speech or language impairment" (18.9%) was the second-largest category of students served in a federally supported program for the disabled after "specific learning disabilities" (50.0%) (US Department of Education, 2002). For students in the 12 through 17 and 18 through 21 age groups, the "speech or language impairment" category was ranked fifth and sixth in size, respectively, after "specific learning disabilities." Interestingly, in a 2011 report entitled *The Condition of Education in the U.S.* issued by the National Center for Education Statistics, it was reported that approximately 22% of children and youth receiving services under IDEA had speech or language impairments (Aud, Hussar, Kena, Bianco, Frohlich, Kemp, & Tahan, 2011). Thus, communication disorders continues to be one of the most prevalent disability types, remaining fairly constant around 3%, with variations of less than 1 percentage point.

There are few reliable data on the general prevalence or incidence of communication disorders among EL populations in the United States. Estimates are generally based on projections from data based on the mainstream population. It is suggested that there is a greater prevalence of communication disorders among the EL population than among white individuals (Benson & Marano, 1994). We know that approximately 11% of native English-speaking students have disabilities (US Department of Education, 2002). The highest reported percentage of ELs with disabilities is lower than that percentage.

Descriptive research has begun to estimate and document the prevalence of ELs with disabilities in American schools (D'Emilio, 2003; Zehler et al., 2003). Prevalence data have suggested a disproportionate representation of ELs with special needs in special education programs (Zehler et al, 2003). Results indicated that 357,325 ELs had disabilities across the US. A second source of prevalence data suggested that ELs with disabilities are probably underrepresented. After averaging the number of ELs with disabilities across all states in a national sample, about 1% of the students were identified as ELs with disabilities (O'Sullivan et al., 1997; Reese et al., 1997). In light of the National Clearinghouse on Bilingual Education's (NCBE) estimate of the national prevalence of ELs (12.7%) and the Office of Special Education Programs' (OSEP) estimate for students with disabilities (10.7%), it would be expected that the number of ELs with disabilities in this national sample might have been higher.

ASHA estimates that 10% of the US population has a disorder of speech, hearing, or language unrelated to the ability to speak English as a native language (Cole, 1989). If the prevalence of communication disorders among racial and ethnic minorities is consistent with that of the general population, then it is estimated that 6.2 million ELs have a communication disorder. For example, the number of children, ages 3 to 21, with disabilities served in the public schools under the Individuals with Disabilities Education Act (IDEA), Part B, in the fall of 2003 was 6,068,802 (in the 50 states, Washington, DC, and outlying areas). Of these children, 1,460,583 (24.1%) received services for speech or language disorders. This estimate does not include children who have speech/language problems secondary to other conditions.

The term communication sciences and disorders has come into consistent use only since the 1980s. The term speech pathology has been used and recognized for much longer (Guilford, 2003; Moeller, 1976). Early pioneers in speech-language pathology came from a variety of disciplines (e.g., education, psychology, linguistics), and the blending of knowledge through research and clinical application in diagnosis and treatment of communication disorders resulted in enhancing the practice of speech-language pathology (Duchan, 2002). The importance of speech-language pathology services has been enhanced by public demand and heightened awareness of communicative needs. During the later decades of the 20th century, federal funding for support of services and for research became available in the US with the passage of legislation that delineated the rights of school-age children. Specifically, educational legislative issues have had a strong impact on the profession, beginning in the 1970s and 1980s when attention was focused on the rights of children from

Table 3–13. Legislative Mandates That Have Influenced the Profession of CSD

Year	Title of Legislative Act	Significance
1975	P.L. 94-142	Increased service to children with communication disorders 6 to 21 years of age
1986	P.L. 99-457 Education for the Handicapped Act P.L. 102-119 (Amended P.L. 99-457) became known as Part H	Increased age range of children who are served from ages 3 to 5 and 6 to 21. Part H mandated that ALL states provide services for 3- to 5-year-olds with special needs
1990	Reauthorization of Education for the Handicapped Act into Individuals with Disabilities Education Act (IDEA)	Later reauthorized again and moved Part H to Part C
2004	Reauthorization of IDEA	Strengthened the role of Naturalistic Environments
2005	No Child Left Behind	Designed to strengthen the academic performance of students whose schools are failing them. Only qualified schools are those receiving Title I funds (low-income schools)

3 to 21 years of age. Table 3–13 provides a summary of federally mandated legislative initiatives that have had an impact on serving school-age students with communication disorders.

Terminology

The term communication disorders encompass speech and language disorders across the life span. A speech disorder is an impairment of the articulation of fluency, speech sounds, and/or voice, whereas a language disorder is the impaired comprehension and/or use of spoken, written, and/or other symbol systems. The disorder may involve the form, content, and/or function of language in communication (ASHA, 2008). Determining the population of children and adults with speech and language disorders has been problematic because there are several populations that may have communication disorders secondary to another disability (i.e., autism, learning disability) (USDOE, 2005). Specifically, when ELs struggle academically, professionals must consider a myriad of variables to determine if a child's learning problems can be attributed to a disorder that is affecting his/her ability to acquire language skills or if the student is progressing through the stages of learning a second language.

Distinguishing between a language difference and the presence of a language disorder is often a demanding task, and requires specific knowledge and competencies to accurately distinguish a communication difference from a disorder. Researchers have described possible indicators of a communication disorder in ELs (Evans, 2001; Kohnert, 2008) and have noted that students with communication disorders often: (a) have difficulty learning language at a normal rate, even with support and assistance in both languages; (b) have gaps in vocabulary and decreased mean lengths of utterance; (c) have difficulties communicating with peers as well as in the home, (d) have difficulty across literacy events, (e) lack organization in the use of language to convey thoughts, and (f) demonstrate poor academic achievement despite adequate academic proficiency in English. Although this list is not exhaustive, it is important to reiterate that language disorders are determined by referencing typical or "normal" language performance. Because typical language abilities serve as the reference point for determining a language disorder, there is a general consensus in the literature that if a student has a language disorder he/she will usually demonstrate problems not only in English but in English and the primary language, or the acquisition of any language (Goldstein, 2004; Kohnert, 2008; Roseberry-McKibben, 2008).

SLPs play a critical role in identifying whether children with limited English proficiency have an underlying communication disorder. This monumental responsibility requires that the SLPs know normal language acquisition, recognize the signs of progressing second language acquisition, and consider the indicators of a communication disorder to better understand ELs with communication disorders (ASHA, 2004).

Summary

In order to understand the larger population to which ELs with special needs belong, this chapter examined several important characteristics of ELs. It looked at definitions and key terms, enrollment data, country of birth, language background, and federal legislation and legal action centered on ELs. Then, in order to build the context for understanding ELs with special needs further, the same parameters were applied to the analysis of ELs in special education programs as well as looking at ELs with communication disorders. At the end of the analysis of ELs, ELs with special needs, and ELs with communication disorders in the school-age population, one idea has become very clear: the notion that English learners are a monolithic group is unmistakably false. We need to ensure that we focus on within-group diversity if we want all ELs to succeed academically, especially under the accountability mandates affirmed in the NCLB Act (2001b).

Chapter 1 concluded with a case study of a student, Rey, who was referred to the speech-language pathologist by his parent and teacher. In order for the SLP and ESOL professional to appropriately and accurately identify and assess Rey, they must share a knowledge base and work collaboratively to identify him as an EL, as well as to determine whether there is a language disorder or a language difference.

This chapter stressed the characteristics of ELs and the legal considerations and mandates that guide the procedures and materials that must be followed to evaluate a student such as Rey. What, then, are the important factors that SLPs and ESOL professionals must consider when working with Rey? IDEA (2004) stipulates that Rey must be assessed using measures that are "culturally and linguistically appropriate." This means that the SLP must use procedures, materials, and protocols that will reduce the likelihood that Rey will be misdiagnosed as having a communication disorder resulting from limited English exposure. The ESOL professional must use appropriate measures to identify Rey as an EL. Both professionals must pool their expertise and resources to determine Rey's language proficiency and use this information in the assessment process. To achieve this, the SLP and ESOL professionals must understand first and second language development, be familiar with basic, typical, developmental features of a student's primary language, and the errors commonly used by ELs in acquiring a second language. The next chapter will discuss first and second language acquisition to provide a framework for distinguishing language disorders from language differences.

References

Alaska Department of Education. (2010). *Data from Guidance for Limited English Proficient (LEP) Student Identification Assessment* and *Data Reports*. Retrieved from http://www.ecd.state.ak.us

Alexander, K., Alexander, M. D., & Alexander, D. (2000). *American public school law* (5th ed.). Belmont, CA: Wadsworth.

American Speech-Language-Hearing Association. (2004). *Knowledge and skills needed by speech-language pathologists and audiologists to provide culturally and linguistically appropriate services* [Knowledge and skills]. Retrieved from http://www.asha.org/docs/html/KS2004-00215.html

American Speech-Language-Hearing Association. (2008). *Incidence and prevalence of communication disorders and hearing loss in children—2008 edition.* Retrieved from http://www.asha.org/research/reports/children.htm

Aud, S., Hussar, W., Kena, G., Bianco, K., Frohlich, L., Kemp, J., & Tahan, K. (2011). *The condition of education 2011 (NCES 2011-033).* US Department of Education, National Center for Education Statistics. Washington, DC: US Government Printing Office.

Ballantyne, K. G., Sanderman, A. R., & Levy, J. (2008). *Educating English language learners: Building teacher capacity.* Washington, DC: National Clearinghouse for English Language Acquisition. Retrieved from http://www.ncela.gwu.edu/practice/mainstream_teachers.htm

Benson, V., & Marano, M. A. (1994). *Current estimates from the National Health Interview Survey, 1993.* Series 10, No. 190. Hyattsville, MD: National Center for Health Statistics.

Bilingual Education Act. (1968). Pub. L. No. 90-247, 81 Stat. 816 (1968).

Birnbaum, B. W. (2008). *English language learners with disabilities: A resource guide for educators.* Lewiston, NY: Edwin Mellen Press.

California Department of Education (n.d.). *Glossary of terms.* Retrieved from http://www.cde.ca.gov/ds/sd/cb/glossary.asp

Capps, R., Fix, M., Murray, J., Ost, J. Passel, J., & Herwantoro, S. (2006). *The new demography of American schools: Immigration and the No Child Left Behind Act.* Washington, DC: Urban Institute.

Castañeda v. Pickard, No. 79-2253. USC (5th, Unit 8) (1981).

Civil Rights Act, Pub. L. No. 88-352, 78 Stat. 241 (1964).

Cole, L. (1989). E pluribus: Multicultural imperatives for the 1990s and beyond. *ASHA Leader,* 65–70.

D'Emilio, T. E. (2003, June). *LEP student participation in special education: Over or under-representation?* Paper presented at the CCSSO Conference on Large-Scale Assessment, San Antonio, TX.

Diana v. State Board of Education, No. C-70-37 (N.D. CA 1970).

Donovan, M. S., & Cross, C. T. (Eds.). (2002). *Minority students in special and gifted education.* National Research Council; Committee on Minority Representation in Special Education. Washington, DC: National Academy Press.

Duchan, J. F. (2002, December 24). What do you know about your profession's history: And why is it important? *ASHA Leader.*

Education for All Handicapped Children Act, 20 U.S.C. § 1400–1485 (1975).

Elementary and Secondary Education Act, Title VII (also known as the Bilingual Education Act), Sections 701 et seq., 20 U.S.C.A., Sections 880b et seq. P.L. 90-247, 81 Stat. 783 (1968).

Evans, J. (2001). An emergent account of language impairments in children with SLI: Implications for assessment and intervention. *Journal of Communication Disorders, 34,* 39–54.

Fernandez, A. T. (1992). Legal support for bilingual education and language-appropriate related services for limited English proficient students with disabilities. *Bilingual Research Journal, 16*(3, 4), 117–140.

Florida Department of Education. (n.d.). *League of United Latin American Citizens (LULAC) et al. v. State Board of Education Consent Decree.* United States District Court for the Southern District of Florida, August 14, 1990. Retrieved from http://www.fldoe.org/aala/cdpage2.asp

Florida Department of Education. (2005). *ESOL English for speakers of other languages. Language enriched pupil (LEP) database and program handbook, 2005–2006.* Tallahassee, FL: Office of Education Information and Accountability Services and the Office of Multicultural Student Language Education (OMSLE). Retrieved from http://www.fldoe.org/aala/pdf/final_lep.pdf

Florida Department of Education. (2011). *Data from 2010–2011 English Language Learners (ELL) Data Base* and *Program Handbook: English for Speakers of Other Languages (ESOL).* Retrieved from www.fldoe.org/aala/pdf/edph10011.pdf

Flynn, K., & Hill, J. (2005). *English language learners: A growing population.* Denver, CO: Mid-continent Research for Education and Learning.

Francis, D., Rivera, M., Lesaux, N., Kieffer, M., & Rivera, H. (2006). *Practical guidelines for the education of English language learners: Research-based recommendations for instruction and academic interventions.* (Under cooperative agreement grant S283B050034 for US Department of Education.) Portsmouth, NH: RMC Research Corporation, Center on Instruction. Retrieved from http://www.center oninstruction.org/files/ELL1- Interventions.pdf

Goldstein, B. A. (2004). Bilingual language development and disorders: Introduction and overview. In B. A. Goldstein (Ed.), *Bilingual language development and disorders in Spanish-English speakers* (pp. 3–20). Baltimore, MD: Brookes.

Guilford, A. (2003). Communication sciences and disorders. In M. A. Richard & W. G. Emener (Eds.), *I'm a people person: A guide to human services professions.* Springfield, IL: Charles C. Thomas.

Hopstock, P. J., & Stephenson, T. G. (2003). *Descriptive study of services to LEP student and LEP students with disabilities. Special topic report no. 1: Native language of LEP students.* Washington, DC: US Department of Education, OELA.

Individuals with Disabilities Education Act (IDEA) of 1997, *Federal Register*, Volume 62, No. 204. Part V, Department of Education, 34 CFR PARTSW 300, 303.

Individuals with Disabilities Education Improvement Act of 2004, Pub. L. 108-446, 108th Congress.

Jose P. v. Ambach, R 557 F. Supp 11230 (E.D.lNl.Y, 1983).

Kohnert, K. (2008). *Language disorders in bilingual children and adults.* San Diego, CA: Plural.

Lau v. Nichols, 414 U.S. 563 (1974).

Matthews, H., & Ewen, D. (2006). *Reaching all children? Understanding early care and education participation among immigrant families.* Washington, DC: Center for Law and Social Policy. Retrieved from ERIC database. (ED489574)

Maxwell, L. A. (2009, January 8). Immigration transforms communities. *Education Week, 20*(17), 1–2.

McCardle, P., Mele-McCarty, J., Cutting, L., Leos, K., & D'Emilio, T. (2005). Learning disabilities in English language learners: Identifying the issues. *Learning Disabilities Research and Practice, 20*(1), 1–5.

Moeller, D. (1976). *Speech pathology and audiology: Iowa organization of a discipline.* Iowa City: University of Iowa Press.

Murdick, N., Gartin, B., & Crabtree, T. (2002). *Special education law.* Upper Saddle River, NJ: Merrill Prentice-Hall.

National Clearinghouse for English Language Acquisition (NCELA). (n.d.). *NCELA state Title III information system.* Retrieved from http://www.ncela.gwu.edu/t3sis/

National Clearinghouse for English Language Acquisition (NCELA). (2006). *The growing numbers of limited English proficient students 1995/1996–2005/2006.* Retrieved from http://www.ncela.gwu.edu/files/uploads/4/GrowingLEP_0506.pdf

National Dissemination Center for Children with Disabilities (NICHCY). (2009). Categories of disability under IDEA. Retrieved from http://nichcy.org/disability/categories

No Child Left Behind (NCLB). (2001a). 20 U.S.C (2001& Supp 2002). Washington, DC: US Department of Education.

No Child Left Behind (NCLB). (2001b). *Title III: Language instruction for Limited English Proficient and immigrant students. 107th Congress, 1st Session, December 13, 2001.* (Printed version prepared by the National Clearinghouse for Bilingual Education). Washington, DC: George Washington University, National Clearinghouse for Bilingual Education.

Office of English Language Acquisition, Language Enhancement, and Academic Achievement for Limited English Proficient Students (OELA). (2008). *Biennial Report to Congress on the implementation of the Title III State Formula Grant Program, School Years 2004–06.* Washington, DC: Author.

O'Sullivan, C. Y., Reese, C. M., & Mazzeo, J. (1997). *NAEP 1996 science report card for the nation and the states.* Washington, DC: National Center for Education Statistics.

Payan, R. M., & Nettles, M. T. (2008). *Current state of English-Language learners in the U.S. K–12 student population. 2008 English Language Learner Symposium.* Princeton, NJ. Retrieved from http://www.ets.org/Media/Conferences_and_Events/pdf/ELLsympsium/ELL_factsheet.pdf

Plyer v. Doe, 47 U.S. 202 (1982).

Reese, C. M., Miller, K. E., Mazzeo, J., & Dossey, J. A. (1997). *NAEP 1996 mathematics report card for the nation and the states.* Washington, DC: National Center for Education Statistics.

Roseberry-McKibben, C. (2008). *Multicultural students with special language needs.* Oceanside, CA: Academic Communication Associates.

Short, D. J., & Fitzsimmons, S. (2006). *Double the work: Challenges and solutions to acquiring language and academic literacy for adolescent English language learners*. New York, NY: Carnegie Corporation.

Tung, R., Uriarte, M., Diez, V., Lavan, N., Agusti, N., Karp, F., & Meschede, T. (2009). *English learners in Boston public schools: Enrollment, engagement and academic outcomes, AY2003-AY2006, final report*. Boston, MA: Mauricio Gastón Institute for Latino Community Development and Public Policy. Retrieved from http://www.gaston.umb .edu/articles/2009%20Final%20ELL%20Report_online.pdf

US Census Bureau. (2011). *Population profile of the United States*. Retrieved from http://www.census.gov/population/www/pop-pro file/profiledynamic.html

US Congress. (1994). *Improving America's Schools Act* (P.L. 103-382), 1994. Retrieved from http://www2.ed.gov/legislation/ESEA/toc.html

US Department of Education. (2001). *Twenty-fourth annual report to Congress on the Implementation of the Individuals with Disabilities Education Act*. Washington, DC: Author.

US Department of Education. (2002). *The condition of education 2002 in Brief, NCES 2002–011*. Washington, DC: Author.

US Department of Education. (2005). *To assure the free appropriate public education of all Americans: Twenty-seventh annual report to Congress on the implementation of the Individuals with Disabilities Education Act*. Retrieved from http://www.ed.gov/about/reports/ annual/osep/2005/index.html

Valdes, G., & Figueroa, R. A. (1996). *Bilingualism and testing: A special case of bias*. Norwood, NJ: Ablex.

Virginia Department of Education. (2009). *Handbook for Educators for Students Who Are English Language Learners with Suspected Learning Disabilities*. Retrieved from http://www.doe.virginia.gov/ instruction/esl/standards_resources/index.shtml

Virginia Department of Education. (2011). *Limited English Proficient Standards: Guidelines for Participation in the Virginia Assessment Program*. Retrieved from http://www.doe.virginia.gov/testing/par ticipation/index.shtml

Y. S. v. School District of Philadelphia, C.A. 85-6924 (E.D. PA 1986).

Yates, J. R., & Ortiz, A. (1998). Issues of cultural and diversity affecting educators with disabilities: A change in demography is reshaping American. In R. J. Anderson, C. E. Keller & J. M. Karp (Eds.), *Enhancing diversity: Educators with disabilities in the education enterprise*. Washington, DC: Gallaudet Press.

Zehler, A. M., Fleischman, H. L., Hopstock, P. J., Pendzick, M. L., & Stephenson, T. G. (2003). *Descriptive study of services to LEP students and LEP students with disabilities. Special topic report no. 4: Findings on special education LEP students*. Arlington, VA: Development Associates.

4

First and Second Language Acquisition: Theoretical and Practical Considerations for SLPs and ESOL Professionals

Introduction

The primary goals of SLPs and ESOL professionals are to address the language development and instructional and literacy needs of ELs (ASHA, 2001a, 2001b, 2010; TESOL, 2001) and to use evidence-based approaches to facilitate the academic success of school-age ELs. To appropriately identify and assess ELs with communication disorders, SLPs and ESOL professionals must understand first (L1) and second (L2) language acquisition theories and stages. They need to know the difference between naturalistic and instructed second language acquisition, the basic constructs of language proficiency, and the influences culture might exert on the acquisition of a second language. Last, SLP and ESOL professionals need to be able to distinguish between a communication difference and a communication disorder when working with ELs (Antunez, 2002; Battle, 2002; Roseberry-McKibben, 2007). We begin with an overview of first language acquisition.

First Language Acquisition

First Language Acquisition Theories

Although there is general agreement on the description of the typical process of acquiring a first language, there are differing theories of how and why the process happens. Three theories are discussed in particular: behaviorist, innatist, and interactionist.

Behaviorist Theory

An early perspective on first language acquisition comes from the school of psychology known as behaviorism. Behaviorists believe that language learning is no different from learning anything else. In this view, all learning results from a process of stimulus and response (Freeman & Freeman, 2004). Children reproduce language, or approximate imitations of what they hear, and are reinforced by rewards, such as attention or response. A child produces an utterance (for example, "milk"), and the parent understands and responds affirmatively by fulfilling the request. Hence, the utterance was rewarded and reinforced. If the utterance is unintelligible or incorrect, the parent corrects the child and the child uses the correct form to obtain the intended outcome. B. F. Skinner, the most well-known of the mid-20th-century behaviorists, hypothesized about first language acquisition in his book *Verbal Behavior* (1957), which was subsequently critiqued by Noam Chomsky (1965), the developer of a linguistic model of first language acquisition that stemmed from a cognitive psychology perspective.

Innatist Theory

Cognitivists view language learning as a more innate process, where children apply inborn rules to language input they receive, forming hypotheses about grammar structures. This theory, also known as innatism or nativism, contrasts with the behaviorist view that new structures are learned by imitating what adults say. Chomsky (1965) refuted this view with the example "goed," which English-speaking children normally say while acquiring the past tense. Clearly they did not learn that term through imitating an adult, because no adult says "goed" rather than "went." Instead, this is evidence that children apply the rule "-ed" for the past tense to the verb stem "go" rather than use the irregular form "went." Interestingly, this process is actually U-shaped, because children often first acquire the irregular form as an unanalyzed chunk, and then once they acquire the "-ed" past tense marker, they apply it to "go" to regularize the irregular verb, and finally they make the distinction that "go" uses an irregular past tense form (Figure 4–1).

The innatist view sees correction of such grammatical errors as unnecessary and ineffective, because children move through the same process with or without correction. Another example of how children apply rules to language is offered by psychologist Jean Berko Gleason's (1958) exploration of children's pluralization of nonsense terms. When shown a cartoon figure and told it was a wug, the children were instantly able to name two of the figures wugs, adding the plural "-s" marker to the nonsense noun. Again, that plural form could not have been an imitation of an adult's use of the plural noun, as it is an invented word (Pinker, 1999). Innatists attribute children's capacity to analyze and construct language forms to an inborn mental facility they term the Language Acquisition Device (LAD).

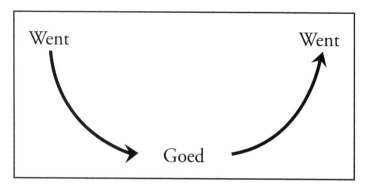

Figure 4–1. *The U-shaped process that children undergo when learning the irregular past tense form of "go."*

Interactionist Theory

A more recent perspective on first language acquisition is the interactionist position. Interactionists believe that the give and take between an adult caregiver and a child is a critical factor in language development. Through what is termed "child-directed speech," adults adjust their language to engage and communicate with children. The characteristics of this speech include slow expression, high pitch, exaggerated intonation, pauses, simple syntax, repetition, comprehension questions, paraphrasing, and a focus on the concrete aspects of the immediate surroundings at the present time (Brown & Attardo, 2000). This position emphasizes the interaction between the learner and the environment as a primary factor in language acquisition.

The three perspectives on language acquisition are summarized in Table 4–1. These theories are compared by: (1) the focus of linguistic input, (2) how each theory accounts for the process of acquisition, (3) the role of the child, and (4) the role of the other people in the social environment (Peregoy & Boyle, 2005).

Stages of First Language Acquisition

The process of normal L1 acquisition goes through predictable stages. In this section we briefly examine the process of acquiring first language and begin with its first stage, the preverbal stage.

Table 4–1. Comparison of Behaviorist, Innatist, and Interactionist Theories of First Language Acquisition

Acquisition Aspects	Behaviorist Perspective	Innatist Perspective	Interactionist Perspective
Linguistic focus	Verbal behaviors (not analyzed per se): words, utterances of child and people in social environment	Child's syntax	Conversation between child and caregiver; focus on caregiver speech
Process of acquisition	Modeling, imitation, practice, and selective reinforcement of correct form	Hypothesis testing and creative construction of syntactic rules using language acquisition device (LAD)	Acquisition emerges from communication; acts scaffolded by caregivers
Role of child	Secondary role: imitator and responder to environmental shaping	Primary role: equipped with biological LAD, child plays major role in acquisition	Important role in interaction, taking more control as language acquisition advances
Role of social environment	Primary role: parental modeling and reinforcement are major factors promoting language acquisition	Minor role: language used by others merely triggers LAD	Important role in interaction, especially in early years when caregivers modify input and carry much of conversational load

Source: From Peregoy, Suzanne F., Boyle, Owen F., *Reading, Writing and Learning in ESL: A Resource Book for K–12 Teachers, MYLABSCHOOL. Edition, 4th Edition,* © 2005. Reprinted by permission of Pearson Education, Inc., Upper Saddle River, NJ.

Preverbal Stages

Newborns are incapable of using language to communicate, but from early on they are involved in the process of L1 acquisition. During the preverbal stage, they are observing facial and vocal expressions. In fact, only a few days after birth, infants are capable of distinguishing their mother's voice, which is verified by babies' heads turning and changing sucking patterns. From birth to 8 weeks, they cry, burp, and cough. At 8 to 20 weeks, they laugh and coo, and their crying differs based on their needs. From 16 to 30 weeks, they repeat vowel or consonant sounds (/o/, /o/, /o/ or / m/, /m/, /m/). The reduplicated babbling stage begins with the repetition of vowel and consonant combinations (/ma/ /ma/ /ma/ /ma/) and continues until infants are approximately 1 year old. Somewhere around 9 months old, infants begin the 9-month-long process of un-reduplicated babbling, which incorporates more consonants as well as stress and intonations (Brown & Attardo, 2000).

Verbal Stages

Children go through predictable stages in acquiring the building blocks of languages: phonology (sounds), morphology (the form of words and units of meaning, such as the addition of "s" to a noun to denote plurality), syntax (word order in phrases and sentences), and semantics (the meaning of an utterance). In phonology, children tend to acquire stops (consonant sounds such as /p/, /t/, and /k/ in English) before liquids (consonant sounds such as /l/ and /r/ in English). Replacing the later-acquired sounds with ones that have already acquired is a common feature of "baby talk," such as saying "weeawee" instead of "really" (Parker & Riley, 2000).

When babies are about 12 months old, they begin to form words. According to Pinker (1994), children begin using the same types of words, half of which are terms for familiar objects, such as "bottle." One word can have different meanings, however. If a child at this stage states "bottle," this could mean "get my bottle" or "fill my bottle." Their vocabulary grows by adding simple adjectives and adverbs and eventually what are called function words, which have a specific grammatical purpose, such as prepositions and articles. Children acquire these grammatical morphemes in a predictable order. In English, the following morphemes are acquired in a regular sequence (Brown & Attardo, 2000):

1. "-ing in the present continuous (smiling)
2. the preposition "in"
3. the preposition "on" (some children acquire "on" before "in")
4. "-s" for plural nouns (dogs)
5. irregular past (had)
6. "-'s" for possessive (Mary's)
7. the verb "be," not in contraction form (I am playing.)
8. articles (a, the)
9. "-ed" for regular past (walked)
10. "-s" for third person simple present tense verbs (she walks)
11. third person present irregular (He marches to bed every night.)
12. auxiliary (also known as helping) verbs, not in contraction form (I have played Go Fish.)
13. the verb "be" in contraction form (She's laughing.)
14. auxiliary verbs in contraction form (I've been to London.)

At about 18 months, children assemble two-word utterances, which is the beginning of eventual sentence formation (syntactic development). "Daddy gone" or "tummy hurt" are examples of such two-word utterances. Pinker (1994) identifies 18 months as a point of rapid vocabulary growth, followed by a period of rapid syntactic growth from the late twos to late threes (Freeman & Freeman, 2004).

Next comes the multiword stage, termed "telegraphic speech" by Brown (1973) because it lacks many function words. An example is "Mommy make cake," meaning "Mommy is making a cake." The most common word order, subject/verb/object, is typically acquired early, whereas questions, negatives, and the passive voice are acquired later. Developing the proper word order for questions and negatives typically involves a predictable process of simplification and word order errors that gradually and finally acquire the proper form. In questioning, for example, children typically use rising intonation to designate a question before they master the correct word order. For example, "Grammy going?" with rising intonation is a common way young children express "Is Grammy going?" For questions using interrogative terms (who, what, etc.), children also go through stages. For instance, "Where Grammy going?" precedes "Where Grammy's going?" which precedes the proper form, "Where is Grammy going?" Similar to questions, negative sentences follow a developmental pattern: (1) "no go"; (2) "I no go"; (3) "I won't go" (Parker & Riley, 2000).

How children begin to understand the meaning and boundaries of words or sentences is known as semantics. The meaning of words is called lexical semantics and the meaning of sentences is called sentence semantics. A common feature of developing lexical semantics is called under- and overextension (Brown & Attardo, 2000). Underextension involves children's assumption that the meaning of a word denoting a concept or category is specific to an item that is part of or possesses a possible characteristic of the concept or category. For example, the verb "fly" applies only to birds (but not airplanes or bumblebees, etc.). Overextension is the opposite of underextension and means overgeneralizing a specific word to include all terms in its class or category. An example would be using the word "dog" to refer to any four-legged mammal. In general, overextension involves categories ("pudding" for all desserts), analogies ("wheel" for anything round), and family resemblances, such as when "rose" is extended to fragrance and a vegetable seedling (Brown &Attardo, 2000).

This section briefly presented the theories of L1 acquisition and outlined the predictable stages children go through in its development. The goal is to establish a basic foundation to be able to compare L1 and L2 processes. Next, the construct of language proficiency, the theories of second language acquisition, stages of second language acquisition, and the similarities and differences between L1 and L2 are discussed.

Second Language Acquisition

Second Language Acquisition and Second Language Proficiency: Defining the Constructs

The term *second language acquisition* (SLA) encompasses many concepts and assumptions. Although the word *second* is used, SLA can incorporate the second, third, fourth, etc., language learned. In other words, *second* refers to any language learned after an individual starts learning the first. In its broadest sense, SLA denotes learning language in different contexts and ways, although there are technical distinctions used for narrower purposes. For example, learning a language where it is the native language of the area, such as English in the US or French in the Canadian province of Quebec, is known as second language learning, but learning a language that is not the native language of the area, such as Japanese in the US, is known as foreign language learning; the latter is typically what high school students engage in when they fulfill a foreign language requirement. However, second language acquisition is also the umbrella term that includes second and foreign language learning, as well as the academic discipline or field of study of these phenomena. This means that those who conduct research and develop theories on how people learn second or foreign languages are called "second language acquisition scholars."

Similar to the technical distinctions for the word *second* in SLA, the word *acquisition* has multiple meanings. In its broadest definition, acquisition refers to any way that a learner develops proficiency in a second language. We can consider two different approaches to learning a second language as being opposite ends of a continuum: on one end is the study of the rules and features of the language and at the other end is "picking up" the language by immersion in a community that speaks a particular language. Undoubtedly, there are many variations and combinations of the two extremes.

The study of bilingual development explores second language acquisition in infants and children. According to Letts (1999), bilingual development complicates the study of second language acquisition due to the variety of factors that lead to the attainment of proficiency in two or more languages. For example, bilingual learners may have parents who speak different languages, they may live in areas where two languages are spoken, or they may be immigrants in a community that speaks a different language than their home language. Letts (1999) describes a rudimentary categorization of two major modes of bilingual development, termed "simultaneous" and "sequential" bilingualism. Simultaneous bilinguals are exposed to both languages in rather equal proportions, beginning at birth. Sequential bilinguals begin acquiring one language before they are exposed to another.

For simultaneous bilinguals, Volterra and Taeschner (1978) identify three stages of development: (1) one lexical (vocabulary) system for both languages; (2) two lexical systems but a simplified and combined syntactic (sentence structure) system; and (3) two separate lexical and syntactic systems. For sequential acquisition, Letts (1999) suggests that younger children go through a process of acquiring an L2 that is similar to acquiring their L1, but that L2 acquisition in older children may be facilitated by formal instruction. Research indicates that children who have had significant input in two languages before the age of three seem to experience minimal interference between the languages (Patterson & Pearson, 2004) and that those who are exposed to L1 during infancy and learn an L2 at a later time show greater diversity in rates and stages of acquisition (Kan & Kohnert, 2005; Kayser, 2002).

An important question to examine at this point is what dimensions define second language proficiency. Cummins (1992, 2000) described two models of language proficiency, the Separate Underlying Proficiency (SUP) and Common Underlying Proficiency (CUP) models (Figure 4–2).

In the Separate Underlying Proficiency (SUP) model, language proficiency in the first language is viewed as entirely separate from proficiency in the second language. Thus, one ramification of this model is that skills learned in the first language will not transfer to the second language. Supporters of this viewpoint suggest that language development activities in the first language will not enhance learning of a second language and often recommend use of English only. Interestingly, there is little evidence to support the SUP model. Roseberry-McKibben (2008) points out that "as children learn their first language, they acquire concepts and strategies that will facilitate the learning of a second language. Concepts are acquired through interaction with the environment. High-quality exposure enhances the learning of concepts that are important for cognitive and linguistic development. As children hear and use their native language in a variety of contexts, they develop the conceptual knowledge and cognitive strategies necessary for success in acquiring new information and linguistic skills" (p. 229).

As an alternative to the SUP model, Cummins offered the Common Underlying Proficiency (CUP) model. Briefly stated,

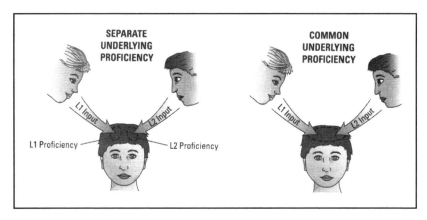

Figure 4–2. *Separate Underlying Proficiency (SUP) (left) and Common Underlying Proficiency (CUP) (right) models.* Source: *From "The Role of Primary Language Development in Promoting Educational Success for Language Minority Students," by J. Cummins, in* Schooling and Language Minority Students: A Theoretical Framework, *by California State Department of Education (Ed.), 1992, Los Angeles: California State University, Evaluation, Dissemination, and Assessment Center. Reprinted with permission.*

Cummins (1992) suggested that in the course of learning one language a child acquires a set of skills and implicit metalinguistic knowledge that can be drawn on when working in another language. This common underlying proficiency (CUP), as he labels such skills and knowledge, provides the basis for the development of both the first language and the second language. It follows that any expansion of CUP that takes place in one language will have a beneficial effect on the other language(s).

The CUP model, then, has major implications for SLPs working with ELs. If a student is not provided with opportunities to strengthen the foundation of the first language, the conceptual foundation necessary for academic success will be underdeveloped. Using the second language for instruction when the first language has not yet been fully developed can provide an unstable foundation and result in low language and literacy competence in both L1 and L2 (Chamberlain, 2005; Cummins, 2000; Cummins, Chow, & Schecter, 2006). This limited performance can at least in part be attributed to limited skills in the first language and lack of opportunities for continued development of skills in that language. However, often this limited performance leads professionals to suspect a language learning disability and the need for special education intervention.

Cummins (1980) introduced two important concepts that have been used to define second language proficiency. They arise from his early work in which he demonstrated his ideas about second language development in a simple matrix (Figure 4–3). These terms are known as Basic Interpersonal Communication Skills (BICS) and Cognitive Academic Language Proficiency (CALP). The distinction between BICS and CALP was introduced to make educators aware of the very different timetable required by immigrant children to acquire conversational fluency in their

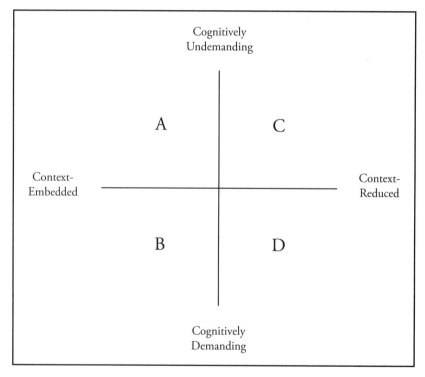

Figure 4–3. *Basic Interpersonal Communication Skills (BICS) and Cognitive Academic Language Proficiency (CALP).* Source: *From "The Role of Primary Language Development in Promoting Educational Success for Language Minority Students," by J. Cummins, in* Schooling and Language Minority Students: A Theoretical Framework, *by California State Department of Education (Ed.), 1992, Los Angeles: California State University, Evaluation, Dissemination, and Assessment Center. Reprinted with permission.*

L2 as compared to grade-appropriate academic proficiency in their L2. Cummins (2000) describes these skills as being on a continuum instead of being discrete and separate entities.

Basic Interpersonal Communication Skills (BICS), or conversational English, are language skills that ELs need to have in order to fully function in social situations. These are cognitively undemanding, context-embedded forms of communication. In context-embedded communication, participants can actively negotiate meaning and they have a shared reality. For example, ELs can be observed to use BICS on the playground, in the lunch room, on the school bus, at parties, playing sports, and talking on the telephone. These language skills usually develop within 6 months to 2 years after arrival in the US. BICS typically occurs in meaningful social contexts and the required language is not specialized. A word of caution for SLPs and ESOL professionals: many problems arise when educators and administrators think that ELs are proficient in English because they demonstrate good social English language skills or BICS.

Cognitive Academic Language Proficiency (CALP), or academic English, refers to formal academic learning. CALP refers to the cognitively demanding, context-reduced forms of communication and does not assume a shared reality. This type of proficiency includes listening, speaking, reading, and writing about subject area content material. CALP is essential for ELs to succeed in school and usually takes from 5 to 7 years to develop. However, research by Collier and Thomas (1995) has shown that if an EL has no prior schooling or has no support in native language development, it may take 7 to 10 years for ELs to catch up to their peers. It is also important to note that academic language acquisition goes beyond the mere understanding of content area vocabulary. It often includes skills such as comparing, classifying, synthesizing, evaluating, and inferring. Table 4–2 summarizes the characteristics of the two concepts that are the foundation of Cummins's (1980) L2 language proficiency framework.

Second Language Acquisition Theories

The road to acquiring a second language is long and arduous and has been the matter of much theoretical debate, especially over the last half of the 20th century. Even now there is no

Table 4–2. *Characteristics of BICS and CALP*

Basic Interpersonal Communication Skills (BICS)	Cognitive Academic Language Proficiency (CALP)

• Conversational fluency: social language
• Includes "silent period" when ELs don't produce oral language but are able to comprehend spoken/written language.
• Lasts 6 months to 2 years
• Involves cognitively undemanding, context-embedded forms of communication
• Vocabulary:
  a. 0–1 year: 1,000 words
  b. 1–2 years: 3,000 words
	• Academic proficiency: school language
	• Lasts 5 to 7 or up to 10 years
	• Refers to cognitively demanding, context-reduced forms of communication
	• Vocabulary:
	  a. 1–5 years: 6,000 words
	  b. 5–7 and even 10 years: 7,000 words +

Source: Adapted from "The Construct of Language Proficiency in Bilingual Education," by J. Cummins, in *Georgetown University Round Table on Languages and Linguistics,* by J. E. Alatis (Ed.), 1980, Washington, DC: Georgetown University Press.

commonly accepted theory of second language acquisition that clearly explains how all learners in all circumstances acquire any language. The second language acquisition community has adapted and proposed various theories to explain second language acquisition; four are presented below and in Table 4–3.

Behaviorism

In the 1950s, when behaviorism was popular, it was applied to second language learning. Behaviorist theory stems from the works of Skinner (1957) and Thorndike (1932). As previously noted, behaviorists view language learning as a result of habit formation (Johnson & Johnson, 1999). Theorists following this approach believe that we are born with a tabula rasa, or blank slate, and that language is learned through a series of stimulus-response behaviors and repeated reinforcements (Brown, 2007). Through imitation, practice, and reinforcement, language

Table 4–3. *Comparison of Behaviorist, Innatist, Interactionist, and Sociocultural Theories of Second Language Acquisition*

Theory	Behaviorist Perspective	Monitor Theory	Interactionist Perspective	Sociocultural Theory
Linguistic focus	Development of new language habits with a focus on L1 and L2 differences	Comprehensible input is essential for L2 acquisition; Acquisition is viewed as different from Learning	Modified Input is essential for L2 acquisition	Zone of Proximal Development is critical for L2
Process of acquisition	Modeling, imitation, practice, and selective reinforcement of correct form	Input that is one level above the actual comprehension level of L2 learners is comprehensible and promotes SLA	Input that is modified, (comprehension checks, clarification requests, paraphrasing, etc.) is comprehensible and facilitates L2 acquisition	Through scaffolding L2 learners move from their zone of actual development to zone of proximal development in their SLA
Role of social environment	Minor role	Minor role	Important role	Vital role

Source: From Peregoy, Suzanne F., Boyle, Owen F., *Reading, Writing and Learning in ESL: A Resource Book for K–12 Teachers, MYLABSCHOOL. Edition, 4th Edition,* © 2005. Adapted by permission of Pearson Education, Inc., Upper Saddle River, NJ.

learning can be achieved (Lightbown & Spada, 1999). Behaviorism helped introduce the idea of contrastive analysis to the field of second language learning. Contrastive analysis is the comparison of two languages to identify similarities and differences (Johnson & Johnson, 1999). According to behaviorists, the differences between two languages can hinder the development of the second language (Lightbown & Spada, 1999).

For behaviorists, second language learning was believed to be about habits. In the learning situation, learners were expected to memorize parts of scripts, which they frequently practiced with a partner. The learners also listened to audiotapes, which were used to help them form habits. The learners did not have to know what their lines or their partners' lines meant, as long as they memorized the words (Ausubel, 1968; Bloomfield, 1942). However, others, including Noam Chomsky (1965), perceived language learning differently. He conceived of another way to explain second language acquisition.

Monitor Theory

As mentioned previously, Chomsky (1965) believed that all people are born with the ability to learn a language. Children are innately predetermined to learn languages, and he observed them doing this within a few short years. Chomsky created the theory of universal grammar, which alleges the existence of a set of basic grammatical elements that are common to all natural human languages and that predetermine how people organize the input. Although Chomsky did not directly address second language acquisition, his L1 theory has had a profound influence on SLA scholars. One such scholar is Stephen Krashen (1981, 1987), who developed the monitor theory. In his view, first and second language acquisition are similar.

Krashen's monitor theory (1981) is one of the most influential and widely accepted second language acquisition theories. This theory consists of five hypotheses in which Krashen offers a comprehensive explanation of the SLA process: the acquisition-learning hypothesis, the natural order hypothesis, the monitor hypothesis, the input hypothesis, and the affective filter hypothesis (Table 4–4).

Table 4–4. Krashen's Theory of Second Language Acquisition

Natural Order Hypothesis	Acquisition–Learning Hypothesis	Monitor Hypothesis	Input Hypothesis	Affective Filter Hypothesis
Language is acquired in a predictable order.	Acquisition is the product of a subconscious process very similar to the process children experience when they acquire their first language. Learning is the product of formal instruction resulting in conscious knowledge about the language	This hypothesis explains the relationship between acquisition and learning The monitor is an internal editor and is a product of conscious learning The monitor plans, edits and corrects L2 when learners have time, focus on form and know the grammar rule	Humans acquire language in only one way — by understanding messages or by receiving "comprehensible input"	Affective factors, such as high motivation, good self-confidence and low anxiety can facilitate second language acquisition Low motivation, low self-esteem, and debilitating anxiety can contribute to the prevention of comprehensible input being used to prevent second language acquisition

Source: Adapted from *Principles and Practices in Second Language Acquisition*, by S. D. Krashen, 1987, New York, NY: Prentice-Hall.

Krashen (1987) formulated the acquisition-learning hypothesis to explain what he believed are two independent systems for developing knowledge of a second language. The first system is through acquisition, which, in nontechnical terms, is the "picking up" of a language. Acquisition is subconscious and does not really address grammar rules. The second system of developing second language competence in a language is through the learning system, which is concerned with grammar rules and being aware of them (Krashen & Terrell, 1983). Each system has different functions. The acquired system is used to produce language. The learned system acts as an evaluator of the acquired system to make sure that what the acquired system is producing is correct.

The second hypothesis is the natural order hypothesis. This hypothesis supports the idea that the rules of language are acquired in a predictable order. This claim is based on the morpheme studies of second language acquirers (Dulay & Burt, 1974). The order is the same regardless of whether the language is learned (through instruction or not). The natural order is part of the acquired system, which is not interfered with by the learned system (Krashen & Terrell, 1983).

The third hypothesis, the monitor hypothesis, explains initiating speech. The learned system is responsible for monitoring the output of the acquired system. Krashen (1987) claimed the monitor could only be used under certain conditions. The learners need time to consciously think about and utilize the appropriate rule. The learner must also be able to pay attention to what is being said and be able to focus on form. Finally, the learner must know the grammar rule in order to apply the rule appropriately (Krashen & Terrell, 1983).

In his fourth hypothesis, the input hypothesis, Krashen (1987) theorized that learners need comprehensible input in order to move through the natural order of acquisition. Learners acquire a second language by "understanding messages, or by receiving 'comprehensible input'" (Krashen & Terrell, 1983). A message that contains structures and vocabulary unknown to the learner can be made comprehensible through the additional support of nonverbal input. As the learner's L2 proficiency increases, less nonverbal input is needed. In order to advance the learner's current knowledge, the language used by the teacher has to include structures and vocabulary at one level higher than what the learner has already acquired. Thus, acquisition for learners with language knowledge "i" can only take place if they are exposed to comprehensible input at a slightly higher level, which Krashen describes as level "i + 1." For example, if "i" is the current acquired linguistic competence, then ELs progress from "i" to "i + 1" by comprehending input that contains "i + 1." The "+1" is symbolic of the new language structures and knowledge that the learner is ready to acquire.

Krashen's final hypothesis, the affective filter hypothesis, explains differences in individual learners. The affective filter can be a potential barrier to second language acquisition. Negative responses to one's environment, such as self-doubt, anxiety, boredom, and any other process, may interfere with the process of learning a second language. This hypothesis accounts for the failure of language acquisition through insufficient input of the appropriate kind or a high affective filter. In other words, the theory states that obstacles to learning a second language can be reduced by providing a low-anxiety environment, sparking the learner's interest, and boosting the learner's self-esteem. In summary, learners must receive comprehensible input and must have a low affective filter for acquisition to take place (Krashen & Terrell, 1983).

In summary, these five hypotheses work together to explain second language acquisition. The process starts with the input hypothesis, which provides the information that the learner needs in order to acquire the language. As the input becomes intake, it makes its way into the developing system, which is the acquisition part of the first hypothesis. The rules that students are taught about the language, metalinguistic knowledge, make up the learning part of the learning-acquisition hypothesis. The learning-acquisition hypothesis has two separate functions. The metalinguistic knowledge of the learning part of the hypothesis becomes the monitor, which corrects output that the learner produces. Any difference that may exist between language learners is explained through the final hypothesis, the affective filter. In order for input to get through to the learner, the affective filter must be low. All of these hypotheses function in concert to produce the language of the learner.

Interactionist Theory

Similar to Krashen (1987), interactionists also believe in the importance of comprehensive input, but they believe that modified interaction is necessary to make language comprehensible. According to Long (1983), modified interaction includes, but it is not limited to, linguistic simplification, conversational modifications such as comprehension checks (efforts made by the L2 native speaker to make sure that the L2 learner understands the meaning of the utterance), clarification requests (efforts made by the L2 learner asking the L2 native speaker to clarify an aspect of the conversation that has not been understood), and self-repetition or paraphrase (efforts made by the L2 native speaker to repeat or paraphrase aspects of the conversation either partially or entirely).

Speakers engaged in conversations negotiate meaning. Negotiation of meaning leads to modified interaction, which consists of various modifications (i.e., linguistic simplification). Long (1983) claims that negotiation for meaning that triggers interactional modifications by the L2 native speaker facilitates acquisition because it connects input, internal learner capacities, particularly selective attention, and output in productive ways. In other words, interactional modifications make input comprehensible and comprehensible input promotes acquisition.

Sociocultural Theory

Related to the interactionist view, which places a great deal of importance on language interaction as a facilitator of second language acquisition, is the concept of the *zone of proximal development (ZPD)* developed by Lev Vygotsky, a Russian theorist and researcher in child development. He viewed language learning as a dynamic process in which external knowledge and abilities in children become internalized. To help explain the way that this social and participatory learning took place, Vygotsky (1962) developed the concept of the zone of proximal development, defined as the difference between what learners can do without help and what they can do with assistance (Figures 4–4 and 4–5).

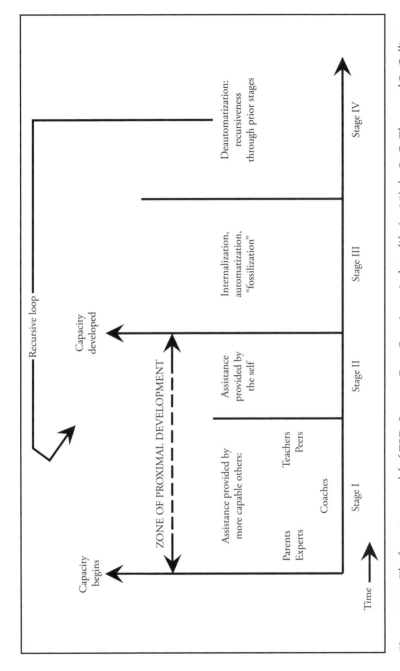

Figure 4–4. *The four-stage model of ZPD. Source: From Rousing minds to life (p. 35), by R. G. Tharp and R. Gallimore, 1988, New York, NY: Cambridge University Press. Copyright 1988 Cambridge University Press. Adapted with permission.*

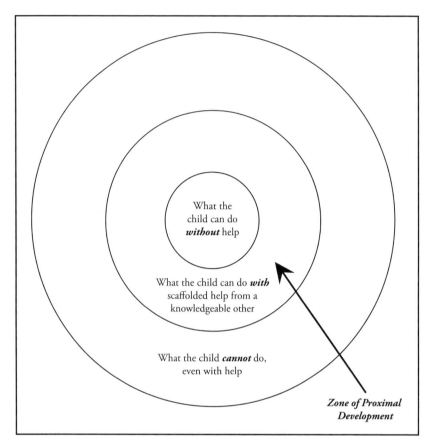

Figure 4–5. *The zone of proximal development.*

The ZPD is where learning can most productively take place. It is the domain of knowledge or skill where the learner is not yet capable of independent functioning, but can achieve the desired outcome given relevant scaffolded help (Mitchell and Myles, 2004). Other theorists have expanded the concept of the ZPD and conceptualize learning as distributed, interactive, contextual, and the result of the learner's participation in a community of practice. Essentially, it is the difference between the child's current level of independent problem solving and the higher level of potential development they gain through problem solving with adult guidance or in collaboration with peers.

This learning can take place in any situation and does not only apply to language learning.

Also, it is important to note that the learning can take place with anyone, as long as that person is more knowledgeable and utilizes scaffolding in order to take the learner to the next level in their learning. The applicability of this theory can be easily demonstrated, whether the tasks are language-based or not. For example, a teacher may assign a task to a group of students in a class. One student may demonstrate some difficulty in answering a question in the assigned task. One of his more knowledgeable peers explains the question to the student and both students decide on an appropriate answer for the problem. This situation highlights one of the key aspects of Vygotsky's ZPD theory, in that one's present ability is taken to the next level with the help of a "knowledgeable other." The example cited above utilized the process of scaffolding.

Scaffolding is the use of dialogue and direction to point out key steps in a process or environment. Also known as "other-regulation," scaffolding is one of the key methods that a teacher, caregiver, or peer can use to teach someone a skill to take the learner to the next level. The ultimate goal of scaffolding, however, is to achieve self-regulation, the ability to function autonomously with no help (Mitchell & Myles, 2004).

The previously discussed theories have all been offered to explain how a second language is acquired. Further information on additional theories can be found in Ellis (2008a).

Individual Factors Affecting Second Language Acquisition

Multiple factors affect the development of second language proficiency. For example, individual differences in learners are a significant factor that has been studied in the field of second language acquisition (Ellis, 2008a). Six major categories believed to be associated with second language acquisition have been discussed in the literature (Walqui, 2000). These include personality, language aptitude, motivation, learning and cognitive styles, language learning strategies, and other factors (anxiety, creativity, willingness to communicate, self-esteem, and learner beliefs) (Dornyei, 2005). Ellis (2008a) identifies four "core" areas of individual differences: language aptitude, motivation, personality, and anxiety. A closer examination of these four areas is necessary to understand individual variations in second language acquisition.

In the area of *language aptitude,* Skehan (1989) notes three abilities, auditory, linguistic, and memory. Studies (Horwitz, 1987; Skehan, 1986a, 1986b, 1990; Harley & Hart, 1997) indicate that language aptitude is a significant factor in second language acquisition, whether the language task is grammar- or communication-focused.

Motivation has also been studied extensively. Two major types of motivation, integrative and instrumental motivation, were identified by Gardner (1980, 2001). Integrative motivation is divided into three main areas, including the degree to which an individual wants to integrate in the L2 language community, attitudes toward the learning context, and the desire to learn the language. A meta-analysis conducted by Masgoret and Gardner (2003) found that integrative motivation is a significant factor in second language acquisition. Complementary to the construct of integrative motivation is Gardner's notion of instrumental motivation. In this case, motivation is determined by the learner's sense of the utility or positive outcomes of learning the second language. Various research studies show that instrumental motivation is a less significant factor in second language acquisition than integrative motivation (Ellis, 2008a).

In the area of *personality*, the concepts of extroversion and introversion have been the subject of study in SLA. Extroversion appears to correlate positively with the development of social language, or BICS (Strong, 1983). This may be due to extroverts' willingness to participate in speaking activities in the classroom (Robson, 1992).

The last individual difference core factor, *anxiety*, affects second language learners in various situations and ways. There are multiple triggers for anxiety regarding listening and speaking a second language. Ellis (2008a) reports that anxiety affects learners differently and to greater or lesser extents, and that this is affected by other individual factors such as motivation and personality.

Stages of Second Language Acquisition

Similar to L1 acquisition, L2 acquisition has predictable stages. In their seminal work about the natural approach, Krashen and Terrell (1983) name these stages and provide a rich description of their characteristics. Depending on learners' first language backgrounds, there may be substages within the sequence. All ELs progress through these four stages, but not at the same rate. Some learners may progress at slower or faster rates due to a variety of factors, including native language, age, and affective factors. Moreover, outcomes vary according to learner characteristics, and the stages are fluid and not discrete. The natural approach divides SLA into four basic stages: preproduction, early production, speech emergence, and intermediate fluency (Table 4–5). Other researchers have described the various levels of acquisition, proposed additional stages (i.e., advanced intermediate fluency; advanced fluency), and noted the length of time it takes an EL to achieve the indicated levels of acquisition (Collier, 2008, 2011; Hoover, Klingner, Baca, & Patton, 2008). TESOL (2006) has also identified five language levels that overlap somewhat with the Krashen and Terrell (1983) levels: Level 1—Starting, Level 2—Emerging, Level 3—Developing, Level 4—Expanding, and Level 5—Bridging. The TESOL levels apply to oral and written language, whereas the Krashen and Terrell levels apply only to oral language. We focus on the stages presented by Krashen and Terrell (1983).

Stage 1—Preproduction

Learners at this stage have experienced 10 hours to 6 months of exposure to English and are beginning to comprehend the language. Most ELs at this level need time to listen and absorb the language before they are required to speak it. This is sometimes referred to as the "silent period." As they move through this stage, ELs' vocabulary includes approximately 500 receptive words (words they can understand but don't use in speaking or writing, and they are beginning to develop BICS (Cummins, 1980). In order for the language learner at this stage to comprehend speech, communication should include lots of panto-

Table 4–5. *Stages of Second Language Development*

1st Stage: Preproduction	2nd Stage: Early Production	3rd Stage: Speech Emergence	4th Stage: Intermediate Fluency
Characteristics • 10 hours to 6 months of exposure to English • language skill—listening (receptive) level • BICS development • English vocabulary—500 receptive words	Characteristics • 6 months to 1 year of English • language skill—continued, mainly listening • BICS development • English vocabulary—1,000 receptive words	Characteristics • 1 to 3 years of English • Student speaks in phrases and short sentences • BICS development • English vocabulary—7,000 receptive words	Characteristics • 3 to 4 years of English • Student engages in dialogue • CALP development • English vocabulary—12,000 receptive words
Sample student behaviors • "silent period" • Has minimal comprehension • Points to or provides other nonverbal responses • Responds to commands	Sample student behaviors • One-word responses • Has limited comprehension • Produces one- or two-word responses or short utterances • Participates using key words and familiar phrases • Uses present-tense verbs	Sample student behaviors • Has good comprehension and demonstrates comprehension in a variety of ways • Can produce simple sentences • Makes grammar and pronunciation errors • Participates in small group activities	Sample student behaviors • Has excellent comprehension • Makes few grammatical errors • Participates in reading and writing activities to acquire new information

Source: Adapted from *The Natural Approach: Language Acquisition in the Classroom,* by S. Krashen and T. Terrell, 1983, Oxford, UK: Pergamon Press.

mime, body language, facial expressions, and gestures. Second language learners can show comprehension nonverbally. For example, they can point to an item, nod to answer simple yes/no questions, and carry out simple commands (e.g., put the apple on the table).

Stage 2 — Early Production

At this stage, learners have been exposed to 3 months to 1 year of English. They can now begin to produce some language, in one- to two-word responses, along with similar nonverbal responses used in stage 1. Their receptive vocabulary consists of about 1,000 words, and as at any other level, about 10% of their receptive vocabulary is expressive (words they regularly use). Learners at this stage can answer yes/no questions, "what" questions that elicit one- to two-word responses ("What is this?"), "who" questions ("Who has the red ball?"), "either/or questions" ("Is this an apple or an orange?") and "where" questions that require a simple phrase response ("Where is the Statue of Liberty?"). Learners begin using formulaic chunks of language, with most of the elements of the chunks remaining unanalyzed. For example, they may be able to use the phrase, "Where've you been?" but they may not be able to understand the function of each word and how the words form a sentence.

Because learners develop expressive skills in English at the early production stage, they can communicate in a simple manner with others. Interacting with language learners and native speakers to solve problems, develop projects, and/or discuss issues, provides opportunities for ELs to develop language skills. Once students have developed basic vocabulary and syntax in English, their progress accelerates. This limited vocabulary and syntax forms the basis on which to build their proficiency, and by understanding and using a few words and phrases, ELs can increase their receptive and expressive abilities in English more independently.

Stage 3 — Speech Emergence

Typically learners' proficiency increases exponentially after 1 to 3 years of exposure to the second language. They use phrases and sentences, and their receptive vocabulary grows to nearly 7,000 words. Questions they can answer include "how" and "why," which require fairly complex responses. They can understand a great deal and can express themselves fairly effectively, although they tend to simplify more complex grammatical structures or produce them with developmental errors. At every stage, when communication breaks down, learners should employ the same strategies as those used in the beginning stages, such as showing a picture, consulting a bilingual dictionary, gesturing and acting out, and so forth.

Stage 4 — Intermediate Fluency

After about 3 to 4 years of exposure to L2, a shift occurs. English language learners begin to develop CALP (Cummins, 1980). Having mastered the knowledge and skills required for social language (BICS), ELs have accumulated approximately 12,000 receptive words. They have gone beyond speaking in phrases and simple sentences to being able to engage in extended discourse. They can answer complex questions that require them to synthesize and evaluate information because they possess adequate academic language proficiency to do so in English. This means that they can write essays, solve complex problems, research and support their positions, and critique and analyze information. Although it may seem that they are able to perform the same activities as native speakers, they continue to need special support until their CALP in the second language is fully developed.

Differences Between First and Second Language Acquisition

Although first and second language acquisition have many commonalities, there are distinct differences. We can consider the degree of commonalities on a continuum, with virtually identical processes for birth through infancy, followed by gradually differing elements that increase incrementally from age 3 to adulthood. In other words, an infant learning two languages simultaneously goes through the same processes for each, but a 3-year-old beginning to learn a second language employs strategies and uses information from the already-acquired first language to build the second. The more mature and proficient the learner, the greater the differences in the processes employed to acquire a second language.

If we look at adolescent and adult learners who are fully proficient in their native languages, we find two main differences between them and their younger counterparts: (1) first language transfer and interference and (2) cognitive development.

The concepts of *transfer* and *interference* are derived from the behaviorist view of language development. Both concepts relate to the influence of the first language on the acquisition of the second. Simply put, transfer is the positive influence from the native language to the second language, and interference is the negative influence. For example, if an Italian speaker reads the word *conversation* in English and infers that it means *conversazione* in Italian, his comprehension of the term is facilitated by transfer from his first language. This positively contributes to comprehension and expression in the second language. Conversely, if a speaker of Italian adds a vowel sound to the end of every consonant-final word in English (as in "She's-ah nice-ah"), that is interference from his native language. Because the majority of Italian words end in vowel sounds, Italian speakers transfer this phonological pattern to English. This can be considered a negative impact on the expression of the second language, as it results in a "foreign" accent and can be perceived as a communication disorder instead of a communication difference. The more developed the native language in the second language learner, the more influence transfer and interference have in the acquisition of the second language. Second language acquisition researcher Rod Ellis (2008b) lists four measures of transfer from the first to the second language: (1) learner errors; (2) positive transfer or facilitation; (3) avoidance; and (4) overuse. Certain of these effects are apparent in productive language, including pronunciation, vocabulary, grammar, and discourse, and/or in the receptive language modalities of reading and listening.

In analyzing transfer through learner errors, care must be taken to ascertain whether they are developmental in nature, meaning that they are common to all learners of L2, regardless of L1, or are a result of transfer from L1. Positive transfer is perhaps more clearly identified, as the learner can often articulate how knowledge of the first language enabled comprehension or expression of the second. Transfer may also be evident in avoidance and overuse of language elements in L2 production (Ellis, 2008a). When learners know that there is a substantial contrast in a particular structure in the first and second languages, they may underuse L2 structure. Conversely, if learners perceive that a particular form in L1 is appropriate in L2, they may use it for all contexts and circumstances.

There is a great range of cognitive capacity between the span of infancy and adulthood, so more fully developed cognitive skills can be applied to acquiring a second language. Clearly, toddlers do not possess the reflective ability to compare linguistic features between their first and second languages, but adolescents and adults have this capability. This means that older children can begin to analyze certain aspects of the second language they are learning, such as when to use which pronoun and why (i.e., "Is it Reese and I or Me and Reese?"). Paying attention to the rules of language is an effective strategy for learners whose cognitive development permits this type of analysis, and it is a hallmark of instructed SLA.

Naturalistic and Instructed Second Language Acquisition

There are different pathways to becoming proficient in a second language. Most similar to the first language acquisition process is what is called *naturalistic second language acquisition.* A typical case of naturalistic SLA is when an adult immigrates to a country without understanding or speaking the language. In the US, for instance, certain industries employ immigrants who cannot speak or understand English in entry-level positions. A group of employees who speak the native language of the new immigrant (let's call him Quan, whose native language is Khmer) often help explain the job responsibilities. Over time, Quan comes into contact with English-speaking workers and supervisors and begins to develop a work-related vocabulary. Outside of work, depending on the extent of the community of speakers of Quan's native language, Khmer, he will begin to develop survival English phrases for shopping, going to the doctor, and other routine needs that may be conducted in English. In other words, if there is a large enough community of Khmer-speaking immigrants, services and businesses may be available in Quan's native language, and there would be less urgency to learn English in order to conduct his daily affairs. As he interacts with English speakers, he will begin to acquire necessary vocabulary, gradually developing the ability to string together simple sentences. This is, in simple terms, the process of naturalistic language acquisition.

As can be seen with the examples of Quan, there are many variables that affect naturalistic second language acquisition. Before we examine these variables and their influence on the rate and ultimate level of second language acquisition, let us look at what the process of naturalistic SLA commonly involves.

Second Language Acquisition Phases and Their Relation to L1 Acquisition

Similar to first language acquisition, naturalistic second language acquisition follows a series of predictable phases, particularly in morphology and syntax. Because those who are learning a second language are already verbal in at least one other language, they do not experience a preverbal phase the way infants who are learning their first language do. In particular, the process of acquiring the phonology of a second language is quite different from acquiring the first. Whereas babies babble new sounds to develop competence in using and combining them, adults typically learn sounds as parts of words. So where a baby will repeat "pa-pa-pa," an adult will learn the word "paper" and will correctly pronounce the sounds that also exist in their native language but will approximate the sounds that do not. This might mean that an Arabic-speaking learner will pronounce it as "baber," /bebɚ/, because Arabic does not have a /p/ sound, and the /b/ sound is the closest approximation. A Spanish speaker may pronounce the /p/ sounds properly but will "tap" the final /r/ sound, /ɾ/, because the retroflex /ɻ/sound used in English is not a feature of Spanish phonology. Clearly, acquiring the phonology of a second language (either naturalistically or through formal instruction) is heavily influenced by the already-acquired phonology of the first language. With babies learning any language, sounds are acquired in an order (i.e., stops before liquids); however, with adults learning a second language, sounds are acquired as the learners are exposed to words that use them, and some sounds that don't exist in the native language or that are used in different combinations or word positions in the native language are not pronounced the way a native speaker would utter them.

Whereas the preverbal stage is limited to first language acquisition, the verbal stages of first and second language acquisition share many commonalities. The acquisition of vocabulary tends to be similar, with frequently used nouns acquired early in first and second language acquisition, probably because of their tangible nature. Of course, nouns used frequently with infants differ from those used frequently with adults. An adult in the workplace will more likely hear the word "paper" before "crib." In addition, adults generally know and understand the concepts for most of the tangible words they learn—if they learn the word "ball," they probably won't assume the moon is also called "ball." However, a concept represented by a word in one language may be represented by two different words in another. For example, the word "know" in English is represented by "conocer" (to know a person) and "saber" (to know a fact) in Spanish and the word "nipote" in Italian means "grandson" and "nephew." These differences can cause confusion or the misuse of a term.

Morphology acquisition is similar in first and second language acquisition. During the 1970s, researchers attempted to determine the acquisition of second language learners from different first language backgrounds (Brown & Attardo, 2000). A general order was established for grammatical markers and function words:

1. Pronouns
2. Articles
3. Copula (be)
4. Present progressive ("-ing")
5. Plural ("-s")
6. Be + verb + "-ing"
7. Regular past ("-ed")
8. Irregular past
9. Irregular plural ("-es")
10. Possessive ("-'s")
11. Third person present ("-s")

Knowing that the first language profoundly affects the acquisition of phonology in the second language, it is surprising that despite various native languages, learners follow the same general sequence of morphological development in their second language (English) (Dulay & Burt, 1980; Kroll & Tokowicz, 2001). Certain morphemes from the list may cluster together at different points in the process (in stages) rather than be acquired individually in a sequence. Additionally, learners from different first language backgrounds may progress from acquiring one morpheme to another at a different rate. Nonetheless, the general order holds true regardless of the native language.

In the area of syntax acquisition, there are also numerous first and second language similarities (Cook, 2008; Dulay, Burt, & Krashen, 1982; Krashen, 1987; Krashen, Scarcella, & Long, 1982; Paradis & Genesee, 1996; Paradis, Genesee, & Crago, 2011). Second language learners begin with one- and two-word statements, often focusing on nouns and verbs and omitting function words. As they develop more competence in the grammar of the second language their sentences become longer, adding prepositions and other function words as well as connecting phrases with conjunctions. Throughout this process, learners produce grammatical errors that are gradually replaced by the correct form in most cases. Questions and negative statements go through the same type of error patterns in SLA as they do during their acquisition in the first language. For example, "How could she have done that" might be stated, "How she can did that?" or in an attempt to avoid making an error in question phrasing, a learner may make a statement with a rising intonation, such as "She came to school late?" With negative statements, second language learners often use "no" when "not" is correct and omit or improperly form the particle "do," such as "I no work on Mondays" instead of "I do not work on Mondays" or state words out of order without the proper grammatical (morphological) markers, such as "She no did laughed at my joke" instead of "She didn't laugh at my joke."

Because learning a second language naturalistically is in many ways similar to the way one learns a first language, many of the same processes and stages occur. Just as first language learners acquire new vocabulary through exposure to real objects and actions and their associated words and phrases, so do L2 learners in naturalistic language learning settings. In addition, the need for communicating different real-life functions, such as requests, providing information, and other communication functions, create a need for first and second language learners to develop comprehension and expression ability through negotiation of meaning.

Naturalistic Second Language Acquisition

Understanding the nature of both naturalistic and instructed second language acquisition has important implications for SLPs. For ELs enrolled in elementary, middle, and high schools in the United States, both naturalistic and instructed second language acquisition are involved. Depending on the grade level and instructional model, ELs may be immersed with native speakers of English, studying subjects such as math, science, and social studies. Under these circumstances, most of their language acquisition is a result of naturalistic learning, where they acquire new vocabulary and structures by understanding academic content that includes multiple means of conveying information, not just language alone. In some schools, ESOL professionals work separately with ELs, providing more focus on the language of instruction to improve comprehensibility as well as to accelerate language development. For example, the ESOL professional might work on science vocabulary and cause and effect sentences to help ELs progress more quickly. This approach comes closer to formal instruction. In a pre-K–12 learning context where English is the language of instruction, it is reasonable to assume that whatever program model that an EL is enrolled in, much more time is spent learning in a naturalistic rather than instructed way. This includes not only subject area classroom instruction but interaction with native speakers of English, in and out of the classroom.

One way to describe the necessary conditions for learning a second language naturalistically is through the information processing concepts of input, interaction, and output (Swain, 1985; Skehan, 1998; Ellis, 2003). Second language acquisition research has demonstrated the importance of each verbal element for language development. Input refers to the information directed toward the learner. The key issue is whether the verbal input is comprehensible to the learner (Krashen, 1981). In other words, if the learner understands the meaning of the input, then she can add the new words and phrases to her linguistic repertoire.

For example, if a teacher told you "siediti" and you did not know Italian, the verbal input would not be comprehensible. However, if the teacher modeled the action of sitting down or gestured by extending and lowering her palm facedown, you would comprehend the term "siediti" as "sit down." After hearing the term a few times and seeing others responding to the command, you would learn the new phrase.

Comprehensible input is necessary but not sufficient for developing proficiency in a second language. A language learner has to do more than just understand—the learner must also express meaning. The expression of information is called output. Although it is normal and even beneficial for second language learners to focus on listening through what is termed a "silent period" (Krashen & Terrell, 1983) in the beginning stages of acquisition, learners in naturalistic settings will often prolong this nonverbal response phase for fear of making pronunciation and grammatical errors. In order for learners to develop speaking skills, it is necessary for them to express meaning in the second language (Swain, 1995).

Communicating in any language requires input (received through listening and reading) and output (produced through speaking and writing), but in real communication input and output do not happen independently. We don't hear input and then speak unrelated output. For example, if you are asked, "What is your name?" (input) you don't state, "It's very hot outside." Input and output in communication are connected. If you sit down with a friend and she asks you if you would like some tea, her question is the input that you need to comprehend. Your answer, "Yes, I would," is your output. The connected exchange of information that occurs in the back and forth between input and output is called interaction, and it is absolutely critical to acquiring a second language. If it was a hot day and you would love a cold drink, you might want to clarify the offer, "Would you like some tea?" with a question of your own, "Is it iced or hot?" Your friend could then provide the necessary detail for you to make your decision. Similarly, those communicating in a second language may not understand a word and can ask for elaboration or explanation, such as "What is a saucer?" to which a native speaker may either point to a saucer or state that it is a dish that goes under a teacup.

Second language learners attempting to use new vocabulary and put together more complicated sentences may make an error that impedes comprehension, at which point the listener can ask for clarification. For example, if an L2 learner states, "Have you shizzor?" and the English speaker replies, "What do you mean? I don't understand what you're asking." The English learner could then reply, "Shizzor, for cutting," while opening and closing his extended index and middle fingers. "Oh, you mean scissors!" would be a likely reply, confirming the correct word. The give and take in these two examples is known as *negotiation of meaning* (Pica, 1994), and its function is critical to language development. Through confirming comprehension of and trying out new ways to express meaning, language learners build their vocabulary and grammar.

Instructed Second Language Acquisition

Depending on the learning environment, instructed SLA can be the sole means of learning a foreign language or a complement to learning a second language naturalistically. Some learners in foreign language contexts have no other means of developing communication skills in the language other than in a formal classroom setting. These language learners' SLA development would then result primarily from instruction, although the proliferation of Internet technologies has broadened the types of opportunities for exposure to a foreign language beyond the classroom. In a second language learning context where the learner is immersed in a community of speakers of the new language, one can learn entirely naturalistically but can benefit from the addition of instructed SLA to the process (Ellis, 2008b).

As a rule of thumb, formal instruction in the second language becomes more important at later ages and grade levels. In a pre-K–12 learning context, language awareness activities that begin in elementary school and progress to formal study of grammar in middle and high school can be very beneficial for English learners.

There are many variations on the approach to instructed SLA, but the vast majority of approaches involve some focus or emphasis on grammar. Ranging from studying grammar rules and practicing examples of the rules to learning dialogues that are organized by grammar points, instructed SLA offers benefits for both the rate of acquisition and ultimate level of attainment. For adults, instructed SLA can speed the process through the various stages of language acquisition. In addition, grammar instruction can help avoid the establishment of errors in the speaker's production. Research shows that learners who study specific grammar points are more likely to acquire the correct form without *fossilizing* an incorrect form (Ellis, 2008b; Pica, 1994; Rowe & Levine, 2006). For example, if Quan learned English without grammar study, he might never move past a particular phase of syntactic errors in questions (e.g., "Why you no come?"), thereby fossilizing.

Fossilization (Selinker, 1972) has also been termed *stabilization* (Long, 1990) to emphasize the possibility of moving beyond the plateau of a non-target-like grammatical form. The notion has important implications for those who work with ELs because when a form becomes fossilized, the learner cannot spontaneously utter it following correction or instruction. Let us look at Quan's question error as it relates to fossilization. If an English speaker corrected Quan and explained how to form the question properly, Quan might understand the rule, but 30 minutes later in conversation with a coworker, Quan would make the same error without realizing it. For SLPs, the important issue is to recognize that some morphological and syntactic errors can hit a plateau that may or may not be overcome with instruction.

Social and Affective Variables in Second Language Acquisition

Second language acquisition occurs in very rich contexts that go beyond linguistic input. In his seminal study, Schumann (1978) proposed that acculturation, defined as the integration of L2 learner with the target language group, can explain second language acquisition in adults who are learning English in naturalistic settings. Because his acculturation model intends to explain the context of naturalistic SLA for adults who are immigrants or want to reside in the target language country for an extended period of time, it does not directly apply to L2 curriculum design or methodology, especially in the case of children who are bilingual or learning another language. However, the social and affective factors that are the basis of Schumann's model affect children just as they affect adults, albeit in different ways and with different degrees of intensity. Therefore, it is very useful to explore the social and affective variables that are related to aspects of second language acquisition.

Schumann's model looks at acculturation as a result of the clustering of two groups of variables: social factors and affective factors. Social factors involve the relationship between two linguistically different groups of people who are in contact: one group consists of people who are learning an L2, and the other group is made up of the native speakers of L2 or the target language group. A number of social factors can, in Schumann's opinion, either promote or hinder contact between two groups with consequences on whether or not the L2 learning group acculturates and consequently acquires L2. Table 4–6 lists and explains the eight social variables that are an integral part of Schumann's acculturation model.

Although the social factors discussed above and in Table 4–6 appear to facilitate second language acquisition, individual variables represented by affective variables might impede the learning of a second language. In the acculturation model, the important affective factors are language shock, culture shock, motivation, and ego permeability, discussed in Table 4–7.

Table 4–6. *Social Factors in Acculturation*

Variable	Characteristics
Social Domination Patterns	• If the L2 learning group is dominant, it will tend not to learn L2. • If the L2 learning group is subordinate, they will tend to resist acculturation and not learn L2. • If the L2 learning group and the L2 group are equal, the contact is likely more extensive with positive influences on L2 acquisition.

Table 4–6. *continued*

Variable	Characteristics
Integration Strategies	• Assimilation: The L2 learning group adopts the values of the L2 group, maximizing contact and L2 acquisition. • Preservation: The L2 learning group rejects the values of the L2 group, minimizing contact and L2 acquisition. • Adaptation: The L2 learning group adapts to the values of L2 group but maintains its own values for intragroup use, with various degrees of contact and L2 acquisition.
Enclosure	• Refers to the degree to which secondary social institutions (school, churches, professions, etc.) are shared by both groups. • Low enclosure: they share many of these institutions, enhancing contact and L2 acquisition. • High enclosure: they have different secondary social institutions, limiting contact and L2 acquisition.
Cohesiveness	• If the L2 learning group is cohesive, there will be separation limiting contact and L2 acquisition.
Size	• If the L2 learning group is large, the intragroup contact will be more prevalent than intergroup contact, limiting L2 acquisition.
Cultural Congruence	• If the two group cultures are similar, then contact is more likely facilitating L2 acquisition
Attitude	• If the two groups have positive attitudes toward each other, this will likely facilitate L2 acquisition.
Intended Length of Residence	• If the L2 learning group intends to reside for a long time in the L2 group area, more contacts are possible with positive influences on L2 acquisition.

Source: Adapted from "The Acculturation Model for Second Language Acquisition," by J. H. Schumann, in *Second Language Acquisition and Foreign Language Learning*, by R. C. Gingras (Ed.), 1978, Washington, DC: Center for Applied Linguistics.

Table 4–7. *Affective Factors in Acculturation*

Variable	Characteristics
Language Shock	• The L2 learners might fear criticism and ridicule when they attempt to speak another language. • Even for young learners, there is wide individual variation in the willingness to tolerate the frustration when trying to use another language in a variety of school activities.
Culture Shock	• Culture shock is the anxiety resulting from entering a new culture. • Adults experience this more than children, but even young L2 learners may be affected by various degrees of culture shock affecting their parents and other members of their community.
Motivation	• Integrative: L2 learners want to learn another language in order to become like the speakers of the other language. • Instrumental: L2 learners want to learn another language for utilitarian purposes. • Integrative motivation is seen more powerful because the L2 learner wants to integrate with L2 speakers, with positive effects on L2 acquisition.
Ego Permeability	• Each person has a language ego that establishes as sense of language limits and boundaries, which are flexible in the early stages of development and become more rigid later. • L2 learners with more permeable language egos will have more success in L2 acquisition.

Source: Adapted from "The Acculturation Model for Second Language Acquisition," by J. H. Schumann, in *Second Language Acquisition and Foreign Language Learning,* by R. C. Gingras (Ed.), 1978, Washington, DC: Center for Applied Linguistics.

The social and affective factors discussed in Schumann's acculturation model work together in determining the success of learning another language. The social factors emphasize the collective distance between two language communities, whereas the affective factors look at perceptions regarding the two languages within individuals. Of the two sets of factors, Schumann suggests that the affective factors may be more important in the success of second language acquisition. L2 learners who perceive a vast psychological distance between themselves and L2 would not likely seek opportunities to develop their proficiency in L2 and might attain an incomplete mastery of the target language.

It is true that Schumann's model was designed with adult immigrants who are learning L2 in a naturalistic way in mind. His model has no direct instructional application. Nevertheless, the social and affective factors that are the basis for his model have an influence on learners engaged in formal language learning as well as on their second language acquisition. It is reasonable to suggest that these factors interact with instructional programs and settings in ways that influence the success of second language teaching, either positively or negatively.

Following a general overview of first and second language acquisition, this chapter now turns to one of the challenging tasks faced by SLP professionals: how to determine whether an EL has a communication disorder or whether they are simply displaying behaviors that are typically associated with normal second language development.

Communication Difference or Disorder?

To understand the differences between a communication difference and a communication disorder, it is important to revisit what constitutes a communication disorder. Communication disorders embrace a wide range of conditions that generate challenges in effective communication. They include speech disorders, which affect the articulation of speech sounds, fluency, and voice, and language disorders, which include impairments in the use of the spoken, signed, or written system. In general, communication disorders are typically classified by their impact on a child's receptive skills (i.e., the ability to understand what is said or to decode, integrate, and organize what is heard) and expressive skills (i.e., the ability to articulate sounds, use appropriate rate and rhythm during speech, exhibit appropriate vocal tone and resonance, and use sounds, words, and sentences in meaningful contexts).

Communication differences are behaviors that are commonly observed among second language learners. For example, ELs at the beginning stages of language proficiency normally produce shorter and less elaborate sentences than their native English-speaking peers; have an underdeveloped vocabulary due to their limited L2 exposure; and a limited capacity for understanding L2 (Paradis, Genesee, & Crago, 2011). Some students, when learning a second language, go through a silent period where they use their receptive skills only; however, this does not mean they do have not expressive skills (Paradis, 2007). When a child is learning a new language he/she will demonstrate differences in sentence structure, speech sound production, vocabulary, and pragmatics. Unfortunately, children with language differences that result from limited experience in using a language are often misidentified as having a communication disorder, and are labeled "language learning disabled" (Roseberry-McKibben, 2008). Table 4–8 presents the common conditions that are associated with receptive and expressive communication challenges (Prelock, Hutchins, & Glascoe, 2008). If we examine the challenges associated with the last category in Table 4–8, specific language impairment, we can easily see how processes typically associated with normal second language acquisition, or language differences, might be interpreted as signs of a communication disorder.

One of the more difficult tasks for SLPs is to determine whether a child is displaying characteristics of normal, typical behaviors for those who are not yet proficient in English or if the child is displaying characteristics of a language disorder. Factors such as language loss, code-switching, and/or interference can confound the issue. For example, code-switching, the practice of switching between a primary and a secondary language or discourse, is a phenomenon that occurs when bilingual speakers substitute a word or phrase from one language with a phrase or word from another language. The sentence "I want a bicycle roja" is an example of code-switching. In this sentence, the English word "red" is replaced with its Spanish equivalent.

Table 4–8. *Disorders Commonly Associated with Receptive and Expressive Communication Problems*

Condition	Expressive Communication Problems	Receptive Communication Problems
Autism	Variability in speech production Use of language in social situations is more challenging than producing language forms Difficulty selecting the right words to represent intended meaning	Difficulty analyzing, integrating, and processing information. Misinterpretation of social cues
Brain Injury	Difficulty in using language appropriately across contexts	Difficulty making connections, inferences and using information to solve problems. Challenges in attention and memory which affect linguistic processing. Challenges in understanding symbolic language and words with multiple meanings.
Hearing Impairment	Limited oral output depending on degree of hearing loss. For oral communicators, vocal resonance, speech sound accuracy, and syntactic structure often affected.	Difficulty with sound perception and discrimination, voice recognition, and understanding of speech.
Intellectual Disability	Production is often below cognitive ability; similar but slower developmental path than typical peers.	Comprehension of language is often below cognitive ability. Difficulty organizing and categorizing information heard for later retrieval.

continues

Table 4–8. *continued*

Condition	Expressive Communication Problems	Receptive Communication Problems
Intellectual Disability *continued*	Tendency to use more immature language forms. Tendency to produce shorter and less elaborated utterances.	Difficulty with abstract concepts.
Specific Language Impairment	Shorter, less elaborated sentences than typical peers. Difficulty in rule formulation for speech sound, word, and sentence productions; ineffective use of language forms in social contexts sometimes leading to inappropriate utterances. Poorly developed vocabulary	Slower and less efficient information processing. Limited capacity for understanding language.

Source: Adapted from "Speech-Language Impairment: How to Identify the Most Common and Least Diagnosed Disability of Childhood," by P. A. Prelock, T. Hutchins, & F. P. Glascoe, 2008, *Medscape Journal of Medicine, 10*(6).

Understanding that L2 learners go through predictable stages of language development with clear characteristics is critical in determining if the child has a communication difference or disorder. The diagnosis of "language learning disabled" should only be used to identify students that have a relatively poor ability in language that cannot be attributed to differences in the child's cultural, linguistic, or educational experiences (Kohnert, 2008). To determine if ELs with communication disorders are eligible to receive services, the Individuals with Disabilities Education Improvement Act regulations published in the Federal Register in 2006 (US Department of Education, 2006) stipulate that the speech and language evaluation of ELs must assess both (all) languages, include the use of culturally appropriate assessment instruments and practices, be conducted by professionals that are familiar with the current best practices literature, and understand the cultural, social, cognitive, and linguistic norms of the child's speech community.

Specifically, in order for an EL to be diagnosed with a communication disorder, he/she must demonstrate delays or difficulties in both (across) languages, demonstrate that the disorder has an adverse affect on their educational performance, and the linguistic behaviors must meet the definition and eligibility requirements of a particular state to be designated as having a "language disorder." For example, in the state of Georgia language impairment is defined as the "impaired comprehension and/or use of spoken language which may also impair the written and/ or other symbol systems and is negatively impacting the child's ability to participate in classroom environment. It may involve, in any combination, the form of language, the content of language, and/or the use of language in communication that is adversely affecting child's communication performance." In the state of Georgia, "language impaired" does not include children who:

- are in normal stages of second language acquisition, unless it is determined that they have a language impairment in their native language
- have regional, dialectic, and/ or cultural differences
- have auditory processing disorders not accompanied by a language impairment
- have anxiety disorders (e.g., selective mutism), unless it is also determined that they have language impairment

What then do SLPs and ESOL professionals need to consider when assessing ELs to ensure they do not mistake a communication difference for a communication disorder? SLPs and ESOL professionals must consider L2 normal processes (i.e., the "silent period," the BICS-CALP gap, and code-switching) and determine if the child is demonstrating behaviors that are characteristic of the normal processes of second language acquisition. The student's performance needs to be compared to the performance of other children who come from a similar cultural, linguistic, and economic background. In diagnosing ELs, extensive information about their home, school, and community needs to be examined alongside test data (Ortiz & Yates, 2002). Professionals who work with the child can provide crucial information about their language and literacy competence. Although the focus of this text is on the role of the SLP and ESOL professional as collaborative partners, it is critical to acknowledge the role of all professionals (i.e., general education teachers, bilingual education teachers, and special education teachers) in native and second language assessment and intervention of ELs (Rosa-Lugo & Fradd, 2000).

Next, it should not be assumed that all EL children have the same language experiences. Some ELs experience language loss or arrested development of their primary language after exposure to English. Language loss occurs as the dominant language (usually English) tends to displace the mother tongue (Brice, Brice, & Kester, 2010). Arrested development occurs as the child ceases to develop L1 while trying to learn L2 (Schiff-Myers, 1992). These two processes, arrested development or language loss, can occur when ELs do not use their primary language. Interestingly, the loss of L1 can occur even in instances when L1 is still used in the home for social interaction by other family members. This may occur when L1 is not valued by the EL or when EL parents encourage the children to become speakers of L2. It is not uncommon for second-generation ELs to become predominantly passive users of their first language. These ELs may respond to their elders in English rather than in their native language.

Language loss has also been attributed to the lack of programs or instructional activities that focus on building conceptual knowledge in the first language (Crawford, 2003). Currently, there are many schools that do not have programs for bilingual students or have transitional programs where the focus is on transitioning into English as quickly as possible. Scholars have discussed some of the deleterious effects of language loss on the development of academic language skills in English (Thomas & Collier, 1997) and transfer of language skills from L1 to English (Cummins, 1984, 1998). Often, language loss may resemble a language learning disability.

Given the length of time it takes to develop academic language proficiency in English, it would seem beneficial for ELs to introduce the learning of L2 as early as possible. However, for many children, the early teaching of subjects in L2 is not preferable. It seems that the more proficient a child is in L1, the easier it will be to learn L2. The level of development of L2 may be influenced by or limited to the level of development of L1 when L2 was introduced. For example, many ELs have never formally developed their L1 and cannot read and write in their home language (i.e., Spanish). Many of these ELs may be dominant in English but have deficits in school performance in English. For many of these children, accessing and mastering the curriculum will be a challenge.

The third consideration for an appropriate separation between a communication difference and a communication disorder is related to the challenges in assessment of ELs in their primary language. There are only a few formal assessment instruments in languages other than English. In addition, some of the assessment instruments are direct translations from English versions, a fact that poses serious threats to the validity of the scores obtained. Moreover, some languages or dialects are only spoken by a minority; therefore, interpreters must be used to assist in the assessment process. However, this is not always a possibility. Interpreters are bilingual individuals who translate written information or who facilitate communication between speakers who do not speak the same language. Parents are often used as interpreters; however, this is not considered a best practice. Criteria to select and use interpreters in the assessment and/or intervention process has been described by several scholars (i.e., Langdon & Cheng 2002; Murphy & Dillon, 2008) and should be used as guidelines in the assessment of ELs.

SLPs and ESOL professionals assessing ELs must keep in mind that there is a great deal of diversity in languages. Additionally, information concerning code-switching and the dialectal variations that the EL hears in the home must be evaluated (Gutierrez-Clellen, Simon-Cereijido, & Leone, 2009). A formal and informal evaluation of the primary language requires not only fluency in the language of the EL but also knowledge about cultural similarities and differences and linguistic variations.

Summary

To provide common ground for the understanding of the fundamental issues in the language acquisition of ELs with a communication disorder, this chapter provided an overview of first and second language acquisition theories and the developmental stages involved in L1 and L2 acquisition. Additionally, recognizing that second language learning is influenced by many non–language related variables, we examined several nonlinguistic factors and discussed how these might affect L2 acquisition. The practical application and the importance of second language acquisition processes was made evident in the discussion of whether observable second language behaviors are indeed examples of communication disorders for ELs, or simply normal language differences all ELs go through during their acquisition of English.

To increase accuracy in disability determinations, professionals must be informed about the possible challenges faced by ELs. These students are required to acquire proficiency in English for both social and academic purposes, learn to read and write English, and obtain background knowledge of mainstream culture to integrate and function effectively in school and achieve the curriculum standards (Cloud, Genesee, & Hamayan, 2009). The next chapter will provide a definition of literacy and provide an overview of literacy development in ELs.

References

American Speech-Language-Hearing Association. (2001a). *Roles and responsibilities of speech-language pathologists with respect to reading and writing in children and adolescents* [Position statement]. Retrieved from http://www.asha.org/docs/html/PS2001-00104.html

American Speech-Language-Hearing Association. (2001b). *Roles and responsibilities of speech-language pathologists with respect to reading and writing in children and adolescents* [Technical report]. Retrieved from http://www.asha.org/docs/html/TR2001-00148.html

American Speech-Language-Hearing Association. (2010). *Roles and responsibilities of speech-language pathologists in schools* [Position statement]. Retrieved from http://www.asha.org/docs/html/PS2010-00318.html

Antunez, B. (2002). Implementing reading first with English language learners. *Directions in Language and Education, 15*. Retrieved from http://www.ncela.gwu.edu/pubs/directions/15.pdf

Ausubel, David P. (1968). *Educational psychology, a cognitive view.* New York, NY: Holt, Rinehart and Winston.

Battle, D. (Ed.). (2002). *Communication disorders in multicultural populations* (3rd ed.). Boston, MA: Butterworth-Heinemann.

Berko-Gleason, J. (1958). The child's learning of English morphology. *Word, 14*, 150–177.

Bloomfield, L. (1942). *Outline guide for the practical study of foreign languages.* Baltimore, MD: Linguistic Society of America.

Brice, A., Brice, R., & Kester, E. (2010). Language loss in English language learners (ELLs). Pedia Staff newsletter. Retrieved from http://www.pediastaff.com/resources-language-loss-in-english-language-learners-ells--february-2010

Brown, H. D. (2007). *Principles of language learning and teaching* (5th ed.). White Plains, NY: Pearson Education.

Brown, R. (1973). *A first language: The early stages.* Cambridge, MA: Harvard University Press.

Brown, S., & Attardo, S. (2000). *Understanding language structure, interaction, and variation: An introduction to linguistics and sociolinguistics for nonspecialists.* Ann Arbor: Michigan University Press.

Chamberlain, S. P. (2005). Recognizing and responding to cultural differences in the education of culturally and linguistically diverse learners. *Intervention in School and Clinic, 40*, 195–211.

Chomsky, N. (1965). *Aspects of a theory of syntax.* Cambridge, MA: MIT Press.

Cloud, N., Genesee, F., & Hamayan, E. (2009). *Literacy instruction for English language learners.* Portsmouth, NH: Heinemann.

Collier, C. (2008). *Handbook for second language acquisition.* Ferndale, WA: CrossCultural Developmental Education Services.

Collier, C. (2011). *Seven steps to separating difference from disability.* Thousand Oaks: CA: Corwin.

Collier, V. P., & Thomas, W. (1995). *Language minority student achievement and program effectiveness. Research summary on ongoing study.* Fairfax, VA: George Mason University.

Cook, V. (2008). *Second language learning and language teaching* (4th ed.). London, UK: Hodder Education.

Crawford, J. (2003). Hard sell: Why is bilingual education so unpopular with the American public? In O. Garcia & C. Baker (Eds.), *Bilingual education: An introductory reader* (pp. 145–164). Clevedon, UK: Multilingual Matters.

Cummins, J. (1980). The construct of language proficiency in bilingual education. In J. E. Alatis (Ed.), *Georgetown University round table on languages and linguistics.* Washington, DC: Georgetown University Press.

Cummins, J. (1984) *Bilingualism and special education.* Clevedon, UK: Multilingual Matters.

Cummins, J. (1992). The role of primary language development in promoting educational success of language minority students. In California State Department of Education (Ed.), *Schooling and language minority students: A theoretical framework.* Los Angeles: California State University, Evaluation, Dissemination, and Assessment Center.

Cummins, J. (1998). *Beyond adversarial discourse: Searching for common ground in the education of bilingual students.* Presentation to the California State Board of Education, Sacramento.

Cummins, J. (2000) *Language, power and pedagogy: Bilingual children in the cross-fire.* Clevedon, UK: Multilingual Matters.

Cummins, J., Chow, P., & Schecter, S. R. (2006). Community as curriculum. *Language Arts, 83,* 297–307.

Dornyei, Z. (2005). *The psychology of the language learner: Individual differences in second language acquisition.* Mahwah, NJ: Lawrence Erlbaum.

Dulay, H., & Burt, M. K. (1974). Natural sequences in child second language acquisition. *Language Learning, 24,* 37–53.

Dulay, H., & Burt, M. K. (1980). On acquisition orders. In S. Felix (Ed.). *Second language development: Trends and issues.* Tubingen, Germany: Narr.

Dulay, H., Burt, M. K., & Krashen, S. (1982). *Language two.* New York, NY: Oxford University Press.

Ellis, R. (2003). *Task-based Language Learning and Teaching.* Oxford, UK: Oxford University Press.

Ellis, R. (2008a). *The study of second language acquisition* (2nd ed.). Oxford, UK: Oxford University Press.

Ellis, R. (2008b). Principles of instructed second language acquisition. *Center for Applied Linguistics Digest,* 1–6. Washington, DC: Retrieved from http://www.cal.org/resources/digest/digest_pdfs/Instructed2ndLangFinalWeb.pdf

Freeman, D. E., & Freeman, Y. S. (2004). *Essential linguistics: What you need to know to teach reading, ESL, spelling, phonics, grammar.* Portsmouth, NH: Heinemann.

Gardner, R. (1980). On the validity of affective variables in second language acquisition: conceptual, contextual, and statistical considerations. *Language Learning, 30*(2), 255–270.

Gardner, R. (2001). Integrative motivation and second language acquisition. In Z. Dornyei & R. Schmidt (Eds.), *Motivation and second language learning.* Honolulu: University of Hawaii Press.

Gutierrez-Clellen, V. F., Simon-Cereijido, G., & Leone, A. E. (2009). Code-switching in bilingual children with specific language impairments. *International Journal of Bilingualism, 13,* 91–109.

Harley, B., & Hart, D. (1997). Language aptitude and second language proficiency in classroom learners of different starting ages. *Studies in Second Language Acquisition, 19,* 379–400.

Hoover, J., Klinmgner, J., Baca, L., & Patton, J. M. (2008). *Methods for teaching culturally and linguistically diverse exceptional learners.* Upper Saddle River, NJ: Pearson.

Horwitz, E. (1987). Linguistic and communicative competence: Reassessing foreign language aptitude. In B. Van Patten, T. Dvorak, & J. Lee (Eds.), *Foreign language learning: A research perspective.* New York, NY: Newbury House.

Johnson, K., & Johnson, H. (1999). *Encyclopedic dictionary of applied linguistics: A handbook for language teaching.* Oxford, UK: Blackwell.

Kan, P. F., & Kohnert, K. (2005). Preschoolers learning Hmong and English: Lexical-semantic skills in L1 and L2. *Journal of Speech, Language and Hearing Research, 48,* 372–383.

Kayser, H. R. (2002). Bilingual language development and language disorders. In D. E. Battle (Ed.), *Communication disorders in multicultural population* (3rd ed., pp. 205–232). Woburn, MA: Butterworth-Heinemann.

Kohnert, K. (2008). *Language disorders in bilingual children and adults.* San Diego, CA: Plural.

Krashen, S. D. (1981). Bilingual education and second language acquisition theory. In California State Department of Education (Ed.), *Schooling and language minority students: A theoretical framework* (p. 51–79). Los Angeles: California State University, Evaluation, Dissemination, and Assessment Center.

Krashen, S. D. (1987). *Principles and practices in second language acquisition.* New York, NY: Prentice-Hall.

Krashen, S., Scarcella, R., & Long, M. (Eds.). (1982). *Child-adult differences in second language acquisition.* Rowley, MA: Newbury House.

Krashen, S., & Terrell, T. (1983). *The natural approach: Language acquisition in the classroom.* Oxford, UK: Pergamon Press.

Kroll, J. F., &Tokowicz, N. (2001). The development of conceptual representation for words in a second language. In J. Nicol (Ed.), *One mind, two languages* (pp. 49–71). Oxford, UK: Blackwell.

Langdon, H. W., & Cheng L. L. (2002). *Collaborating with interpreters and translators: A guide for communication disorders professionals.* Eau Claire, WI: Thinking Publications.

Letts, C. (1999). Becoming bilingual. In B. Spolsky & R. E. Asher (Eds.), *Concise encyclopedia of educational linguistics.* Oxford, UK: Pergamon.

Lightbown, P., & Spada, N. M. (1999). *How languages are learned.* Oxford, UK: Oxford University Press.

Long, M. H. (1983). Native speaker/non-native speaker conversation and negotiation of comprehensible input. *Applied Linguistics, 4*(2), 126–141.

Long, M. H. (1990). Maturational constraints on language development. *Studies on Second Language Acquisition, 12*(3), 251–285.

Masgoret, A., & Gardner, R. (2003). Attitudes, motivation, and second language learning: A meta-analysis of studies conducted by Gardner and associates. *Language Learning, 53*, 123–163.

Mitchell, R., & Myles, F. (2004). *Second language learning theories.* New York, NY: Hodder Arnold.

Murphy, B. C., & Dillon, C. (2008). *Interviewing in action in a multi-cultural world* (3rd ed.). Belmont, CA: Thomson Higher Education.

Ortiz, A. & Yates, J. (2002). Considerations in the assessment of English language learners referred to special education. In A. Artiles & A. Ortiz (Eds.), *English language learners with special education needs. Identification, assessment and instruction* (pp. 65–86). McHenry, IL: Center for Applied Linguistics and Delta Systems.

Paradis, J. (2007). Bilingual children with specific language impairment: Theoretical and applied issues. *Applied Psycholinguistics, 28*, 551–564.

Paradis, J., & Genesee, F. (1996). Syntactic acquisition in bilingual children. *Studies in Second Language Acquisition, 18*, 1–25.

Paradis, J., Genesee, F., & Crago, M. (2011). *Dual language development and disorders.* Baltimore, MD: Brookes.

Parker, F., & Riley, K. (2000). *Linguistics for non-linguists: A primer with exercises.* Needham Heights, MA: Allyn & Bacon.

Patterson, J. L., & Pearson, B. Z. (2004). Influences, contexts and processes. In B. A. Goldstein (Ed.), *Bilingual language development and disorders in Spanish-English speakers* (pp. 77–104). Baltimore, MD: Brookes.

Peregoy, S. F., & Boyle, O. F. (2005). *Reading, writing and learning in ESL: A resource book for K–12 teachers, MYLABSCHOOL Edition* (4th ed.). Upper Saddle River, NJ: Pearson.

Pica, T. (1994). Questions from the language classroom: Research perspectives. *TESOL Quarterly, 28*, 49–79.

Pinker, S. (1994). *The language instinct: How the mind creates language.* New York, NY: William Morrow.

Pinker, S. (1999). *Words and rules: The ingredients of language.* London, UK: Weidenfeld & Nicholson.

Prelock, P. A., Hutchins, T., & Glascoe, F. P. (2008). Speech-language impairment: How to identify the most common and least diagnosed disability of childhood. *Medscape Journal of Medicine, 10*(6).

Robson, G. (1992). *Individual learner differences and classroom participation: A pilot study.* Unpublished paper, Temple University, Japan.

Rosa-Lugo, L. I., & Fradd, S. (2000). Preparing professionals to serve English-language learners with communication disorders. *Communication Disorders Quarterly, 22*(1), 29–42.

Roseberry-McKibben, C. (2007). *Language disorders in children. A multicultural and case perspective.* Boston, MA: Allyn & Bacon.

Roseberry-McKibben, C. (2008). *Multicultural students with special language needs* (3rd ed.). Oceanside, CA: Academic Communication Associates.

Rowe, B. M., & Levine, D. P., (2006). *A concise introduction to linguistics.* Boston, MA: Pearson Education.

Schiff-Myers, N. (1992). Considering arrested language development and language loss in the assessment of second language learners. *Language, Speech, and Hearing Services in Schools, 23*, 28–33.

Schumann, J. H. (1978). The acculturation model for second language acquisition. In R. C. Gingras (Ed.), *Second language acquisition and foreign language learning.* Washington, DC: Center for Applied Linguistics.

Selinker, L. (1972). Interlanguage. *International Review of Applied Linguistics in Language Teaching, 10*, 209–232.

Skehan, P. (1986a). Cluster analysis and the identification of learner types. In V. Cook (Ed.), *Experimental approaches to second language acquisition.* Oxford, UK: Pergamon.

Skehan, P. (1986b). Where does language aptitude come from? In P. Meara (Ed.), *Spoken language.* London, UK: Centre for Information on Language Teaching.

Skehan, P. (1989). *Individual differences in second language learning.* London, UK: Edward Arnold.

Skehan, P. (1990). The relationship between native and foreign language learning ability: Educational and linguistic factors. In H. Dechert (Ed.), *Current trends in European second language acquisition research.* Clevedon, UK: Multilingual Matters.

Skehan, P. (1998). *A cognitive approach to language learning.* Oxford, UK: Oxford University Press.

Skinner, B. F. (1957). *Verbal behavior.* Acton, MA: Copley.

Strong, M. (1983). Social styles and second language acquisition of Spanish-speaking kindergartners. *TESOL Quarterly, 17*, 241–258.

Swain, M. (1985). Communicative competence: Some roles of comprehensible input in its development. In S. Gass & C. Madden (Eds.),

Input and second language acquisition (pp. 235–252). Rowley, MA: Newbury.

Swain, M. (1995). Three functions of output in second language learning. In G. Cook & B. Seidlhofer (Eds.), *Principles and practice in the study of language: Studies in honor of H. G. Widdowson*. Oxford, UK: Oxford University Press.

Teachers of English to Speakers of Other Languages (TESOL). (2001). *Position statement on language and literacy development for young English language learners*. Retrieved from http://tesol.org/s_tesol/ bin.asp?CID=32&DID=371&DOC=FILE.PDF

Teachers of English to Speakers of Other Languages (TESOL). (2006). *PreK–12 English language proficiency standards*. Alexandria, VA: TESOL.

Tharp, R. G., & Gallimore, R. (1988). *Rousing minds to life*. New York, NY: Cambridge University Press.

Thomas, P., & Collier, V. (1997). *School effectiveness for language minority students*. Washington, DC: National Clearinghouse for Bilingual Education.

Thorndike, Edward L. (1932). *The fundamentals of learning*. New York, NY: Teachers College, Columbia University.

US Department of Education. (2006, August 14). Rules and regulations. *Federal Register, 71*(156): 46540–46845.

Volterra, V., & Taeschner, T. (1978). The acquisition and development of language by bilingual children. *Journal of Child Language, 5*, 311–326.

Vygotsky, L. (1962). *Thought and language*. Cambridge, MA: MIT Press.

Walqui, A. (2000). Contextual factors in second language acquisition. *ERIC Clearinghouse on Language and Linguistics*. Retrieved from http://www.cal.org/resources/digest/0005contextual.html

5

Literacy Development in a Second Language

Introduction

Regardless of specialization or academic preparation, all teachers and professionals who work with students are "teachers" of literacy. Literacy development provides the perfect venue for collaboration between SLPs and ESOL professionals. Language is the foundation of literacy and plays a very important role in the academic achievement of ELs, with or without communication disorders. In order for ELs with communication disorders to be successful, it is imperative that the two categories, SLPs and ESOL professionals, collaborate fully in developing language and literacy skills of ELs with communication disorders (ASHA, 1998, 2001a, 2001b, 2010). Their collaboration will ensure that ELs with communication disorders are appropriately identified and that evidence-based interventions are provided for the purpose of decreasing the "at risk for literacy development" likelihood for the student (ASHA, 2002).

ESOL professionals are first and foremost literacy teachers because the ESOL curriculum strongly emphasizes the development of English language and literacy for ELs (TESOL 2001, 2010). In the area of EL literacy, the academic preparation of ESOL teachers makes them aware of the differences between literacy (i.e., reading and writing) in L1 and literacy in L2 (TESOL, 2007). Some of the key issues in L2 literacy are language transfer, background knowledge, affective factors, and the importance of oral language in literacy development.

The importance of oral language development underlines the pivotal role of the SLP-ESOL collaboration. In this partnership SLPs can provide critical information and support ESOL professionals when ESOL professionals have ELs with communication disorders in their classrooms (ASHA, 1998). ESOL teachers have a very good knowledge of the English literacy issues and challenges pertaining to the EL general student population, but they might not be as prepared to address specific issues linked to the literacy development of ELs with communication disorders. This is where the contribution of the SLP is invaluable. In 2001 the American Speech-Language-Hearing Association (ASHA) published several documents addressing literacy and the roles and responsibilities of SLPs in the development of reading and writing among children and adolescents, and particularly for younger children who have communication disorders (ASHA 20001a, 2001b, 2001c, 2002). These documents specified the role of SLPs in literacy in the area of prevention, identification, assessment, collaboration, and advocacy (ASHA, 2002) and noted their unique contributions to literacy instruction. Within this framework, specifically in the area of prevention, the Response to Intervention (RtI) process and its focus on optimizing student performance prior to being declared a special education student provides the SLP with an excellent opportunity to make greater use of their expertise in language and literacy (Ehren, 2005; Ehren, Montgomery, & Whitmire, 2006).

SLPs have acquired a great deal of information in their academic training about English literacy challenges related to communication disorders. Their knowledge of language and its subsystems (phonology, morphology, syntax, semantics, and pragmatics), their training in language development and acquisition, as well as communication processes and disorders, combined with their skills in using diagnostic-prescriptive approaches to assessment and intervention, are particularly valuable in the educational context (Ehren & Murza, 2010; Spracher, 2000). Depending on the educational placement of the EL student, the ESOL professional might have the primary role of facilitating oral language skills and the general education teacher for teaching reading and writing. An SLP can complement and augment the skills and knowledge of these, and other, professionals, who also have unique perspectives, knowledge, and skills. These professionals can include general education teachers, bilingual education teachers, ESOL professionals, reading specialists, literacy coaches, and special education teachers. For example, SLPs are able to provide a solid analysis from their perspective of the English language demands present in the textbooks, language of instruction in the classroom, and grade- and age-level curriculum expectations for ELs.

If we are to describe the role of each element of the SLP-ESOL pair as it relates to ELs with communication disorders, we can say that SLPs have detailed knowledge about communication disorders and general EL knowledge, whereas ESOL professionals have detailed EL knowledge and general knowledge about communication disorders. The SLP-ESOL collaboration vis-à-vis ELs with communication disorders encompasses the entire educational cycle of this student population. This collaboration starts with the correct identification and appropriate placement of ELs with communication disorders, a process that should determine whether the student demonstrates normal characteristics and processes found in students acquiring English as a second language or a communication disorder. The very nature of this fundamental question points out that an accurate identification and placement is not possible without the full involvement of SLPs and ESOL professionals, and other school professionals (Rosa-Lugo & Fradd, 2000).

Once EL students with communication disorders are identified and placed in appropriate programs to include English language development programs, the SLP-ESOL team should work together in providing the best instruction and intervention strategies (Collier, 2010; Echevarria & Vogt, 2011). These strategies should target the specific literacy challenges of ELs with communication disorders and should incorporate best literacy development practices during ESOL classes and speech and language therapy sessions. Finally, the SLP-ESOL team should work closely in the assessment of ELs with communication disorders. Classroom-based and large-scale assessments should measure the literacy development of this student population to determine whether the intervention has proven effective and to routinely monitor progress (Klingner, Mendez Barletta, & Hoover, 2008). The importance of measuring academic and English language development for all students is a critical and unavoidable requirement of the No Child Left Behind Act (NCLB), making the collaboration between SLPs and ESOL professionals crucial.

Literacy: Definition and Attributes

The definition of literacy has evolved over the past century. Literacy has traditionally been defined as the ability to read and write. Today the definition has been expanded. The Workforce Investment Act of 1998 defines literacy as "an individual's ability to read, write, speak in English, compute and solve problems at levels of proficiency necessary to function on the job, in the family of the individual, and in society" (ASHA, 2008). This is a broader view of literacy than just an individual's ability to read. As new information and technology have increasingly shaped our society, the skills needed to function successfully have gone beyond reading and literacy and has come to include the skills listed in the current definition of literacy (National Institute for Literacy, n.d.). The relationship between language and literacy and the connection between spoken and written language are addressed in ASHA's position statement *Roles and Responsibilities of Speech-Language Pathologists Related to Reading and Writing in Children and Adolescents.* Specifically, the document establishes the connection between spoken and written language and points out that:

A. Spoken language provides the foundation for the development of reading and writing;
B. Spoken and written language have a reciprocal relationship, such that each builds on the other to result in general language and literacy competence; and
C. Instruction in spoken language can result in growth in written language, and instruction in written language can result in growth in spoken language (ASHA, 2002).

One possible way of operationalizing the construct of literacy is by examining literacy attributes. Walmsley (2008) defines literacy attributes as what students should know, do, understand, and have experienced. In other words, *knowing* means that students should "know what" (e.g., knowledge of vocabulary, background knowledge, etc.) and "know how" (e.g., strategies of inferring meaning of an unknown word). *Doing* means that students should have constant engagement in literacy behaviors, such as independent reading, and *understanding* means that students should be able to make sense of many types of texts, either literary or informational. The last part of the definition, *have experienced*, means that students should accumulate literacy and continue to increase these experiences over time. Literacy attributes are based on the Communication Triangle, a concept developed by Kinneavy (1969) (Figure 5–1).

The Communication Triangle illustrates the basic relationships between the encoders, or those who originate communication; the decoders, or those who receive the communication; and the reality, or the knowledge shared by the encoder and

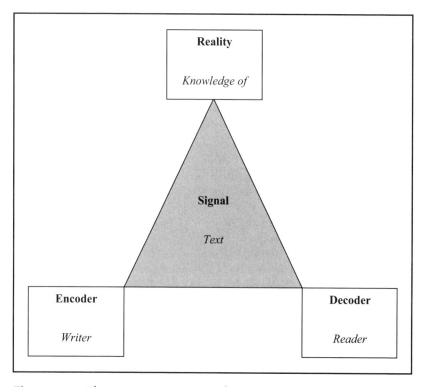

Figure 5–1. *The Communication Triangle. Source: Adapted from "The Basic Aims of Discourse," by J. E. Kinneavy, 1969, College Composition and Communication, 20(5), 297–304. Published by National Council of Teachers of English.*

decoder. Central to the entire triangle is the medium used to convey the message, or the signal. It is important to note that these relationships occur in a social context and have a crucial role in defining and sometimes constraining the types of communication that typically take place, the ways language is used, and the perceived appropriateness and correctness of the conveyed message. Using the Communication Triangle, literacy attributes are defined in three major areas: receptive language, expressive language, and background knowledge (Walmsley, 2008). Receptive language focuses on understanding meaning that is read, heard, or viewed. Expressive language focuses on creating meaning through writing, speaking, and/or drawing. Finally, background knowledge is the knowledge that is necessary to understand and create meaning (Table 5–1). Because of the importance assigned to reading and writing, we will concentrate our attention on these two domains, and the importance of background knowledge for reading and writing in a second language.

Table 5–1. *Literacy Attributes*

Area	Domains

Receptive Language	Reading—can make sense of what it is read
	   – understands what is read
	   – decodes fluently
	   – understands different types of text
	   – understands big ideas
	   – understands vocabulary
	   – applies comprehension strategies
	   – reads extensively
	
	Listening—can make sense of what it is heard
	   – is a critical and responsive listener
	
	Viewing—can make sense of what is observed
	   – is a critical and responsive viewer

Expressive Language	Writing—can express ideas in written form
	   – communicates ideas effectively
	   – demonstrates effective language/style
	   – organizes and develops writing adequately
	   – uses appropriate mechanics
	
	Speaking—can express ideas in spoken form
	   – communicates ideas effectively
	
	Representing—can express ideas in a variety of media (drawing, photography, etc.)
	   – communicates ideas effectively

Background Knowledge	Knowledge of the world *– understands the world around and beyond himself/herself*

Source: Data from *Closing the Circle: A Practical Guide to Implementing Literacy Reform, K–12*, by S. A. Walmsley, 2008, San Francisco, CA: Jossey-Bass.

Receptive Language: The L2 Reading Domain

Reading: Definition and Purpose

Reading is a cognitive process that involves the comprehension of written messages. During this process, the reader not only receives, but also interprets language that is encoded in print. It is very important to emphasize the interdependence of the three literacy attributes as noted by Walmsley (2008). Reading comprehension takes place when the reader decodes the information contained in the text in written form and utilizes background knowledge to integrate and interpret the decoded information.

Why do readers read? There are many purposes for reading. Readers read for enjoyment, to locate specific information, or to learn new information. Let us focus on two other important purposes of reading: reading for comprehension and reading to learn. When readers read novels, or newspaper articles, they read for enjoyment or pleasure. In that case, readers read for general comprehension or to get the "gist" of the text. Readers who read for pleasure are not preoccupied with remembering all the important details for a later recall task.

To develop proficiency in casual reading and related comprehension takes time, but this type of reading and comprehension is usually an effortless process. It does not mean that reading for comprehension is easy; rather, fluent readers have achieved reading fluency as a result of considerable (in both time and quantity) extended reading, which ultimately lead to automaticity of reading processes, such as word recognition, meaning formation, and strategies for constructing meaning for unknown words. Reading for comprehension is essential and provides the foundation for other reading purposes, such as reading to learn. In academic contexts, probably the most important purpose for reading is reading to acquire new information. However, it is not the only purpose of academic reading. Many times, EL and non-EL students read to search for specific information. In that case, they skim and scan through texts to find out, for example, a specific date a historical event occurred, or the name of the person who wrote a famous novel, or the researchers who created a life-saving medicine. Nevertheless, most of the time students read to learn new information with the purpose of using it in a related academic task either immediately following the reading or in the near future.

Reading to learn involves not only the comprehension of the main themes or ideas presented in a text, but also the recall of the critical supporting ideas and details. The need to process all this information in an attempt to learn results in a slower rate of reading fluency in comparison to reading fluency associated with general comprehension. When students read to learn, in addition to reading for understanding the main idea of a text, they use supporting information, create outlines that organize information by cause and effect and/or compare and contrast, and use their prior knowledge consciously.

Reading in L1 and L2: Similarities and Differences

Early literacy development in a first language is well documented for young children. We have information about young children's early literacy development in English, Spanish, and other languages (Peregoy & Boyle, 2005). However, there is a need for research that documents early literacy development in English as a second language (Lesaux & Siegel, 2003). Specifically, information is lacking about students who have never had literacy instruction in their first language (Freeman, Freeman, & Mercuri, 2002). Yet, research has demonstrated that English reading and writing development processes are essentially similar for both English learners and native English speakers (Edelsky, 1981; Hudelson, 1984). Although many aspects of reading and writing development are basically similar for English learners and native English speakers, there are important differences. To obtain information about reading in L1 and L2 literacy research has posed the following questions: Is reading in L1 similar to reading in L2? Do ELs go through the same processes when they read as non-ELs?

Several researchers have supported a reading universal hypothesis, which affirms that reading processes in L2 are very similar to reading processes in L1 (Goodman & Goodman, 1994; National Reading Panel, 2000). Goodman (1979) has stated that reading processes are very much the same in all languages, and variation occurs simply due to specific characteristics of the writing system particular to one language, or perhaps its grammatical structure. There are, indeed universals of reading abilities, as identified by Grabe (2009). The first one relates to the cognitive nature of reading. All readers utilize pattern-recognition skills, working memory, and long-term memory. Therefore, reading in L1, as well as reading in L2, is a cognitive process.

Second, all writing systems are based on spoken language and phonological decoding is an essential element of reading in all languages, including those that do not use alphabetical script. Research that has focused on reading in Chinese has shown that phonological awareness is a predictor of Chinese abilities. For example, one aspect of phonological awareness in Chinese, syllable awareness, seems to be very strongly related to the ability to read Chinese characters (Chow, McBride-Chang, & Burgess, 2005). When comparing alphabetical and nonalphabetical languages, ELs whose L1 is alphabetical, e.g., Spanish or French, seem to be better at acquiring the letter-to-sound correspondence of English than ELs whose first language is non-alphabetical (Bialystok, 2001). Alphabetical languages have a much stronger letter-to-sound correspondence. After ELs acquire an alphabetical system in their L1, their phonological awareness will transfer to an alphabetical L2, even when the sound-to-letter relationship is not clear, as is the case in English.

The third universal of reading abilities is the extent to which transfer in L2 reading is facilitated by the similarities between L1 and L2. When L1 and L2 share similar linguistic properties, L2 reading comprehension is vastly improved. For example, in a research study conducted by Muljani, Koda, and Moates (1998), Indonesian students speaking Indonesian Bahasa were faster in English word recognition than Chinese students were because of their previous alphabetical experiences, especially when the English words conformed to the syllable structures of their L1. Finally, reading processes in all languages rely on background knowledge and culture socialization in order to make sense of print and incorporate the new information into existing knowledge and linguistic systems.

There is strong evidence of similarities between reading in L1 and reading in L2, but not an absolute congruence between the two. The fundamental difference between the two processes is revealed in the nature of L2 reading. Reading in L2 involves two languages. They continuously interact and make reading in L2 more complex than reading in L1 (Koda, 2007). In most cases, ELs who start reading in L2 already bring to the reading process their L1 language background. However, L2 reading is not just a transfer of ELs' first language abilities (Durgunoglu, 1998; Leafstedt & Gerber, 2005; Mathes et al., 2007). Although L1 plays an important role in L2 reading proficiency, many issues of L2 reading development are often associated with L2 language proficiency, L2 language and print exposure, and L2 processing skills development. In fact, these issues are the important differences between reading in L1 and reading in L2.

In a survey of many years of research on L2 reading, the National Literacy Panel on Language-Minority Children and Youth (August & Shanahan, 2006) synthesized nearly 300 studies into a number of important findings on L2 reading. Their review of studies showed that first and second language speakers learning to read can develop word-level literacy, i.e., decoding and spelling, at equal levels. A disparity exists, however, in text-level skills. For example, L2 readers do not attain reading comprehension at the same level as L1 readers. They also found that second language oral proficiency is essential for L2 reading comprehension. This includes vocabulary knowledge, listening comprehension, syntactic skills, and metalinguistic knowledge. The panel determined that second language readers have additional factors involved in reading comprehension in the L2, such as L1 literacy and L2 oral proficiency. Certain errors occur because of differences between L1 and L2; however, research has also demonstrated that literacy skills in L1 facilitate L2 literacy development (Calderon, 2007; Cardenas-Hagan, Carlson, & Pollard-Durodola, 2007; Vaugh et al., 2006). Some language transfer issues are more likely to affect L2 literacy development than others and at certain stages of literacy development. Understanding how the first language of Spanish speakers, the majority of ELs in the United States, is different from English can shed light on this issue.

Contrasting the Spanish sound system with the English sound system illustrates how the native language can transfer to the L2, resulting in errors in reading and spelling (Bear, Invernizzi, Templeton, & Johnston, 2004). For example, there are English vowel sounds that do not exist in Spanish, such as the vowels /æ/, as in the word "man," or /ɛ/, as in "pen." English let-ters that represent different sounds in Spanish are another area of contrast. For example, the letter "a" as in "cake" is represented by the sound /e/ in Spanish and, similarly, the letter "e" as in "bean" is the sound /i/ in Spanish.

In addition to L1 transfer, sociocultural variables have an effect on reading (August & Shanahan, 2006). Six variables were identified in their review of studies: immigration status, discourse/interactional characteristics, other specific sociocul-tural variables, parent and family influences, district, state, and federal policies, and language prestige. The research indicated that mediating home/school interaction differences improves students' engagement in classroom instruction. In addition, cul-turally familiar texts facilitate comprehension, although it is a weak predictor compared to proficiency in the language of the text. Moreover, it was found that schools do not take full advan-tage of parents' potential contributions.

In terms of instructional factors in ELs' literacy develop-ment, it appears that the same components of literacy instruction that apply to first language learners apply to second language learners, particularly at the word level. Interestingly, instruc-tional practices that are successful with both L1 and L2 learners do not improve literacy skills for ELs as much as their Eng-lish-speaking peers. The exception to this finding is vocabulary instruction, which seems to yield greater benefits for ELs than native speakers.

Oral English proficiency is necessary for reading in Eng-lish, and literacy instruction should include the development of listening and speaking skills. Research has demonstrated this because L2 learners with strong L1 reading skills do not read at the same levels in English as their native-speaking peers. A commonality between L1 and L2 readers is the basic sequence of the development of reading skills, beginning with decoding and moving to comprehension at later stages. Throughout this sequence, vocabulary instruction is critical. Taking advantage of ELs' native language oral proficiency has been shown to benefit their L2 reading development — specifically, instructing ELs to read in their native language leads to better outcomes in reading in English at both the elementary and secondary levels.

Learning to Read and Reading to Learn: A Key Distinction

There are more differences than similarities between reading in L1 and reading in L2 (Anderson, 2008; National Reading Panel, 2000). Although the National Reading Panel Report (2000) did not focus on preventing reading failure in ELs, they did identify effective practices in five areas of reading instruction: phonemic awareness, phonics, fluency, vocabulary, and text comprehension. Related to the findings identified by the National Literacy Panel, Anderson (2008) identified six key factors that influence L2 literacy for ELs: literacy in L1, oral language proficiency in L2, age of arrival in US, expectations of the school experience, types of L2 readers, and parents' educational levels. Language professionals need to know how literate ELs are in L1 and their level of oral fluency in English. Oral proficiency, discussed later in this chapter, is an asset in developing reading proficiency.

Anderson and Nunan (2008) depict the learning/reading continuum, as shown in Figure 5–2. For L1 readers, grades K–3 mark the "learning to read" period; once L1 readers are in fourth grade and beyond, they are "reading to learn." For L2 readers, we can't assume that reading has been fully developed in K–3. Regardless of the age of the learner, when working with ELs at beginning levels of language proficiency, all professionals involved in literacy need to assist students to learn to read. From intermediate levels of language proficiency on, these professionals can also aid in reading to learn.

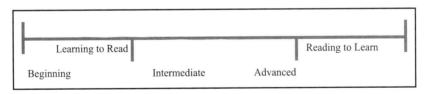

Figure 5–2. *Learning/reading continuum.* Source: *From* Practical English Language Teaching: PELT, *by N. Andersen & D. Nunan, 2008, New York, NY: McGraw-Hill, p. 58. Copyright 2008 by the McGraw-Hill Companies. Reprinted with permission.*

According to Anderson (2009), there are four similarities and ten differences in L1 and L2 readers. Similarities in L1 and L2 reading processes include the involvement of:

◆ the reader, text, and context;
◆ metacognitive strategies;
◆ bottom-up (for example, decoding) and top-down (for example, inferential reasoning) strategies; and
◆ language systems with systematic and rule-governed structures.

Differences include:

◆ specific language system contrasts;
◆ vocabulary knowledge in L1 and L2;
◆ language awareness in L1 and L2;
◆ the amount of time necessary to learn to read;
◆ reading rate (L2 readers read more slowly);
◆ motivation;
◆ oral English proficiency;
◆ background knowledge;
◆ learning context; and
◆ position on the literacy continuum.

The general characteristics of first and second language learners are summarized and contrasted in Table 5–2.

We have noted the importance of literacy in L1 and language proficiency in L2 reading research. Given the importance of the relationship between these two necessary key components, this chapter explores that relationship; however, it asserts that these components are not sufficient for EL reading proficiency in L2.

L2 Reading: Language Problem (Short-Circuit/ Threshold Hypothesis) or Reading Problem (Interdependence Hypothesis)?

There are important differences between reading in L1 and reading in L2. To address this question scholars have posed the following question: when ELs struggle with reading in a sec-

Table 5–2. *Differences in Learning to Read Between L1 and L2 Readers*

L1 (English-speaking) Literacy Learners	L2 (English learners) Literacy Learners
Developing communicative competence in one-language system	Developing communicative competence in two-language systems
Can comprehend and express information orally in language of literacy development	Different degrees of ability to comprehend and express information orally in language of literacy instruction
May already possess precursor literacy skills in language of literacy development	May already possess precursor literacy skills in L2 that can be transferred to L1 literacy
Use a set of strategies to improve comprehension in language of instruction	Use a set of strategies that may include L1 to improve comprehension in language of instruction
Knows only one language system	May experience negative transfer (interference) from the native language when it contrasts with the L2; may experience positive transfer from native language (e.g., cognates) or may be more sensitive to language issues due to knowledge of two systems

Source: From *Reading in a Second Language: Moving from Theory to Practice*, by W. Grabe, 2009, New York, NY: Cambridge University Press, pp. 648–650. Copyright 2009 by Cambridge University Press. Adapted with permission.

ond language, is that due to a language problem or a reading problem? In other words, do EL readers have comprehension problems when reading in English because of low proficiency in English or because of poor reading skills in their first language?

According to Alderson (1984), ELs who have been exposed only to English instruction have experienced low academic achievement and literacy levels in both languages. In contrast, ELs who have been exposed to instruction in both their L1 and English have demonstrated high academic and cognitive achievement. Additionally, instruction in ELs' native language has positively influenced ELs' academic development in English and has facilitated transfer of academic skills and knowledge across languages.

To address whether a difficulty with L2 reading is a language problem or a reading problem, two hypotheses have been proposed: the short circuit hypothesis or linguistic threshold hypothesis (Cummins, 1976) and the linguistic interdependence hypothesis (Cummins, 1979). The short circuit hypothesis or linguistic threshold hypothesis identifies language proficiency as the key factor in determining the success of reading tasks in L2. This hypothesis suggests that EL readers must achieve a certain level of English proficiency in order to be able to comprehend what they read in L2. Even if EL readers have strong literacy skills in their first language, those skills do not necessarily translate to reading skills in English. Thus, a lack of English language knowledge will hinder access to English language reading knowledge. Several studies are summarized in Table 5–3 and have explicitly investigated the influence of second language proficiency on second language reading.

Although there is evidence to support a relationship between language proficiency in L2 and reading ability in L2, there are a variety of complicating factors. Reading is a complex process and the concept of linguistic threshold is not easy to operationalize, isolate from other factors, or quantify. To operationalize the concept of linguistic threshold one has to consider that reading in English is a very dynamic process and differs depending on whether ELs are children, adolescent, or adults. What a young EL is able to transfer from L1 into L2 is very different from what an adult EL can transfer, both in quantity and quality. These considerations require more research that will account for all the aspects of the ever-changing relationship between L2 proficiency and L2 reading.

The second hypothesis is the linguistic interdependence hypothesis (Cummins, 1979). This hypothesis disputes the claim that difficulty reading in L2 is purely a language problem. According to this hypothesis, proficiency in reading in a second language is shared with the reading ability ELs have in their first language. The premise is that when ELs reading in the first

Table 5–3. Research Evidence for the Linguistic Threshold Hypothesis

Study	Description
Yamashita (2002)	241 Japanese students participated in the study, which examined L1 literacy, L2 language proficiency, and L2 reading. L1 literacy and L2 language proficiency accounted for 40% of reading ability in L2. Additionally, the L2 language proficiency was a much stronger predictor of L2 reading comprehension than literacy in L1.
Schoonen, Hulstijn, and Bossers (1998)	The study, which involved 274 adolescent Dutch students, looked at the relationship among L1 reading abilities, L2 vocabulary, metacognitive knowledge, and L2 reading. The researchers found that, at lower levels of English proficiency, knowledge of English vocabulary is a very strong predictor of English reading ability. At high proficiency levels in English, metacognitive knowledge, which involves awareness of and knowledge one's own thinking processes, was a much stronger predictor of reading ability in English.
Lee and Schallert (1997)	809 adolescent Korean students learning English participated in the study. The study examined the influence of L1 reading proficiency and L2 language proficiency on L2 reading comprehension and found that 56% of L2 reading comprehension was explained by L2 language proficiency and only 30% by L1 literacy. Also, the study revealed higher correlations between L1 and L2 reading and higher levels of L2 proficiency than at lower levels.
Perkins, Brutten, and Pohlman (1989)	The study had 174 Japanese students and looked at the relationship among L1 literacy, L2 language proficiency, and L2 reading. The findings revealed strong correlations between proficiency in L2 and comprehension in L2, and weak correlations between L1 and L2 literacy.

language attain a certain level of proficiency, then that reading proficiency will transfer to L2 reading (Cummins, 1979; 2000). In other words, ELs who are literate in their first language simply need to learn English words and sentences, because cognitive skills required to be a proficient reader in English will transfer from the first language into English. At the core of this hypothesis is the belief that second language reading skills are fundamentally interdependent or the same as the skills ELs already have as a result of acquiring their L1 reading skills. Table 5–4 summarizes several studies that investigated the relationship between L1 reading skills and L2 reading comprehension.

These two hypotheses can have positive and negative influences on educational decisions made about ELs. If we concur with the linguistic threshold hypothesis and consider language proficiency as the most important factor in achieving reading proficiency in L2, then ELs would need to have a strong command of spoken English prior to initiating reading instruction in English. However, if we agree with the linguistic interdependence hypothesis and consider second language reading simply as a transfer of first language reading skills, then ELs will not need instruction in second language reading because ELs who are literate in their L1 can become literate in English with little effort.

To better understand the initial question of whether a difficulty with second language reading is a language problem or a reading problem, Bernhardt and Kamil (1995) reframed the question as follows: How much English language knowledge do ELs have to have in order to make their L2 literacy knowledge work? What should be the extent of EL literacy in L1 so that ELs can make their English language knowledge work? Reframing the question in this way eliminates the potential dichotomy between the two hypotheses and addresses the issue of accountability. The question then is: how much does second language knowledge and (not "or") first language literacy account for EL reading performance in English?

An L2 Reading Model

Restating the second language reading question and focusing on accountability allows us to acknowledge the contribution of

Table 5–4. *Research Evidence for the Linguistic Interdependence Hypothesis*

Study	Description
van Gelderen, Schonnen, Stoel, de Glopper, and Hulstijn (2007)	This study investigated the relationship between reading comprehension development of 389 Dutch adolescents in Dutch and English. Students' reading comprehension, their linguistic and metacognitive knowledge, and processing efficiency were measured. The findings showed a very strong relationship between L1 and L2 reading comprehension, L1 reading proficiency being a much stronger predictor of reading comprehension in English than the other variables assessed.
Durgunoglu (1998)	The study looked at 46 first graders enrolled in two bilingual classes in the United States. The data revealed that 47% of the variance in English (L2) phonological awareness was explained by Spanish (L1) phonological awareness. Additionally, Spanish phonological awareness and letter recognition explained 84% of the variance in English spelling performance. Strong correlations were reported between Spanish word recognition and English word recognition and Spanish spelling and English word recognition.
Verhoeven and Aarts (1998)	188 Turkish-speaking students learning Dutch participated in this study, which examined the relationship between school literacy and functional literacy. The functional literacy assessment was based on newspapers, maps, application forms, letters, etc. The analysis of data showed that the literacy level in Turkish has an effect on literacy level in Dutch.
Umbel and Oller (1994)	This study looked at vocabulary acquisition processes of 102 English-Spanish first, third, and sixth graders who were native speakers of Spanish. The findings showed that Spanish vocabulary knowledge represented 27% of the variance in English vocabulary knowledge, making Spanish receptive vocabulary development the stronger predictor of English receptive vocabulary scores.

each component of L2 reading performance. Research conducted with this focus has suggested that contribution of L2 knowledge to L2 reading is approximately 30%, whereas the contribution of L1 literacy to L2 reading proficiency is between 14% and 21% (Bernhardt & Kamil, 1995; Bossers, 1991; Brisbois, 1995; Carrell, 1991; Hacquebord, 1989). Undeniably, these two variables (L2 proficiency and L1 literacy) account for a very important part of the variance in second language reading; however, they do not capture the entire spectrum of the development of second language reading at different proficiency levels. They do, however, emphasize that more research needs to be conducted to account for the remaining 50%. Bernhardt (2005) has proposed a compensatory processing approach that takes these critical considerations into account. His model offers an explanation of how established knowledge sources assist or even take over when other knowledge sources are not adequate or do not exist. Bernhardt's compensatory model, illustrated in Figure 5–3, has three dimensions: L1 literacy, L2 knowledge, and unexplained variance. For emerging L2 readers, the contribution of each element is almost equal. However, when ELs move to a more advanced level of L2 literacy and become readers acquiring L2 literacy, L1 literacy contributes 20% to L2 reading comprehension, whereas L2 knowledge contributes 30% to reading comprehension. The remaining 50% consists of unexplained variance, such as interest, motivation, engagement, and so forth.

The Relationship Between Oral Language Proficiency and Reading Proficiency for ELs and ELs with Communication Disorders

In the discussion of Bernhardt's reading model, we noted that L2 knowledge explains a significant part of L2 reading competence. Additionally, the findings of the National Literacy Panel on Language-Minority Children and Youth (August & Shanahan, 2006) revealed the importance of oral language proficiency in developing literacy in the second language. To better understand the relationship between oral language proficiency and reading proficiency for ELs and ELs with communication disorders, this chap-

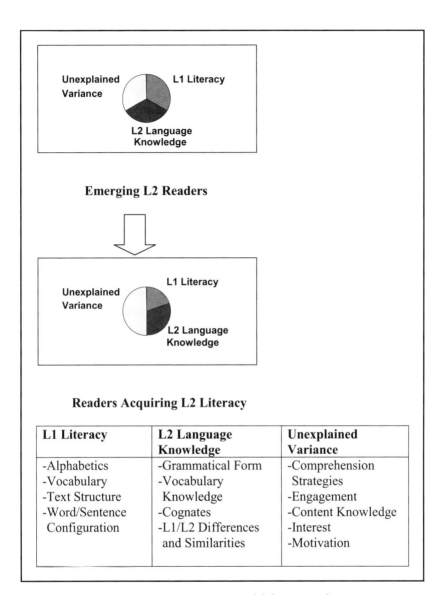

Figure 5–3. *Bernhardt's compensatory model for L2 reading.* Source: *From "Progress and Procrastination in Second Language Reading," by E. Bernhardt, 2005,* Annual Review of Applied Linguistics, 25, *p. 140, Figure 2. Copyright 2005 by Cambridge University Press. Adapted with permission.*

ter examines the research on oral proficiency in L1 and literacy in L2. Table 5–5 summarizes research on word-level skills (word and pseudoword reading in English), and Table 5–6 lists studies focusing on text-level skills (reading comprehension in English).

Based on the evidence found in Table 5–5, it is important to note that L1 phonological processing skills are closely related

Table 5–5. L1 *Oral Proficiency and L2 Word-Level Skills*

Study	Description
Mumtaz and Humphreys (2002)	The participants were 7- and 9-year-old Urdu-English bilingual students. The study found that rhyme detection and phonological memory in Urdu correlated significantly with word-level reading skills in English.
Gottardo, Yan, Siegel, and Wade-Woolley (2001)	The participants were Cantonese-speaking EL students in grades 1 through 8. Phonemic awareness in Cantonese correlated significantly with word and pseudoword reading skills in English.
Gholamain and Geva (1999)	The participants were Farsi-speaking ELs in grades 1 through 5. Verbal working memory and rapid automized naming, assessed in the first language (Farsi), accounted for significant variance in the students' word and pseudoword reading scored in English, in spite of the orthographic differences between the two languages.
Abu-Rabia (1997)	The participants were Hebrew-speaking tenth grade ELs. The study found that L1 oral language proficiency did not correlate with the ELs' performance on English word reading tasks, such as word attack and word recognition.
Da Fontoura and Siegel (1995)	The participants were Portuguese-speaking ELs attending a Portuguese heritage language program The study found that L1 did not correlate with English word or pseudoword reading.

to the development of reading skills in English. However, oral proficiency in ELs' native language does not correlate with English reading skills. Most of the studies in Table 5–6 examining the influence of L1 oral proficiency (measured through self-ratings or language use) and English reading comprehension

Table 5–6. *Oral Proficiency in L1 and L2 Text-Level Skills*

Study	Description
Nguyen, Shin, and Krashen (2001)	The study examined the relationship between first language oral proficiency and reading outcomes and did not find a relationship between L1 proficiency and general L2 reading achievement.
Dufva and Voeten (1999)	The study focused on English reading comprehension skills of third grade Finnish-speaking students who were learning English in school. The study reported that the students' listening comprehension skills in Finnish assessed in first grade had an indirect effect on English reading comprehension scores and the students' phonological memory, assessed in second grade, correlated significantly with English reading comprehension.
Royer and Carlo (1991)	The participants were middle school Spanish-speaking ELs in a transitional bilingual education program. The study found no significant correlation between the students' Spanish listening comprehension skills and their English reading comprehension.
Buriel and Cardoza (1988)	The participants were ninth grade Spanish-speaking EL students. The study looked at the relationship between self-reports of L1 proficiency and English reading comprehension. For first- and second-generation Mexican American high school ELs, there were no significant relationships between L1 proficiency and English reading comprehension. For third-generation Mexican American students, there were negative relationships between L1 proficiency and English reading.

found little or no relationship between the two. However, there have been studies that noted that phonological memory and other components are directly associated with the development of English reading comprehension (Dufva and Voeten, 1999).

Another dimension of oral proficiency worthy of investigation with regard to literacy development in L2 is oral proficiency in a second language. Three studies that focus primarily on speakers of Spanish are used to discuss the relationship between reading in English and English oral language. The first study investigated the relationship between Spanish oral language proficiency, Spanish phonological awareness, and English word and pseudoword reading skills (Durgunoglu, Nagy, & Hancin-Bhatt, 1993). English language proficiency was measured in three areas of oral language: morphology, syntax, and semantics. The results of this study revealed that English language proficiency was not a statistically significant predictor of effective English word and pseudoword reading. However, Spanish phonological awareness was significant for beginning L2 readers. Gottardo (2002) also studied the relationship between language skills in L2 (semantic and syntactic processing and phonological awareness) and word reading skills of Spanish-speaking ELs. This study showed that English oral proficiency correlated significantly with ELs' performance on English word reading tasks.

In a different study, Quiroga, Lemos-Britten, Mostafapour, Abbott, and Berninger (2002) examined first-grade Spanish-English bilinguals who had not had systematic reading instruction in Spanish. The study found that there was a modest correlation between ELs' oral proficiency in English and their word and pseudoword reading in English. Moreover, the researcher found a strong correlation between phonological awareness and English word and pseudoword decoding in the case of a phoneme-deletion task.

One possible explanation of the discrepancy in the findings presented in the first study and the findings of the second and third study is offered by Geva (2006). In the first study, the children were in a transitional bilingual program and the assumption is that they had fewer opportunities to develop their English language skills. In contrast, the ELs in the second and third studies were taught exclusively in English and presumably had more opportunities to develop their English proficiency.

Studies that focus on the relationship between L2 oral language proficiency and reading ability in L2 in ELs with communication disorders are necessary. It is well-known that a large number of ELs are overrepresented in specific special education categories (e.g., learning disabilities, speech and language impairments) because they demonstrate limited English proficiency. It is recommended that professionals who work with ELs be familiar with the characteristics of the second language acquisition process and consider how these often mirror the characteristics of a learning disability (Gonzales, 2007; Kohnert, 2008; Paradis, 2005; Roseberry-McKibben & O'Hanlon, 2005). Professionals should be familiar with the behaviors commonly observed among students learning a second language and students with communication disorders to prevent inappropriate identification and mislabeling of ELs.

It is important to note that ELs' rate of English oral language proficiency differs by the age of introduction to English and their use of English. In general, according to MacSwan and Pray (2005), Spanish-speaking ELs entering kindergarten with little or no English become orally proficient in English by the time they reach fourth or fifth grade. When looking at the length of time required to become proficient in English, Pray (2003) found no statistical differences between bilingual students enrolled in special education and bilingual students enrolled in general education programs. Pray (2009) also looked at oral language use among ELs diagnosed with a learning disability and ELs in general education. All the participants in the study were native speakers of Spanish. The errors in the oral tasks performed by the two groups in both Spanish and English were categorized as syntactic errors ("The car white is going fast"), morphological errors ("ated," "a elephant"), and lexical errors (using the word "can" when the item was a bottle). In the case of oral performance in Spanish, the findings revealed that 95% of all students showed a Spanish morphological error ratio of 5% or less and a lexical error ratio of 2% or less. Error ratio was defined as the ratio of the number of erroneously rendered items to the total number of items. Only one participant who was diagnosed as having a learning disability showed an error ratio of more than 10%. However, that participant made no English lexical errors and had only a 3% morphological error ratio in English. This particular case showed that some children in special education may experience a loss in their first language while making important gains in the second language.

Specific to English oral performance, all students demonstrated an English morphological error ratio of 5% or less, and an English lexical error ratio of 3% or less. It is interesting to note that one student diagnosed with a learning disability had an English morphological error rate of 7% (which could be considered within the range of normal performance parameters) but did not have morphological errors in Spanish oral production. This study pointed out that there were significant differences between ELs in special education and ELs in general education: ELs who were diagnosed with a learning disability made proportionally more errors than ELs enrolled in general classrooms. However, 95% of all ELs regardless of their status showed an English morphological error ratio of less than 6% and a lexical error rate of less than 3%. In other words, according to the data collected on their English oral proficiency, a vast majority of the ELs participating in the study showed they had mastered the fundamentals of English morphology and syntax.

Although there is a paucity of studies that address the language of instruction and the impact on oral L1 in general (e.g., Kan & Kohnert, 2005) or studies that examine the English oral proficiency of ELs with communication disorders, researchers have provided preliminary and essential data on factors to consider when working with students at risk for language and literacy development (Gutierrez, Restrepo, Bedore, Pena, & Anderson, 2000; Restrepo, 1998; Restrepo & Kruth, 2000; Restrepo et al., 2010; Simon-Cereijido & Gutierrez-Clellen, 2007). For example, in a qualitative study conducted by Gutierrez-Clellen and DeCurtis (1999), the Spanish word definition skills of Spanish-speaking children with and without language impairment were compared. Their findings revealed several differences in word definition skills between Spanish-speaking students with and without language impairment (LI). Children without LI had the tendency to use formal definitions more than children with LI. The study also showed a large variation within the groups. Formal definitions represented between 10 and 70% of the word definitions generated by the students without LI, and these were attributed to individual school experiences. Therefore, the limited use of formal definitions by students with LI was proposed to be related to differences in access to educational opportunities that facilitate language development.

This study offers two important recommendations in the area of assessment. First, language tests should include in their word definition tasks nouns that are concrete and familiar. Often tests do not include such words and really are measures of vocabulary knowledge and not vocabulary definition skills. Moreover, many tests emphasize the correctness of the word definition, meaning the focus is on the content of the definition associated with the word to be defined. Instead, tests should take into account the quality or communicative adequacy of the definitions produced by students. There is a need for an evaluation protocol that will consider how well the definitions meet expectations for specificity and relevance, and the amount of information contained in the word definitions produced by students. This will help determine whether more emphasis is necessary on definition skill development or content development and which instructional strategy would yield better results with ELs.

Expressive Language: The Writing Domain

Writing: Definition and Purposes

Writing has been defined as the act of creating original text using the individual's intellectual and linguistic resources, rather than using someone else's text, a prepared list of words to create sentences or stories, filling in the blanks, or practicing handwriting. Writing is made of letters or symbols that are imprinted on a surface to represent the sounds of a language (Hudelson, 1988). Writing is a tremendous challenge for ELs. They are required to develop novel ideas and express these ideas using new words that they are often learning in the new language. Current research has provided insight about children's native language writing development (August & Shanahan, 2006; Li & Edwards, 2010). From early childhood, children work to make sense of written language. They make predictions about how written language works and create texts based on these predictions. The text changes as the child's understanding of and predictions about written language evolve (Peregoy & Boyle,

2005). Studies of the writing development of native speakers influenced other researchers to investigate the writing development of ELs. The most general conclusion reached by researchers (Edelsky, 1986; Hudelson, 1986, 1987; Samway, 1987; Urzua, 1987) is that the process of writing is similar for first and second language writers. Hudelson (1988) offers the following conclusions about writing development in ELs: (1) they can write and create their own meaning as they are learning English; (2) they can respond to the works of others and use another learner's responses to their work to make substantive revisions in their writing; (3) texts produced by ELs are similar to those produced by young native speakers; (4) they approach writing and develop as writers differently from one another; (5) the classroom environment has a significant impact on their development as writers; (6) culture may affect the writers' view of writing, of the functions or purposes for writing, and of themselves as writers; and (7) the ability to write in the native language facilitates ELs' writing in several different ways. Native language writing provides learners with information about the purposes of writing. Writing ability in the native language provides ELs with linguistic and nonlinguistic resources that they can use as they approach second language writing. In addition, ELs apply the knowledge about writing gained in first language settings to second language settings.

Grabe (2001) proposed six purposes of writing. First, we write to learn the mechanical production aspect, to practice motor coordination. For this purpose, minimal fluency is required. Copying sentences from a textbook simply to learn and practice the shape of letters is an example. Second, we write to list, repeat, or paraphrase. This is not composing, it is simply stating knowledge. One example is when we write extended notes to ourselves. The third purpose of writing is to understand, remember, and summarize processes that require composing and recounting. Fourth, we write to solve problems, learn, and synthesize. When we do engage in that type of task we compose and transform already available text. The fifth purpose of writing is to critique, persuade, or interpret. Academic writing where we use evidence selectively but appropriately is an illustration of this purpose. The sixth purpose of writing is to create an aesthetic experience. Fiction writers and poets adhere to this sixth purpose. They compose in new ways and do not follow writing conventions to the letter; however, the results are effective.

Britton (1975) describes three kinds of writing that are similar to those proposed by Grabe (2001). The three kinds of writing are transactional, expressive, and poetic.

> Transactional writing is used "to get things done." Its purpose is to inform, advise, persuade, or instruct. In short, it is a means to an end. A second category is expressive. This is language "close to the self," often a kind of "thinking aloud" on paper. It reflects the writer's immediate thoughts and feelings; it is relaxed and familiar rather than formal; and allows the writer to take risk. We frame the tentative first drafts of new ideas . . . where in times of crisis . . . we attempt to work our way towards some kind of a resolution. A third category, the poetic, is language used as an art form, and it exists for its own sake. (Britton, 1975, p. 88)

Similarities and Differences Between Writing in L1 and L2

Just like reading in a second language, writing in a second language is different than writing in a first language. Scott (1991) articulated a very important distinction between L1 and L2 writing. When writing in L1, we create ideas and then find the words to express them. In a L2 writing process, we do the opposite; we look at the available words in L2 and then we generate ideas based on them. ELs, new to English, usually experience some challenges in expressive written language with vocabulary, syntax, and idiomatic expressions. ELs also may not have had the exposure to written English that comes from reading or being read to. Therefore, they may not understand the way that English conventionally translates into the written form. Some ELs may have experience writing in their native language that can facilitate writing in English. Research has suggested that ELs are able to read and write in the second language prior to having obtained proficiency over the phonological, syntactic, and semantic systems of spoken English (Hudelson, 1984; Peregoy & Boyle, 1991).

At first, the two processes look very similar because writers in both L1 and L2 follow similar protocols in developing their ideas on paper: they all plan, write, and revise. For example,

Matsumoto (1995) interviewed four Japanese university professors on the strategies they used when writing a research paper in English. The analysis of data showed that those writers followed the same processes and used the same strategies across L1 and L2 writing. Beare (2000) investigated the inventory of strategies used to plan and generate content for proficient bilingual writers and whether the writing strategies in L1 writing differed from L2 writing in the context of generating content and planning. Her findings indicated that bilingual writers used the same strategies in L1 as in L2 writing (brainstorming, writing drafts, rereading, etc.). According to Berman (1994), writers transfer their skills from L1 to L2, indicating that writers' thoughts are not restricted to a particular language and are able to transfer across languages. Consequently, because many ELs come with writing skills in their first language, they are able to transfer those skills when they write in English. In an experimental study, Berman (1994) found that ELs' success in transferring writing skills was assisted by their grammatical proficiency in the target language, which was English.

In light of the similarities between writing in L1 and writing in L2, L2 writing practitioners might be inclined to simply adopt practices from L1 writing when teaching L2 writing. However, there are important differences that need to be taken into account so SLPs and ESOL professionals can make sound decisions in adapting practices that work for native English speakers to ELs and ELs with communication disorders.

Silva (1993) examined the distinct nature of second language writing in a meta-analysis of approximately 70 research reports that examined over 27 different first languages. The findings were divided into two categories: the writing process and written text features. In terms of the writing process, Silva's (1993) analysis showed that, overall, when writing in the second language, L2 writers did less planning than L1 writers. More attention was devoted to generating writing material, but it was more difficult and time-consuming. A lot of time was dedicated to understanding the topic and many of the generated ideas were not found in the final written product. In the actual production of written text in L2, the task was more laborious, less fluent, and less productive. L2 writers spent more time going back to the outline or prompt, and consulting a dictionary when it was allowed. L2 writers wrote at a slower rate and generated fewer words of written text. An examination of the last stage in the writing process, "reviewing," it was revealed that L2 writers did less rereading of and reflecting on the written text. Similar patterns and strategies were reported in L1 and L2 reading, but revisions in L2 were less frequent compared with revisions in L1. The L2 revision was more difficult and focused more on grammar and less on mechanics (e.g., spelling).

The analysis of written text features showed various differences in fluency, accuracy, quality, and structure. For fluency, the majority of research evidence pointed out that L2 writing is less fluent than L1 writing. The research also showed that L2 writers made more errors in their writing, rendering it less accurate than writing in L1. Additionally, a large number of studies reviewed by Silva (1993) stated that L2 writers were less effective and received lower overall scores when their writing was graded holistically by native English speakers. The findings discussing the differences in structure between L1 and L2 writing are summarized in Table 5–7.

In summary, L2 writing research shows that L2 writing is distinct from L1 writing. Although general composing processes are similar in L1 and L2, L2 composing is more difficult and less effective. Writing production in L2 is more time-consuming but less fluent and productive. L2 writers review and reread their writing less, revise more, and such revisions are done with more difficulty. L2 texts are less fluent, contain more language errors, and are not as effective as the texts generated by proficient English writers. Reader orientation of L2 texts is often considered less acceptable and appropriate. In terms of style, L2 writing is simpler in structure and distinct stylistically. The clauses are longer but fewer, and there is more coordination and less subordination. Overall, L2 texts show less lexical control, variety, and sophistication.

The Structure of English Writing: A Contrastive Rhetoric Approach

In his seminal study that set the foundation for the discipline of contrastive rhetoric, Kaplan (1966) described the thought

Table 5–7. *L1/L2 Differences in Written Structure*

Category	Findings
Argument Structure	L2 writers did not state and support their position fully and had the tendency to develop their arguments by restating their position. L2 arguments had fewer paragraphs and connectors, and contained more errors. Some L2 writers preferred a "situation + problem + solution + conclusion" pattern versus the "claim + justification + conclusion" pattern of native English speakers.
Narrative Structure	L2 narratives often began in the middle of the story, omitted essential elements of the story, had less action and more focus on mental states. Also, many L2 narrative patterns in English were closer to the participants' L1 narrative patterns.
Reader Orientation	L2 writing contained fewer and a smaller range of attention-getting devices. They also used fewer sentences that signaled a following theme, overspecified their themes and underestimated their readers' knowledge by introducing information readers considered obvious.
Stylistic Features	L2 writing was found to be less complex, less mature, and less appropriate from a stylistic perspective. Many L2 writers used a more direct, explicit, and authoritative tone. They also used strong modals (will, should, must), and showed less variety in stylistic devices (fewer interrogative sentences, less analogy, less parallel structure, and more repetition of ideas)
Cohesion	L2 writers used more conjunctive ties and fewer synonyms and collocations.

Source: Data from "Toward an Understanding of the Distinct Nature of L2 Writing: The ESL Research and its Implications," by T. Silva, 1993, *TESOL Quarterly, 27*(4), 657–677.

pattern of native and nonnative English writers. He based his assumptions on the comparison and contrast of written samples generated by the two populations. According to Kaplan (1966), the pattern of English rhetorical organization is linear in nature.

English writing is organized around a central idea, or a thesis statement. Every part of the writing is expected to be directly related to the thesis statement and should progress in a straight line from the beginning to the end. Kaplan noted four other organizational patterns, very different from the linear English model. These are the Semitic, Oriental, Romance, and Russian organizational patterns (Figure 5–4).

The first pattern discussed by Kaplan (1966) is the Semitic pattern. This pattern is characterized by parallel constructions, as seen from this English example generated by an Arabic-speaking student: "The first problem is that we import many things from other countries and we cannot depend on ourselves in producing the things we need and we import different kinds of food, electric materials, cars and clothes."

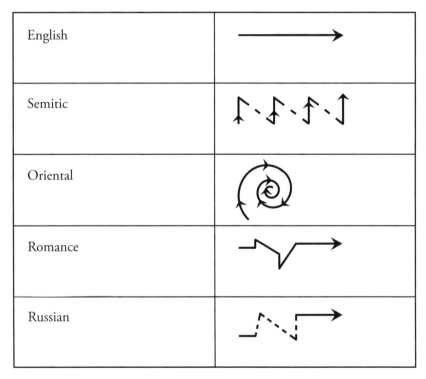

Figure 5–4. *Kaplan's rhetorical organization patterns.* Source: *Data from "Cultural Patterns in Intercultural Education," by R. B. Kaplan, 1966,* Language Learning, 16, 1–20.

The second pattern, the Oriental pattern, is present in Indonesian, Chinese, or Korean, and the writing topic is examined from a variety of points, but never directly. Freedom to digress is a characteristic of Romance- and German-language writers. Digression introduces extraneous material into the writing, with the purpose of providing additional information, suggesting alternative possibilities in considering an issue, or simply inserting humor in the text. However, English academic writing may consider digression as being irrelevant to the topic or inappropriate to the context, because it violates the linearity of English writing conventions. The last pattern, the Russian rhetorical organization, is similar to the Romance pattern, but with more amplification of subordinate elements.

The fact that English rhetorical style is represented by a linear line does not imply it is superior to other rhetorical organizations. It simply emphasizes the idea that each language has its own way of organizing reality, similar to the uniqueness of each culture. Culture is not universal in the sense of uniformity and each culture views the same reality differently. Rhetorical organization, based on logic, is not universal and varies from culture to culture and sometimes even within the same culture. Even Kaplan has modified his initial position: he no longer views rhetorical patterns as reflective of a certain way of thinking but rather as a result of different writing conventions that are taught (Kaplan, 2000). The idea that writing patterns can be learned is key. Therefore, in the case of Spanish-speaking ELs who are literate in Spanish, they need to learn the new linear convention of English academic writing. This does not mean that they have to abandon their preferred forms of expression but they should learn when that style of writing is required in specific contexts and necessary for specific tasks. We provide another example of linearity and directness of the English rhetorical style by contrasting it with the Korean language.

Before comparing linearity in English and linearity in Korean, it is essential to operationalize the construct of linearity. In general, linearity is defined as a progression that supports a thesis without digression. This definition needs to be further explored and more rhetorical parameters need to be added for a more effective contrastive analysis of the rhetorical organization employed by the two languages. Monroy and Scheu (1997) established several guidelines for a linear rhetorical pattern common to the organization of English writing (Table 5–8).

In contrast, the Korean rhetorical organization uses a different, more nonlinear pattern (Eggington, 1987). The nonlinear Korean style originated from the "qi-cheng-zhuan-he" (起承轉合) style in Chinese. A similar pattern can also be found in Japanese writing ("ki-sho-ten-ketsu"). The Korean version, "ki-sung-chon-kyul," has four stages: beginning, development, turn, and end. In Korean, the main idea is presented late in the essay, whereas the thesis in an English essay is expected to be introduced very early. It is important to note that writing conventions might change in time within the same culture. For example, in China, the structure described above is increasingly losing its influence

Table 5–8. *Guidelines for Establishing Linearity of Discourse*

Thematic Unit	A single thesis connects the whole text together. Multiple theses influence linearity negatively.
Thematic Progression	A direct relationship between all the different thematic sentences that link every paragraph with the main thesis.
Paragraph Unity	Paragraphs have one controlling idea which is developed by expanding, qualifying, and illustrating it.
Personal Tone	The use of one point of view and pronouns that refer to the subject.
Interparagraph Cohesion	Paragraphs are linked to each other in evident ways and they all adhere to the thesis.
Concreteness	The use of concrete words and less reliance on abstract words.
Sentence Simplicity	The presence of simple or coordinated sentences and the lack of overuse of complex or subordinated sentences.

Source: Data from "Reflejo cultural en los estilos de hispanohablantes estudiantes de inglés como LE. Consideraciones pedagógicas," by R. Monroy & D. Scheu, in *Estudios de Lingüística Aplicada y Literatura. Homenaje Póstumo al Prof. Juan Conesa,* 1997, pp. 201–221, Murcia, Spain: Universidad de Murcia.

over mainland Chinese students writing in Chinese. A survey of contemporary Chinese textbooks on composition showed that the prescriptive advice given in these texts reflected a linear English rhetorical style more than the traditional Chinese style (Kirkpatrick, 1997).

Korean style is not only nonlinear, but also indirect. In other words, the writing is not developed in a straight line proceeding from a statement of the thesis or central idea followed by elaboration. Instead, the subject is looked at indirectly, a process done by examining issues not directly related to the main idea.

How do we translate the insights obtained through contrastive rhetoric to the practice of teaching ELs how to write in a second language? Matsuda (1997) proposed a model of L2 writing that goes beyond the background of ELs and accounts for the complexity of factors that contribute to the organization of texts written by ELs in a second language.

Contrastive Rhetoric and the Practice of Teaching Second Language Writing: Matsuda's Dynamic Model

Matsuda's (1997) model, represented in Figure 5–5, emphasizes the dynamic nature of writing in L2. The context of the writing act includes not only the writer, but also the reader. This context is created as a result of the interaction between the writer and the reader and realized through L2 text. The key components of this dynamic model are the backgrounds of the writer and the reader, the shared discourse community, and the interaction of the elements of L2 writing: the EL writer, the EL-generated text and the EL/native English speaker (NES) reader.

The first feature, represented by the writer's and reader's backgrounds, includes more than language, culture, and education experiences. These sources of influence are undoubtedly important, but there are other influences that might influence a writer's decisions, such as dialect, socioeconomic status, knowledge of the subject matter, and membership to various L1 and L2 discourse communities. The background of both the writer and the reader is a very complex notion and almost escapes a comprehensive definition. However, what is important here is to understand the complexity of background and the fact that it is

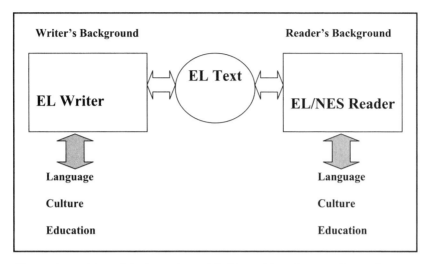

Figure 5–5. *Matsuda's dynamic model of L2 writing.* Source: *From "Contrastive Rhetoric in Context: A Dynamic Model of L2 Writing," by P. K. Matsuda, 1997, Journal of Second Language Writing, 6(1), p. 52, Figure 2. Copyright 1997 by Elsevier. Adapted with permission.*

a contributing element to the dynamic nature of L2 writing due to its flexibility. For example, ELs who have been exposed to the conventions of English writing and have a good command of the linguistic aspect of the language might be able to generate L2 writing that is very close to the one produced by NESs who are proficient writers. From a different background perspective, EL teachers who have been exposed to a variety of EL-generated texts might be able to react differently to linguistic and structural errors in their students' texts than an average NES reader with limited EL contact.

The discourse community, the second feature of the model, is shared by both the writer and the reader. Discourse is a construct defining all forms of communication that contribute to a particular form of thinking. Swales (1990) defines a discourse community as a community that has an agreed set of common goals and ways of communication among its members. As a member of a discourse community in their own native language, literate ELs share (with their readers) one or more writing genres and specific languages (i.e., vocabulary) that serve the goals of that particular discourse community.

To gain access to the L2 discourse community, ELs need to acquire relevant content and discourse expertise in L2, regardless of their linguistic, cultural, or educational background. For example, ELs can negotiate their access to an L2 discourse community by learning the rhetorical patterns of English or other discourse conventions specific to the target language. The process is not unidirectional, though. The EL/NES reader can also help enlarge the shared aspect of the L1 and L2 discourse communities by becoming more and more accustomed to L2-generated texts that exhibit different assumptions, experiences, and levels of L2 discourse expertise.

The last important feature of the model is represented by the bidirectional interaction between the three principal elements of the L2 reading model: the EL writer, the EL text, and the EL/NES reader. The writer influences and is influenced by the participation in the L2 discourse community, an experience that will become part of the EL writer's background. The EL text can be seen as a virtual world in which the writer and the reader meet, building a shared reality. To make L2 writing effective, L2 texts should reflect the EL writer's understanding that acquiring the organizational patterns in L2 is a necessary, but not sufficient, condition for successful L2 writing. Consequently, the text should reflect the fact that the writer knows and understands not only the reader's background but also the writing genres in the discourse community shared by both the writer and the reader.

ELs are not solely responsible for gaining membership to existing L2 discourse communities. NES readers might also experience a process of revisiting their own backgrounds as a result of reading an EL-generated English text. The presence of L2 texts may cause the NES reader to gain a new perspective and reevaluate and incorporate new discourse patterns into their own background.

ELs with Communication Disorders and Writing in English: A Focus on Morphology

The majority of studies that examine the acquisition of literacy in a second language have been conducted with typically developing EL students (Bialystok, Luk, & Kwan, 2005; Carlo et al.,

2004; Genesee, Lindholm-Leary, Saunders, & Christian, 2005; Paez, Tabors, & Lopez, 2007). As a consequence, there is a very limited body of research exploring the acquisition of language and literacy skills of ELs with communication disorders, specifically in the area of writing. Studies that focus on non-EL students who have communication disorders usually provide us with information on the connection between language and reading disorders, literacy development of students with specific special needs (e.g., deaf and hard of hearing (DHH), specific learning impairment (SLI), or students from low-income backgrounds or high-risk populations; see Catts, 1993; Gillam & Johnston, 1992; Hengst & Johnson, 2008; Roseberry-McKibben, 2008).

In one study focusing on the literacy levels of students who are deaf or hard of hearing (DHH), researchers found that high school graduates were functionally illiterate, with a reading and writing proficiency of a third- or fourth-grade student (Waters & Doehring, 1990).

In term of language usage, studies have found that students who were DHH showed considerable delays in their written language. Their written language was characterized with many nouns and verbs and too few adverbs, pronouns, prepositions, and adjectives (McAnally, Rose, & Quigley, 1994; Simmons, 1962). One study reported that students with hearing loss frequently used the same descriptors at age 18 as they did at age 10 when asked to depict an item (McCombs & McCombs, 1969).

In terms of language disorders, most research has been focused on morphological and phonological aspects of second language discrepancies. The importance of phonology and oral language development has been discussed previously in the chapter. The focus now shifts to morphological development, which plays a very important role in the writing domain.

Most of the studies in the area of morphology have looked at ELs with specific language impairment (SLI) and found that ELs with SLI are very similar to their monolingual NES peers with SLI. For example, Paradis, Crago, Genesee, and Rice (2003) investigated the morphological skills of French-English simultaneous bilinguals (bilinguals who are learning two languages at the same time) with SLI and compared them with the skills of French and English monolingual students with SLI. Related to verb tenses and accuracy of tense markers, their findings showed that the bilingual children in their study did not display more profound deficits in the use of these grammatical morphemes than their monolingual peers. They concluded that bilinguals were not more impaired than monolinguals simply because they were simultaneously acquiring two languages.

There are important differences between the language produced by ELs with SLI and ELs without SLI. Jacobson and Schwartz (2002) looked at a number of studies that analyzed the speech of Spanish-speaking ELs with SLI in an attempt to create a profile that could be used for future research or that could be shared among researchers. They reported that conflicting findings in their research and in the literature made it difficult to create a profile of morphological difficulty for that population of students. However, they observed that the morphological problems of Spanish-speaking ELs with SLI included decreased use of function words, such as articles, and difficulty with third person verb inflections and noun plural inflections. Spanish-speaking children between the ages of 5 and 7 with SLI who were living in the United States used fewer articles than their age-matched control groups. However, no discrepancies in tense marking or increased use of infinitive forms were found. The lack of general consensus on the profile of morphological acquisition of ELs with SLI emphasizes the need for more research in this important area of language acquisition.

An important point that needs to be made here is related to the dilemma SLPs and ESOL professionals face when analyzing EL errors. They must ascertain whether the errors occur as a result of normal language development or if the errors are indicative of language impairment. The presence of morphological errors in writing and speech does not mean that ELs have an SLI, as pointed out by Paradis (2005). Regardless of their L1 background, beginning EL students will make morphological errors, which could extend into their second year of speaking English. Examples of such morphological errors are morphemes that mark the grammatical category tense, such as auxiliary verbs and verb inflections (for example, "-s" for the third person singular).

As a general characteristic, ELs will interchange the correct use of a morpheme with the omission of a morpheme in their writing and speech, but they will become proficient in using them over time. These characteristics also describe typical

English-language learning. However, they overlap with the characteristics of monolingual students with SLI. As a consequence, it is challenging to determine whether beginning EL morphological errors are due to second language learning processes or to specific language impairment. Therefore, it is vital that SLPs and ESOL professionals exercise caution in the presence of morphological errors and not consider them a marker of SLI in beginning ELs.

Background Knowledge and Its Contribution to Second Language Literacy

Schema: Definition and Examples

There are several definitions of schema (schemata or schemas in plural form) that can be traced back to Plato, who proposed the theory of ideal types that exist in the human mind, and Kant, who emphasized the importance of background knowledge in comprehending a literary text. However, the origin of the majority of definitions of schema can be traced to Bartlett, who defined schema as an active organization of past responses to past experiences (Bartlett, 1932).

Rumelhart (1980) proposed that schema theory is a theory about how knowledge is represented and how this representation makes possible the use of knowledge in a specific way. According to schema theory, all knowledge is packed into units called schemata. In addition to the knowledge itself, these units also contain information or directions on how these units of knowledge should be used. One example of schema is provided by Davis (1991), as seen in Figure 5–6.

Carrell (1983) identifies two categories of schema: formal schema and content schema. Formal schema, also called textual or discourse schema, refers to the organizational forms and rhetorical structure of the text. It includes syntax, semantics, and all other linguistic knowledge, as well as text genre and background knowledge on how the text should be organized rhetorically. Content schema refers to knowledge beyond the linguistic knowledge. It includes the reader's culture and world knowledge, as well as any kind of information related to a

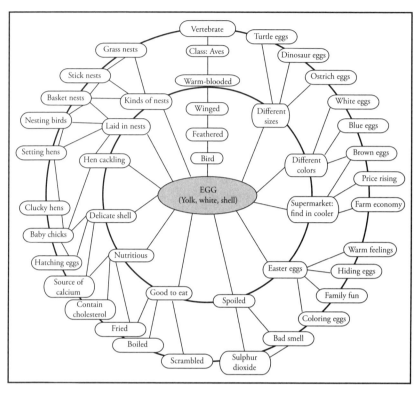

Figure 5–6. *Example of schema.* Source: *Adapted from* Cognition and Learning: A Review of the Literature with Reference to Ethnolinguistic Minorities, *by P. M. Davis, 1991, Dallas, TX: Summer Institute of Linguistics, p. 21. Copyright 1991 by SIL. Reprinted with permission.*

particular topic. Deaux and Wrightsman (1988) propose a model that explains how schema operates, as seen in Figure 5–7.

Schema Theory and Reading Comprehension in a Second Language

Research in the area of schema theory and its influence on L2 reading comprehension has concluded that there is a very strong relationship between the reader's schema and the ability to understand a text. Thus, EL readers may fail to make sense of a text if their schema cannot easily fit within the content of the English text they are reading.

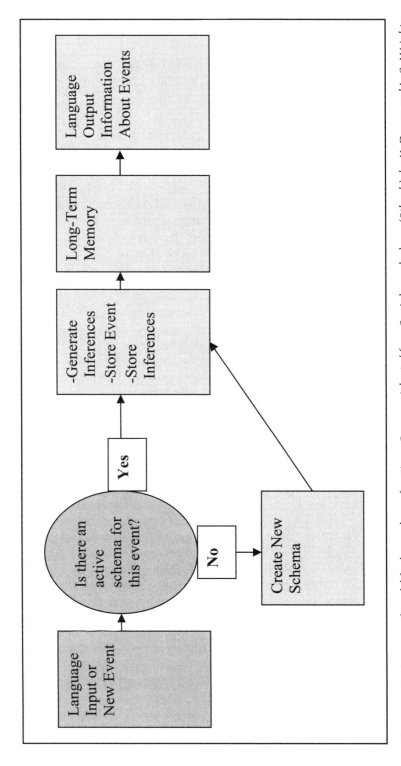

Figure 5–7. *A proposed model for how schema functions. Source: Adapted from Social psychology (5th ed.), by K. Deaux and L. S. Wrightman, 1988, Pacific Grove, CA: Brooks/Cole. Copyright 1988 by Wadsworth, a part of Cengage Learning, Inc. Reprinted with permission.*

Several studies reviewed by Al-Issa (2006) have shown the influence of content schema on L2 reading comprehension. We previously defined content schema as the degree to which L2 readers are familiar with the subject matter of the text they are trying to understand. Carrell (1981) studied the effect of cultural origin of the reading materials on EL comprehension and recall. Two groups of students, Chinese and Japanese, participated in the study. They were asked to read stories in English that had been translated from Chinese, Japanese, French, and American Indian folktales. The study showed that ELs ranked the comprehensibility of the texts as low in the case of stories where story schemata differed drastically from that of their own culture. When asked to recall these stories in writing, their rewriting of the stories was also ranked low in comprehensibility by American native speakers.

Similar to Carell's results, Johnson (1981) found similar relationships between EL cultural background and their reading comprehension of English texts. The study looked at the language complexity and the cultural origin of prose (Iranian and American folktales) on the reading comprehension of EL students of Iranian origin. The findings revealed that the cultural origin of the story had a more significant effect on reading comprehension than the level of language complexity.

Winfield and Barnes-Felfeli (1982) conducted a study with twenty intermediate EL students, half of them Hispanic. The participants were asked to read a sixth-grade level passage of two texts translated into English: *Don Quixote* and a text from the Japanese Noh theater. After analyzing ELs' responses generated through a written recall task of the two texts, the researchers concluded that the non-Hispanic students performed consistently on both texts, but the Hispanic students exhibited a much greater range of vocabulary and scored much higher on *Don Quixote*. The researchers proposed that familiar material increases reading fluency in a second language for ELs as a possible explanation for the differences between Hispanic and non-Hispanic students.

The idea of familiar material was expanded by Krashen (1993), who came up with two ways to activate the ELs' content schemata. The first strategy was called free voluntary reading. It referred to an accountability-free (no follow-up comprehension tests) reading activity in which ELs select and read texts that are of interest to them. One important possible result of this strategy was that reading these books would build the familiarity necessary to read more advanced books. The second strategy was to have ELs read school texts in their first language. By doing that, they would construct the knowledge base necessary to understand the material in the second language. If the content of the reading material were familiar in the ELs' first language, the reading selection in English would be easier to understand.

Based on these studies, it is clear that ELs' content schema has a very important influence on their comprehension of English texts. Al-Issa (2006) proposed 12 questions that can be used to guide SLPs and ESOL professionals select reading materials for their EL students and EL students with communication disorders:

1. Will my students be interested in reading such materials?
2. Will these materials be relevant to my students' English proficiency levels?
3. What content knowledge is to be extracted from these materials?
4. Will these materials cause cultural conflicts in the classroom?
5. How can I motivate my students and involve them in reading such materials?
6. What kinds of prereading, reading, and postreading activities and materials can be designed to increase my students' understanding of these materials?
7. Do the reading materials provide students with sufficient background information about the content of the text?
8. How much time and freedom am I giving my students to exercise their understandings of the materials?
9. Am I being sensitive to my students' hidden comprehension problems?
10. Am I helping my students become more aware of the fact that reading is a highly interactive process?
11. Are my students changing their attitudes about reading?
12. Am I allowing my students to become independent, self-directed readers?

Schema Theory and Writing Proficiency in a Second Language

In the discussion on the influence of schema on L2 reading comprehension, this chapter focused on one dimension of schema, content schema. We now turn our attention to another type of schema, formal schema, to determine if it influences the English writing proficiency of ELs. We defined formal schemata as the knowledge about discourse structure, which may include linguistic and rhetorical organization knowledge. In term of rhetorical organization, we have seen the influences that L1 can have on L2 writing when we compared English rhetorical organization with the rhetorical patterns of several language groups.

Several studies are relevant to the study of form schema in EL writing. For example, Hinds (1990) looked at the differences of rhetorical structures in English and East Asian languages. The analysis of English writing samples generated by Asian students revealed a tendency to use an inductive writing approach, which places the thesis statement at the end of the essay. Because the traditional pattern of English writing is more deductive in nature, it will be more challenging for most English-speaking readers to understand the competent writing of these ELs due to the placement of the thesis statement at the beginning of the essay. The reason for this lack of comprehensibility is not based on lack of language clarity, but more likely due to a mismatch between the writers' approach of organizing text and the readers' expectations.

Similarly, a study conducted by Reid (1996) suggested that ineffective EL writers might employ a formal schema in English that is different from that of NESs. The study examined how well NES and EL student readers and writers could predict and produce appropriate second sentences that followed the topic sentence in a paragraph of academic American English. The findings revealed that NES writers were able to predict the second sentences twice as often as EL writers. The researcher attributed this difference to the fact that NESs have more complete formal schemata than ELs. Therefore, NESs were better equipped to identify and fulfill the expectations of US academic readers.

Based on the research done on contrastive rhetoric and on empirical studies that focused on the importance of schema in second language writing ability, the building of formal schema has a very important place in the second language pedagogy. Why should SLPs and ESOL professionals concentrate on teaching the academic English rhetorical form for ELs and ELs with communication disorders? Xiao (2008) provides three reasons. First, form is relatively stable, predictable, and teachable. Even though it has individual variations, it will not change abruptly. Knowing how to organize their academic texts in English will help ELs take control of English literacy in general and make them more effective writers and readers.

Second, the form of textual structure can serve as an advanced organizer for ELs. Once they create the structure of their essay or any other kind of academic writing, ELs will be able to concentrate on selecting the appropriate vocabulary and grammar they need for expressing their ideas on paper. They will not need to worry about organization any longer, thus freeing more cognitive resources for this more linguistic-oriented task. Finally, as was previously noted, second language literacy research has found that many problems that EL writers encounter can be directly related to English academic form. Because writing forms and styles differ vastly across cultures, these differences can have a negative effect on the perceived effectiveness of ELs' writing in English. If the text written by ELs does not contradict the expectations of the English rhetorical style, the message the text is trying to convey will be better understood, thus increasing the perceived effectiveness of the EL text.

Summary

The reciprocal and multiple relationships between spoken and written language make it appropriate for SLPs and ESOL professionals to play an integral role in helping children become literate. These roles are implemented in collaborative partnerships with other professionals (general education teachers, bilingual education teachers, special education teachers, reading teachers, literacy coaches) who have expertise in the development of reading and written language and vary with settings and the experience of those involved. The knowledge of how the fundamentals of literacy apply to the instruction of ELs and ELs with communication disorders is a sine-qua-non condition for SLPs and ESOL professionals who are contributing to their L2 literacy. Therefore, this chapter provided a definition of literacy and discussed the operations of the construct of literacy, placing a strong emphasis on L2 reading, L2 writing, and schema, and how these operations contribute to the literacy development of ELs and ELs with communication disorders. The following chapter comprehensively examines the assessment instruments and procedures that are in place for ELs, from the incipient stages of placement to the final stages of exiting or dismissal.

References

Abu-Rabia, S. (1997). Verbal and memory working skills of bilingual Hebrew-English speaking children. *International Journal of Psycholinguistics, 13*(1), 25–40.

Alderson, J. C. (1984). Reading in a foreign language: A reading problem or a language problem? In J. C. Alderson & A. H. Urquhart (Eds.), *Reading in a foreign language*. London, UK: Longman.

Al-Issa, A. (2006). Schema theory and L2 reading comprehension: Implications for teaching. *Journal of College Teaching and Learning, 3*(7), 41–48.

American Speech-Language-Hearing Association. (1998). *Provision of instruction in English as a second language by speech-language pathologists in school settings* [Position statement]. Retrieved from http://www.asha.org/docs/html/PS1998-00102.html

American Speech-Language-Hearing Association. (2001a). *Roles and responsibilities of speech-language pathologists with respect to reading and writing in children and adolescents* [Technical report]. Retrieved from www.asha.org/policy

American Speech-Language-Hearing Association. (2001b). *Roles and responsibilities of speech-language pathologists with respect to reading and writing in children and adolescents* [Position statement]. Retrieved from www.asha.org/policy

American Speech-Language-Hearing Association. (2001c). *Roles and responsibilities of speech-language pathologists with respect to reading and writing in children and adolescents* [Guidelines]. Retrieved from www.asha.org/policy

American Speech-Language-Hearing Association. (2002). *Knowledge and skills needed by speech-language pathologists with respect to reading and writing in children and adolescents* [Knowledge and skills]. Retrieved from www.asha.org/policy

American Speech-Language-Hearing Association. (2008). *Communication facts: Special populations: Literacy — 2008 edition.* Retrieved from http://www.asha.org/research/reports/literacy.htm

American Speech-Language-Hearing Association. (2010). *Roles and responsibilities of speech-language pathologists in schools* [Professional issues statement]. Retrieved from http://www.asha.org/docs/html/PI2010-00317.html

Anderson, N. J. (2008). *Practical English language teaching: Reading.* New York, NY: McGraw-Hill.

Anderson, N. J. (2009). ACTIVE reading: The research base for a pedagogical approach in the reading classroom. In Z. Han & N. J. Anderson (Eds.), *Second language reading research and instruction: Crossing the boundaries.* Ann Arbor: University of Michigan Press.

Andersen, N., & Nunan, D. (2008). *Practical English language teaching: PELT.* New York, NY: McGraw-Hill.

August, D., & Shanahan, T. (Eds.) (2006). *Developing literacy on second-language learners: Report of the National Literacy Panel on language-minority children and youth.* Mahwah, NJ: Lawrence Erlbaum.

Bartlett, F. C. (1932). *Remembering: A study in experimental and social psychology.* Cambridge, UK: Cambridge University Press.

Bear, D. R., Invernizzi, M., Templeton, S., & Johnston, F. (2004). *Words their way: Word study for phonics, vocabulary, and spelling instruction* (3rd ed.). Upper Saddle River, NJ: Pearson Prentice-Hall.

Beare, S. (2000) *Differences in content generating and planning processes of adult L1 and L2 proficient writers.* PhD thesis, University of Ottawa, Canada.

Berman, R. (1994). Learner's transfer of writing skills between languages. *TESL Canada Journal, 12*(1), 29–46.

Bernhardt, E. (2005). Progress and procrastination in second language reading. *Annual Review of Applied Linguistics, 25*, 133–150.

Bernhardt, E., & Kamil, M. L. (1995). Interpreting relationships between L1 and L2 reading: Consolidating the linguistic threshold and the linguistic interdependence hypotheses. *Applied Linguistics, 16*, 15–34.

Bialystok, E. (2001). *Bilingualism in development: Language, literacy, and cognition.* New York, NY: Cambridge University Press.

Bialystok, E., Luk, G., & Kwan, E. (2005). Bilingualism, biliteracy, and learning to read: Interactions among languages and writing systems. *Scientific Studies of Reading, 9*, 43–61.

Bossers, B. (1991). On thresholds, ceilings, and short circuits: The relation between L1 reading, L2 reading, and L1 knowledge. *AILA Review, 8,* 45–60.

Brisbois, J. (1995). Connections between first- and second-language reading. *Journal of Reading Behavior, 24*(4), 565–584.

Britton, J. (1975). *The development of writing abilities.* London, UK: Macmillan.

Buriel, R. & Cardoza, D. (1988). The relationship of Spanish language background to achievement. In J. R. Garcia, J. C. Rodriguez, & C. Lomas (Eds.), *In times of challenge: Chicanos and Chicanas in American Society.* Houston, TX: University of Houston Press.

Calderon, M. (2007). *Teaching reading to English language learners, Grades 6–12.* Thousand Oaks, CA: Corwin Press.

Cardenas-Hagan, E., Carlson, C. D., & Pollard-Durodola, S. D. (2007). The cross-linguistic transfer of early literacy skills: The role of initial L1 and L2 skills and language of instruction. *Language, Speech, and Hearing Services in Schools, 38,* 249–259.

Carlo, M. S., August, D., McLaughlin, B., Snow, C. E., Dressler, C., Lippman, D. N., Lively, T. J., & White, C. E. (2004). Closing the gap: Addressing the vocabulary needs of English language learners in bilingual mainstream classrooms. *Reading Research Quarterly, 39,* 188–215.

Carrell, P. L. (1981). Culture-specific schemata in L2 comprehension. In R. Orem & J. Haskell (Eds.), *Selected papers from the Ninth Illinois TESOL/BE Annual Convention, First Midwest TESOL Conference* (pp. 123–132). Chicago, IL: TESOL/BE.

Carrell, P. L. (1983). Some issues in studying the role of schemata or background knowledge in second language comprehension. *Reading in a Foreign Language, 1,* 81–92.

Carrell, P. L. (1991). Second language reading: Reading ability or language proficiency? *Applied Linguistics, 12,* 159–179.

Catts, H. W. (1993). The relationship between speech-language impairments and reading disabilities. *Journal of Speech and Hearing Research, 36,* 948–958.

Chow, B. W., McBride-Chang, C., & Burgess, S. (2005). Phonological processing skills and early reading abilities in Hong Kong Chinese kindergarteners learning to read English as a second language. *Journal of Educational Psychology, 97*(1), 81–87.

Collier, C. (2010). *RtI for diverse learners.* Thousand Oaks, CA: Corwin.

Cummins, J. (1976). The influence of bilingualism on cognitive growth: A synthesis of research findings and explanatory hypotheses. *Working Papers on Bilingualism, 9,* 1–43.

Cummins, J. (1979). Linguistic interdependence and the educational development of bilingual children. *Review of Educational Research*, *49*, 222–251.

Cummins, J. (2000). *Language, power, and pedagogy: Bilingual children in the crossfire*. Philadelphia, PA: Multilingual Matters.

Da Fontoura, H. A., & Siegel, L. S. (1995). Reading, syntactic and working memory skills of bilingual Portuguese-English Canadian children. *Reading and Writing: An Interdisciplinary Journal*, *7*, 139–153.

Davis, P. M. (1991). *Cognition and learning: A review of the literature with reference to ethnolinguistic minorities*. Dallas, TX: Summer Institute of Linguistics.

Deaux, K., & Wrightman, L. S. (1988). *Social psychology* (5th ed.). Pacific Grove, CA: Brooks/Cole.

Dufva, M., & Voeten, M. J. M. (1999). Native language literacy and phonological memory as prerequisites for learning English as a foreign language. *Applied Psycholinguistics*, *20*, 329–348.

Durgunoglu, A. Y. (1998). Acquiring literacy in English and Spanish in the United States. In A. Y. Durgunoglu & L. Verhoeven (Eds.), *Literacy development in a multilingual context: Cross-cultural perspective* (pp. 135–146). Mahwah, NJ: Lawrence Erlbaum.

Durgunoglu, A. Y., Nagy, W. E., & Hancin-Bhatt, B. J. (1993). Cross-language transfer of phonological awareness. *Journal of Educational Psychology*, *85*, 453–465.

Echevarria, J., & Vogt, M. (2011). *Response to intervention (RtI) and English learners. Making it happen*. Boston, MA: Pearson.

Edelsky, C. (1981). From "JIMOSALCO" to "7 naranjas se calleron e el arbol-est-trite en lagrymas": Writing development in a bilingual program. In B. Cronnel (Ed.), *The writing needs of linguistically different students* (pp.63–98). Los Alamitos, CA: Southwest Regional Laboratory.

Edelsky, C. (1986). *Writing in a bilingual progam: Habia una vez*. Norwood, NJ: Ablex.

Eggington, W. (1987). Written academic discourse in Korea. In U. Connor, & R. B. Kaplan (eds.), *Implications for effective communication in writing across languages: Analysis of L2 text* (pp. 153–167). Reading, MA: Addison-Wesley.

Ehren, B. J. (Ed.). (2005). Responsiveness to intervention and the speech-language pathologist [Special issue]. *Topics in Language Disorders*, *25*(2), 120–131.

Ehren, B., Montgomery, J., & Whitmire, K. (2006). Responsiveness to intervention: New roles for speech-language pathologists. In ASHA (Ed.), *New roles in response to intervention: Creating successful schools and children* (pp. 3–8). Rockville, MD: ASHA. Retrieved from http://www.asha.org/uploadedFiles/slp/schools/prof-consult/rtiroledefinitions.pdf

Ehren, B., & Murza, K. (2010). The urgent need to address workforce readiness in adolescent literacy intervention. *Perspectives on Language Learning and Education, 17*, 93–99.

Freeman, Y. S., Freeman, D. E. & Mercuri, S. (2002). *Closing the achievement gap: How to reach limited formal schooling and long term English language learners*. Portsmouth, NH: Heinemann.

Genesee, F., Lindholm-Leary, K., Saunders, W., & Christian, D. (2005). English language learners in U.S. schools: An overview of research findings. *Journal of Education for Student Placed at Risk, 10*(4), 363–385.

Geva, E. (2006). Second-language oral proficiency and second-language literacy. In D. August & T. Shanahan (Eds.), *Developing literacy on second-language learners: Report of the National Literacy Panel on language-minority children and youth*. Mahwah, NJ: Lawrence Erlbaum.

Gholamain, E. & Geva, E. (1999). Orthographic and cognitive factors on the concurrent development of basic reading skills in English and Persian. *Language Learning, 49*, 183–217.

Gillam, R. B., & Johnston, J. R. (1992). Spoken and written language relationships in language/learning impaired and normally achieving school-age children. *Journal of Speech and Hearing Research, 25*, 1303–1315.

Gonzales, D. (2007). *Evaluating bilingual students for eligibility as speech/language impaired: A handbook for evidence-based decision-making*. Houston, TX: Region 4 Education Service Center.

Goodman, K. S. (1979). Psycholinguistics universals in the reading process. *Journal of Typographic Research, 4*, 103–110.

Goodman, K. S., & Goodman, Y. (1994). To err is human: Learning about language processes by analyzing miscues. In R. B. Ruddell, M. R. Ruddell, & H. Singer (Eds.), *Theoretical models and processes of reading* (pp. 104–123). Newark, DE: International Reading Association.

Gottardo, A. (2002). Language and reading skills in bilingual Spanish-English speakers. *Topics in Language Disorders, 23*, 42–66.

Gottardo, A., Yan, B., Siegel, L. S., & Wade-Woolley, L. (2001). Factors related to English reading performance in children with Chinese as a first language: More evidence of cross-language transfer of phonological processing. *Journal of Educational Psychology, 93*(3), 530–542.

Grabe, W. (2001). Notes toward a theory of second language writing. In T. J. Silva & P. K. Masuda (Eds.), *On second language writing*. Mahwah, NJ: Lawrence Erlbaum.

Grabe, W. (2009). *Reading in a second language: Moving from theory to practice.* New York, NY: Cambridge University Press.

Gutierrez-Clellen, V. F., & DeCurtis, L. (1999). Word definition skills in Spanish-speaking children with language impairment. *Communication Disorders Quarterly, 21*(1), 23–31.

Gutierrez-Clellen, V. F., Restrepo, M. A., Bedore, L., Peña, L., & Anderson, R. (2000). Language sample analysis: Methodological considerations. *Language, Speech, and Hearing Services in Schools, 31*, 88–98.

Hacquebord, H. (1989). *Reading comprehension of Turkish and Dutch students attending secondary schools.* Groningen, Germany: RUG.

Hengst, J., & Johnson, C. J. (2008). Writing and communication disorders across the life span. In C. Bazerman (Ed.), *Handbook of research on writing: History, society, school, individual, text* (pp. 471–484). New York, NY: Lawrence Erlbaum.

Hinds, J. (1990). Inductive, deductive, quasi-inductive: Expository writing in Japanese, Korean, Chinese & Tai. In U. Connors & A. Johns (Eds.), *Coherence in writing: Research and pedagogical perspectives* (pp. 87–109). Alexandria: TESOL.

Hudelson, S. (1984). "Kan yu ret an rayt en ingles" Children become literate in English as a second language. *TESOL Quarterly, 18*, 221–238.

Hudelson, S. (1986). Children's writing in ESL: What we've learned, what we're learning. In P. Rigg & D. S. Enright (Eds.), *Children and ESL: Integrating perspectives.* Washington, DC: TESOL.

Hudelson, S. (1987). The role of native language literacy in the education of language minority children. *Language Arts, 64*, 827–841.

Hudelson, S. (1988). *Children's writing in ESL.* Washington, DC: ERIC Clearinghouse on Languages and Linguistics.

Jacobson, P. F., & Schwartz, R. G. (2002). Morphology in incipient bilingual Spanish-speaking preschool children with specific language impairment. *Applied Psycholinguistics, 23*, 23–41.

Johnson, P. (1981). Effects on reading comprehension of language complexity and cultural background of a text. *TESOL Quarterly, 15*(2), 169–181.

Kan, P. F., & Kohnert, K. (2005). Preschoolers learning Hmong and English: Lexical-semantic skills in L1 and L2. *Journal of Speech, Language, and Hearing Research, 48*, 372–383.

Kaplan, R. B. (1966). Cultural patterns in intercultural education. *Language Learning, 16*, 1–20.

Kaplan, R. B. (2000). Contrastive rhetoric and discourse analysis: Who writes what to whom? When? In what circumstances? In S. Sarangi & M. Coulthard (Eds.), *Discourse and social life.* Edinburgh, UK: Pearson Education.

Kinneavy, J. E. (1969). The basic aims of discourse. *College Composition and Communication, 20*(5), 297–304.

Kirkpatrick, A. (1997) Traditional Chinese text structures and their influence on the writing in Chinese and English of contemporary mainland Chinese students. *Journal of Second Language Writing, 6*(3), 223–244.

Klingner, J. K., Mendez Barletta, L., & Hoover, J. (2008). Response to intervention models and English language learners. In J. Klingner, J. Hoover, & L. Baca (Eds.), *Why do English language learners struggle with reading?* (pp. 37–56). Thousand Oaks, CA: Corwin.

Koda, K. (2007). Reading and language learning: Crosslinguistic constraints on second language reading development. In K. Koda (Ed.), *Reading and language learning* (pp. 1–44). Special issue of *Language Learning Supplement, 57*, 1–44.

Kohnert, K. (2008). *Language disorders in bilingual children and adults*. San Diego, CA: Plural.

Krashen, S. (1993). *The power of reading: Insights from the research*. Englewood, CO: Libraries Unlimited.

Leafstedt, J. M., & Gerber, M. M. (2005). Crossover of phonological processing skills: A study of Spanish-speaking students in two instructional settings. *Remedial and Special Education, 26*, 226–235.

Lee, J., & Schallert, D.L. (1997). The relative contribution of L2 language proficiency and L1 reading ability to L2 reading performance: A test of the threshold hypothesis in an EFL context. *TESOL Quarterly, 31*, 713–739.

Lesaux, N. K., & Siegel, L. S. (2003). The development of reading in children who speak English as a second language. *Developmental Psychology, 36*, 1005–1019.

Li, G., & Edwards, P. (Eds.). (2010). *Best practices in ELL instruction*. New York, NY: Guilford Press.

MacSwan, J., & Pray, L. (2005). Learning English bilingually: Age of onset of exposure and rate of acquisition among English language learners in a bilingual education program. *Bilingual Research Journal, 29*, 653–678.

Mathes, P. G., Pollard-Durodola, S., Cardenas-Hagen, E., Linan-Thompson, S., & Vaugh, S. (2007). Teaching struggling readers who are native Spanish speakers: What do we know? *Language, Speech, and Hearing Services in Schools, 38*, 260–271.

Matsuda, P. K. (1997). Contrastive rhetoric in context: A dynamic model of L2 writing. *Journal of Second Language Writing, 6*(1), 45–60.

Matsumoto, K. (1995). Research paper writing strategies of professional Japanese EFL writers. *TESL Canada Journal, 13*(1), 17–27.

McAnally, P. L., Rose, S., & Quigley, S. P. (1994). *Language learning practices with deaf children*. Austin, TX: Pro-Ed.

McCombs, M., & McCombs, Z. (1969). Descriptive style of deaf children. *Volta Review, 71*, 23–26.

Monroy, R., & Scheu, D. (1997). Reflejo cultural en los estilos de hispanohablantes estudiantes de inglés como LE. Consideraciones pedagógicas. In *Estudios de Lingüística Aplicada y Literatura. Homenaje Póstumo al Prof. Juan Conesa* (pp. 201–221). Murcia, Spain: Universidad de Murcia.

Muljani, D., Koda, K., & Moates, D. (1998). The development of word recognition in a second language. *Applied Psycholinguistics, 19,* 99–113.

Mumtaz, S., & Humphreys, G. (2002). The effect of Urdu vocabulary size on the acquisition of single word reading in English. *Educational Psychology, 22,* 165–190.

National Institute for Literacy. (n.d.). *Frequently asked questions.* Retrieved from http://www.nifl.gov/nifl/faqs.html

National Reading Panel. (2000). *Report of the National Reading Panel: Teaching children to read: An evidenced-based assessment of the scientific research literature on reading and its implications for reading instruction* (NIH Publication No. 00-4769). Washington, DC: US Government Printing Office.

Nguyen, A., Shin, F., & Krashen, S. (2001). Development of the first language is not a barrier to second-language acquisition: Evidence from Vietnamese immigrants to the United States. *International Journal of Bilingual Education and Bilingualism, 4*(3), 159–164.

Paez, M. M., Tabors, P. O., & Lopez, L. M. (2007). Dual language and literacy development of Spanish-speaking preschool children. *Journal of Applied Developmental Psychology, 28*(2), 85–102.

Paradis, J. (2005). Grammatical morphology in children learning English as a second language: Implications of similarities with specific language impairment. *Language, Speech, and Hearing Services in Schools, 36,* 172–187.

Paradis, J., Crago, M., Genesee, F., & Rice, M. (2003). French-English bilingual children with SLI: How do they compare with their monolingual peers? *Journal of Speech, Language, and Hearing Research, 46,* 113–127.

Peregoy, S., & Boyle, O. (1991). Second language oral proficiency characteristics of low, intermediate and high second language readers. *Hispanic Journal of Behavioral Sciences, 13*(1), 35–47.

Peregoy, S. & Boyle, O. (2005). *Reading, writing and learning in ESL* (4th ed.). New York, NY: Pearson.

Perkins, K., Brutten, S., & Pohlman, J. (1989). First and second language reading comprehension. *RELC Journal, 20,* 1–9.

Pray, L. (2003, April). *A comparison of the rate of English acquisition of general education and special education second language learners.* Paper presented at the national conference of the American Educational Research Association, Chicago, IL.

Pray, L. (2009). Comparison of oral language usage among English language learners diagnosed with a learning disability and those in general education. *International Multilingual Research Journal, 3,* 110–119.

Quiroga, T., Lemos-Britten, Z., Mostafapour, E., Abbott, R. D., & Berninger, V. W. (2002). Phonological awareness and beginning Spanish-speaking ESL first graders. Research into practice. *Journal of School Psychology, 40*(1), 85–111.

Reid, J. (1996). U.S. academic readers, ESL writers, and second sentences. *Journal of Second Language Writing, 5*(2), 129–161.

Restrepo, M. A. (1998). Identifiers of predominantly Spanish-speaking children with language impairment. *Journal of Speech, Language, and Hearing Research, 41,* 1398–1411.

Restrepo, M. A., Castilla, A., Schwanenflugel, P., Neuharth-Pritchitt, S., Hamilton, C., & Arboleda, A. (2010). Effects of a supplemental Spanish oral language program on sentence length, complexity, and grammaticality in Spanish speaking children attending English only preschools. *Language Speech and Hearing Services in Schools, 41,* 3–13.

Restrepo, M. A., & Kruth, K. (2000). Grammatical characteristics of a bilingual student with specific language impairment. *Journal of Children's Communication Development, 21,* 66–76.

Rosa-Lugo, L. I., & Fradd, S. (2000). Preparing professionals to serve English language learners with communication disorders. *Communication Disorders Quarterly, 22,* 29–42.

Roseberry-McKibben, C. (2008). *Increasing language skills of students with low income backgrounds.* San Diego, CA: Plural.

Roseberry-McKibben, C., & O'Hanlon, I. (2005). Nonbiased assessment of English language learners: A tutorial. *Communication Disorders Quarterly, 26,* 178–185.

Royer, J. M., & Carlo, M. S. (1991). Transfer of comprehension skills from native to second language. *Journal of Reading, 34,* 450–455.

Rumelhart, D. (1980). Schemata: The building blocks of cognition. In R. J. Spiro & W. F. Brewer (Eds.), *Theoretical issues in reading comprehension.* Hillsdale, NJ: Erlbaum.

Samway, K. (1987). *The writing processes of non-native English speaking children in the elementary grades.* Unpublished doctoral dissertation, University of Rochester, New York.

Schoonen, R., Hulstijn, J., & Bossers, B. (1998). Metacognitive and language-specific knowledge of native and foreign language reading comprehension: An empirical study among Dutch students in grades 6, 8, and 10. *Language Learning, 48,* 71–106.

Scott, V. M. (1991) *Write from the start: A task-oriented developmental writing program for foreign language students.* Paper presented at the Southern Conference on Language Teaching, Valdosta, GA.

Silva, T. (1993). Toward an understanding of the distinct nature of L2 writing: The ESL research and its implications. *TESOL Quarterly*, *27*(4), 657–677.

Simon-Cereijido, G., & Gutierrez-Clellen, V. (2007). Spontaneous language markers of Spanish language impairment. *Applied Psycholinguistics*, *28*, 317–339.

Simmons, A. (1962). A comparison of type-token ration of spoken and written language in deaf and hard of hearing children. *Volta Review*, *84*, 81–95.

Spracher, M. M. (2000, April 25). Learning about literacy: SLPs play key role in reading, writing. *ASHA Leader*.

Swales, J. M. (1990). *Genre analysis: English in academic and research settings*. New York, NY: Cambridge University Press.

Teachers of English to Speakers of Other Languages (TESOL). (2001). *Position statement on language and literacy development for young English Language Learners*. Retrieved from http://tesol.org/s_tesol/bin.asp?CID=32&DID=371&DOC=FILE.PDF

Teachers of English to Speakers of Other Languages (TESOL). (2007). *Position statement on teacher credentialing for teachers of English to speakers of other languages in primary and secondary schools*. Retrieved from http://tesol.org/s_tesol/bin.asp?CID=32&DID=8863&DOC=FILE.PDF

Teachers of English to Speakers of Other Languages (TESOL). (2010). *Position paper on Language and literacy development for young English Language Learners (ages 3–8)*. Retrieved from http://tesol.org/s_tesol/bin.asp?CID=32&DID=13010&DOC=FILE.PDF

Umbel, V. M., & Oller, D. K. (1994). Developmental changes in receptive vocabulary in Hispanic bilingual school children. *Language Learning*, *44*(2), 221–242.

Urzua, C. (1987). You stopped too soon: Second language children composing and revising. *TESOL Quarterly*, *21*, 279–304.

van Gelderen, A., Schonnen, R., Stoel, R., de Glopper, K., & Hulstijn, J. (2007). Development of adolescent reading comprehension in language 1 and language 2: A longitudinal analysis of constituent components. *Journal of Educational Psychology*, *88*, 477–491.

Vaughn, S., Linan-Thompson, S., Mathcs, P. G., Cirino, P., Carlson, C. D., Pollard-Durodola, S.D., . . . Francis, D. J. (2005). Effectiveness of Spanish intervention for 1st grade English language learners at risk for reading difficulties. *Journal of Learning Disabilities*, *39*, 56–73.

Verhoeven, L., & Aarts, R. (1998). Attaining functional biliteracy in the Netherlands. In A. Y. Durgunoglu & L. Verhoeven (Eds.), *Literacy development in a multilingual context: Cross-cultural perspectives* (pp. 111–133). Mahwah, NJ: Lawrence Erlbaum.

Walmsley, S. A. (2008). *Closing the circle: A practical guide to implementing literacy reform, K–12.* San Francisco, CA: Jossey-Bass.

Waters, G. S., & Doehring, D. G. (1990). Reading acquisition in congenitally deaf children who communicate orally: Insights from and analysis of component reading, language, and memory skills. In T. H. Carr & B. H. Levey (Eds.), *Reading and its development.* San Diego, CA: Academic Press.

Winfield, F. E. & Barnes-Felfeli, P. (1982). The effects of familiar and unfamiliar cultural context on foreign language composition. *Modern Language Journal, 66,* 373–378.

Xiao, Y. (2008). Building formal schemata with ESL student writers: Linking schema theory with contrastive rhetoric. *Asian EFL Journal, 32,* 13–40.

Yamashita, J. (2002). Mutual compensation between L1 reading ability and L2 language proficiency in L2 reading comprehension. *Journal of Research in Reading, 25,* 81–95.

6

An Interdisciplinary Approach to the Assessment of English Learners

Introduction

As accountability for both SLPs and ESOL professionals has increased with federal and state legislation, the focus on student performance makes the collaboration of these two professionals critical. ESOL professionals and SLPs each have expertise that can address the impact of language differences and second language acquisition on student learning to promote efficient and effective outcomes for ELs with communication disorders. To ensure that ELs are receiving quality, culturally responsive services and being accurately identified as having a communication disorder, it is essential that these two professionals collaborate with each other as well as with different professional partners (e.g., administrators, teachers, support services personnel, parents/guardians) in the assessment process.

However, collaboration does not just happen. It needs a framework and a starting point. Friend and Cook (2009) define collaboration as "a style for direct interaction between at least two coequal parties voluntarily engaged in shared decision making as they work toward a common goal" (p. 6). In schools, collaboration usually includes a number of individuals representing different disciplines, across different levels of the organization. Essentially, collaboration includes a shared purpose, unambiguous definitions, delineation of roles, and shared leadership (Briggs, 1991; Friend & Cook, 2009). An important step in collaboration is to understand the unique contributions of each professional and how each can complement and augment those made by other professionals who also have unique perspectives and skills in working with ELs and ELs with communication disorders (Rosa-Lugo & Fradd, 2000; Pena & Quinn, 2003; Spencer, 2005).

ASHA's 2010 position paper outlines the roles and responsibilities of SLPs in schools in prevention, assessment, intervention, and program design. Applied to ELs, one role of the SLP is to reduce disproportionate referrals of ELs to special education by using preventive evidence-based practice (EBP) approaches. In the absence of improvement by using EBP strategies, SLPs are responsible for identifying and implementing appropriate assessment methodologies and approaches to accurately identify whether the performance of an EL is reflective of a true disorder.

TESOL's 2007 position paper addresses the identification of ELs with special needs and the role of the ESOL professional and bilingual educator. The position paper highlights their expertise in applying culturally responsive and comprehensible instruction. Specifically, both position papers emphasize the importance of purposeful collaboration in identifying ELs with special needs, developing goals, and identifying appropriate services and instruction for ELs (ASHA, 2010; TESOL, 2007).

Knowledge of professional roles and responsibilities in assessing ELs has the potential to lead to shared common goals and equal responsibility for decision making and program planning (Rosa-Lugo & Fradd, 2000). To address the interdisciplinary nature and appropriate assessment of ELs, this chapter will discuss the role of the ESOL professional in the identification and assessment of ELs. It is the goal of this chapter to provide information so SLPs will be more familiar with the assessment procedures and instruments used by ESOL professionals in the assessment and identification of EL students. In particular, we discuss the importance of assessing "language proficiency" and how the assessment of language proficiency impacts the identification, placement, and exit of ELs from special programs. Finally, accountability assessment and modifications and accommodations for ELs and ELs with communication disorders are discussed.

Identification Practices and Protocols for English Learners

Procedures for Identification and Placement of ELs

Before we discuss the identification and placement protocols for ELs with communication disorders, it is beneficial to look at the procedures that are in place for the identification and placement of the general EL population. The policies in Florida, California, and Minnesota to identify ELs will serve as examples.

Florida

In Florida, the identification and placement of ELs is based on the steps outlined in the Consent Decree (*League of United Latin*

American Citizens (LULAC) et al. v. State Board of Education et al. Consent Decree, 1990). The Consent Decree (also known as the META or ESOL Consent Decree) of 1990 is the state of Florida's framework for compliance with federal and state laws regarding the education of ELs. It addresses the civil rights of these students, with the primary right being that of equal access to comprehensible instruction (Florida Department of Education, 2001, 2011). This settlement agreement states how Florida is to address the needs of its EL students. According to the Consent Decree, when parents enroll their children in school, they are asked to complete a home language survey (HLS). The purpose of the HLS is to determine whether or not their children speak a language other than English at home. A series of questions are posed to obtain information on language acquisition and proficiency in order to guide educators to make an informed decision about whether or not a student needs EL services. An example of what a typical HLS might look like can be seen in Figure 6–1.

Home Language Survey

To be completed for all students enrolling in the district.

School:_____   Date:_____

Name of person completing this survey: (Please Print)

_____

Student's Name:_____

Date of Birth:_____   Grade:_____

Figure 6–1. Generic example of a Home Language Survey. continues

1. Is a language other than English used in the home? Yes___ No___

2. Did the student have a first language other than English? Yes___ No___

3. Does the student most frequently speak a language other than English? Yes___ No___

4. What is the predominant language spoken in the home by the parent(s)/guardian(s)?

_____

5. What is the country of national origin of the student?

_____

6. If the student was born in another country, what is his/her date of entry in the United States?

_____

7. Number of years of school outside the U.S._____

8. Number of years of school inside the U.S._____

_____   _____
Signature of person completing this survey   Date

Relationship to student: (Circle One) Mother Father Guardian Self

_____
Signature of translator (if necessary)

Figure 6–1. continued

227

This survey (or a similar one) is the first protocol used to identify potential ELs in Florida. If the answers on the HLS reveal that the student speaks another language, then the school personnel responsible for testing ELs is informed that a potential EL student has registered to attend the school. After the notification, the student's English language proficiency must be assessed within 20 days of entry in the school using specific state-approved tests.

Students may also be referred to a Limited English Proficiency (LEP) team or committee by a parent or teacher to determine if the student meets the criteria to be identified as an EL. The criteria to be identified as an EL is determined by results on an English language measure and at least two of the following criteria: proficiency test; previous educational and social experiences; student interview; written recommendation and observation by current and previous instructional and supportive services staff; level of mastery of basic competencies or skills in English and/or home language according to appropriate criterion-referenced standards; and previous or current grades and test results.

California

California does not have a Consent Decree as we have seen in Florida's case, but the steps of identification and placement of ELs are somewhat similar to Florida. California state law (EC sections 313 and 60810) and federal law (Title I and Title III of the Elementary and Secondary Education Act [ESEA]) require that local educational agencies (LEAs) administer a test of English language proficiency (e.g., listening, speaking, reading, and writing) to newly enrolled students whose primary language is not English (California Department of Education, n.d.). Additionally, upon enrollment in a California public school it is required that a primary home language determination is made for all students in kindergarten through grade 12 (K–12). An HLS is used to obtain this information (California Department of Education, n.d.a).

Minnesota

The identification and placement procedures for ELs in Minnesota are not identical to Florida and California but share similarities. All students, regardless of perceived native language, require a home language questionnaire upon initial registration in the district. In addition to the HLS, a teacher referral may be used to indicate possible EL status. The decision to identify a student as an EL is based on multiple measures, including an appropriate combination of teacher judgment, parental input, assessment of academic achievement, and assessment of English proficiency skills in speaking, listening, reading, and writing for students in grades K through 12. If an EL student does not demonstrate proficiency in one or all of the three areas assessed, then the student meets the state's criteria for EL services and is placed in a program designed for ELs. Parents are notified within 10 days of enrolling the student in an instructional program for ELs. The parent notification includes the student's English proficiency level in speaking, reading, and writing, the amount of time and type of EL service to be provided, and parent procedures for refusal of service (Minnesota Department of Education, 2011).

As illustrated in the above examples, an HLS is used by each of these states to identify ELs and determine which students should be tested more thoroughly for special language programs (bilingual or ESL). Most HLSs have a series of questions that survey the language(s) spoken in the home and to identify the first language learned by the child. Although many states use HLSs to identify ELs, there is variation across states in the specific measures that are used to determine eligibility for identification and placement in an instructional program for ELs.

Instruments and Techniques Used for EL Identification and Placement

Common to Florida, California, and Minnesota is the use of home language surveys and language proficiency tests as a means of identifying and placing ELs in programs that will help them transition from limited English proficiency to full English proficiency. Nationally, a variety of instruments and techniques are used by K–12 school districts to assess and identify ELs, including home language surveys, achievement tests, and criterion-referenced tests (Table 6–1; Rhodes, Ochoa, and Ortiz, 2005).

We have discussed the HLS and noted its use in identifying ELs. However, it is not the only protocol used by school districts to identify ELs. The second most commonly used instruments to identify and place ELs in appropriate instructional programs

Table 6–1. *EL Identification Instruments and Protocols Nationwide*

Identification Technique	Number of States
Home language survey	46
Language proficiency test	45
Student records	40
Teacher observations	40
Parent information	38
Achievement tests	36
Informal assessment	34
Referral	34
Student grades	34
Teacher interview	31
Criterion-referenced test	20
Other	13

Source: Adapted from *Assessing Culturally and Linguistically Diverse Students: A Practical Guide*, by R. L. Rhodes, S. H. Ochoa, & S. O. Ortiz, 2005, New York, NY: Guilford Press.

are measures of language proficiency. In Chapter 3 we discussed Title I of NCLB, which requires states to test the oral language, reading, and writing skills of ELs each year to determine their language proficiency in English. Title III is even more focused on language proficiency. First, it defines English language proficiency according to comprehension, listening, speaking, reading, and writing skills. Next, Title III requires annual English language testing to assess the progress of ELs learning English and to determine their level of English proficiency. To monitor the progress of ELs and their growth in English proficiency, a variety of tests have been used. Their use by SLPs and ESOL and bilingual professionals are key in determining the communicative competence of an EL.

Assessing ELs' Language Proficiency for Identification and Placement

Traditionally, language proficiency has been measured using discrete-point assessment measures that yield a proficiency score in each language assessed. Often students are determined to be proficient in a language when they are able to understand and speak with a rudimentary level of conversational fluency. Many tests that measure language proficiency focus solely on listening and speaking skills and do not provide information about the child's functional use of language and their skill in using language across social demands. The absence of information about the child's language competence in reading and writing also provides a limited view of the student's language capabilities. Nonetheless, there are students that have no formal schooling or who have interrupted formal education that would perform poorly if they were required to read and/or write in their first language (Calderón, 2007). Professionals must remember that a student's level of proficiency will depend on the aspect of language that is being assessed. For this reason, professionals must recognize that formal language proficiency tests do not always provide a comprehensive view of a student's language capabilities (Ortiz & Yates, 2002).

Several tests have been commonly used to determine whether ELs need to be placed in an instructional program for ELs. These include the IDEA Language Proficiency Test (IPT) (2005), the Language Assessment Scales-Links (LAS Links) (Indiana Department of Education, 2006), and the Woodcock-Muñoz Language Survey—Revised Normative Update (WMLS-R NU) (Schrank, Wendling, Alvarado, & Woodcock, 2010). The WMLS-R NU is a revision of the Woodcock-Muñoz Language Survey—Revised (WMLS-R, 2005) (Woodcock, Muñoz-Sandoval, Ruef, & Alvarado, 2005) and features updated norms, and a computer software scoring and interpretive program that links student performance on this measure with specific evidenced-based educational interventions. The instruments noted above are often administered by a designated professional in the school system (e.g., ESOL professional, general education teacher, bilingual teacher), as designated by policies and procedures (Loop, 2002). In addition to these three tests, many states currently use the WIDA ACCESS (Assessing Comprehension and Communication in English State-to-State for English Language Learners) Placement Test (W-APT) (2007a) developed by the World-Class Instructional Design and Assessment (WIDA) consortium. To better understand these assessment measures we provide a brief overview of each of the tests and their use and importance in determining language proficiency and identifying ELs.

IDEA Language Proficiency Tests (IPT)

The IPT (2005) is a nationally normed series of language proficiency assessments for ELs in grades pre-K–12. It is currently available for students in English and Spanish in a paper-based format and an online format. This test is widely used in many districts and schools across the nation to determine if a student is a non-English speaker, a limited English speaker (LES), or a fluent English speaker (FES) or competent language learner. To determine an ELs' oral, reading, and writing proficiency in English the IPT is administered according to a students' age and grade level. The Pre-IPT is used for ELs aged 3, 4 and 5; the IPT I is used for ELs in grades K–6; and the IPT II is used for ELs in grades 7–12. Two examples of an oral task from the IPT II for Level A (the levels range from A to F) are provided below:

Example 1. (Examiner points to a picture of a dog and a horse) Tell me what these animals are.

Example 2. Point to the astronaut at the bottom left corner of the picture.

The IPT also evaluates a students' oral, reading, and writing proficiency using specific tests organized by grade level. ELs in grades K–1 take the Early Literacy test; ELs in grades 2 and 3 take the IPT I; ELs in grades 4 through 6 take the IPT II; and ELs in grades 7 through 12 take the IPT III. Reading tasks ranging from vocabulary in context to reading for life skills are found in the IPT II Reading test. An example of a *vocabulary in context* reading task is presented below. This measure is often used by an ESOL professional to identify and place an EL, monitor the progress of an EL, or to redesignate a students' language proficiency.

Tom _____ to the store to buy bread.
- A. laughed
- B. added
- C. skated
- D. rested

Language Assessment Scales-Links (LAS Links)

The LAS Links test (Indiana Department of Education, 2006) is designed to place students upon initial entry into appropriate instructional programs. The LAS Links addresses the four language domains of speaking, listening, reading, and writing. The LAS Links consists of short placement tests, two summative test forms (Forms A and B) for each grade span, one Spanish form, and three parallel benchmark assessment forms. Instructional guidance binders are available for teacher use and to augment professional development/training. The LAS Links assessment is divided into five grade level spans: Primary (K–1), Early Elementary (2–3), Elementary (4–5), Middle School (6–8), and High School (9–12). A rubric is used to grade students' responses. An example of the rubric is presented in Table 6–2.

A combination of the LAS Links test and results are used by ESOL and bilingual professionals: (a) for English language development; (b) to monitor student progress; (c) to link results to teaching strategies; and (d) to create remedial instruction to ensure the successful academic achievement of ELs in all English academic settings.

Woodcock-Muñoz Language Survey—Revised Normative Update (WMLS-R NU)

The Woodcock-Muñoz Language Survey—Revised Normative Update (WMLS-R NU) (Shrank, Wendling, Alvarado, & Woodcock,

Table 6–2. *LAS Links Speaking Rubric*

Score	Descriptor	Example
0	No response in English, response only in home language, or response does not relate to the prompt, including "I don't know."	**Student response to any task:** I don't know.
1	Response relates to the prompt but does not satisfy the task. Lack of sentence form, errors in grammar and vocabulary, and insufficient vocabulary interfere with communication. Response consists of at least one on-topic English word. If a text prompt is given, a single-word response may not be a repetition of the prompt.	**Grade:** 3 **Picture prompt:** A man who is sitting in a wheelchair is feeding a couple of birds. **Teacher prompt:** Tell me what is happening in the picture. **Student response:** A man in a wheelchair.
2	Response satisfies the task and is in sentence form (subject/predicate) with errors in grammar and/or vocabulary or insufficient vocabulary not typical of a native speaker.	**Grade:** 1 **Picture prompt:** A boy is eating vegetables. **Teacher prompt:** Tell me what is happening in the picture. **Student response:** That boy is eating with broccolis and carrots.
3	Response satisfies the task, is in sentence form, and is spoken with the vocabulary, grammar, and ease of expression of a native speaker.	**Grade:** 10 **Picture prompt:** A girl is at the doctor's office and the doctor is consulting her. **Teacher prompt:** Tell me what is happening in the picture. **Student response:** The doctor is checking the little girl's heart.

Source: Adapted from Academic Language Programs Department—LAS Links. Retrieved from http://www2.yisd.net/education/components/docmgr/default.php ?sectiondetailid = 162164&catfilter = 10502#showDoc

2010) provides a norm-referenced measure of reading, writing, listening, and comprehension. The WMLS-R NU features two English forms and one Spanish form and is comprised of several sets of individually administered tests that provide a broad sampling of proficiency in oral language, language comprehension, reading, and writing (Table 6–3).

The WMLS-R NU, with age norms from 2 to 90+ and grade norms available for kindergarten through graduate school, primarily measures language skills that are predictive of success in situations characterized by Cognitive Academic Language Proficiency (CALP) requirements. This test situates students in one of six levels of CALP, ranging from Level 1: Negligible to Level 6: Very Advanced, and provides a picture of student strengths and weaknesses in specific aspects of English academic language proficiency. The WMLS-R NU also generates qualitative information (e.g., a Language Exposure Questionnaire, a Language Use Questionnaire, and a Test Session Observations Checklist) that provides useful information about language proficiency (Shrank, Wendling, Alvarado, & Woodcock, 2010).

The WMLS-R NU is often used by the ESOL or bilingual professional to: (a) assess the level of English language proficiency (ELP); (b) measure CALP; (c) determine eligibility for ESL services; (d) plan instructional programs; (e) monitor progress; and (f) evaluate program effectiveness.

WIDA ACCESS Placement Test (W-APT)

The World-Class Instructional Design and Assessment (WIDA) ACCESS Placement Test (W-APT) (2007a) is another tool used to measure English language proficiency for students who recently arrived in the US or in a particular school district. The purpose of the W-APT is to: (a) identify students who may be candidates for English as a second language (ESL) and/or bilingual services; (b) determine the academic English language proficiency level of students new to a school or to the US school system in order to determine appropriate levels and amounts of instructional services; and (c) accurately assign students identified as ELs to one of the three tiers for ACCESS for ELs (i.e., A, B, or C) (WIDA, 2007a).

Table 6–3. The Woodcock-Muñoz Language Survey—Revised Normative Update (WMLS-R NU, 2010)

Test Component	Descriptor	Example
Picture Vocabulary	Oral language, including language development and lexical knowledge	Identify pictured objects; expressive semantic task at single-word level.
Verbal Analogies	Reasoning using lexical knowledge	Listen to three words of an analogy and then complete the fourth word, e.g., a is to b and c is to ?
Letter-Word Identification	Letter-word identification skills	Identify presented single letters or single words.
Dictation	Prewriting skills, ability to respond in writing to a variety of questions	Draw lines, write letters, and/or words.
Understanding Directions	Listening, lexical knowledge, working memory	Listen to audio-recorded instructions and follow directions by pointing at objects.
Story Recall	Listening, meaningful memory, expressive language	Recall stories heard from audio recordings.
Passage Comprehension	Reading	Rebus and pictures, multiple choice items with pointing, and reading passages for comprehension and completion.

Source: Adapted from *Woodcock-Muñoz Language Survey—Revised Normative Update (WMLS-R NU)*, by F. A. Schrank, B. Wendling, C. Alvarado, & R. Woodcock, 2010, Itasca, IL: Riverside.

The test, developed by the WIDA 19-state consortium, is an individually administered test that addresses the academic English language proficiency (ELP) standards at the core of the

WIDA consortium's approach to instructing and evaluating the progress of ELs (WIDA, 2007b).

The WIDA consortium was founded in 2002 with the purpose of meeting the requirements of the NCLB for ELs with standards and assessment instruments. This assessment provides information about the ELP level of ELs in kindergarten through grade 12 in the skill areas of listening, speaking, reading, and writing and discriminates across the full proficiency range of the WIDA ELP scale. The WIDA framework recognizes the continuum of language development within the four domains, with six English language proficiency levels ranging from Level 1: Entering (reflecting only rudimentary knowledge of and skills in English) to Level 6: Reaching (the level at which students can succeed academically in English on par with their English-proficient peers in speaking, listening, reading, and writing).

The individually administered test adapts to the test taker's ability level and is considered fully adaptive. For example, if the test taker performs well on a test item of moderate difficulty, then the test taker is presented with a more difficult test item. Likewise, if the test taker performs poorly, they are presented with a simpler test item. The speaking subtest of the W-APT requires approximately 15 minutes to administer and is scored using a rubric. The listening and reading subtests take 20 minutes to administer and are scored using an answer key. The writing subtest takes 30 minutes to administer and is scored using a rubric. For example, for the writing section of the W-APT, test raters use a rubric organized around the six levels of language proficiency developed by WIDA (WIDA, 2007c). This rubric (available at http://title-iii.pbworks.com/f/Writing+Rubric.pdf) is used to measure three components of writing: linguistic complexity, vocabulary usage, and language control. The use of this rubric on an authentic student response is highlighted in an example provided in Figure 6–2 (WIDA, 2007c). Here, the EL was required to generate a list of important details associated with an event and then use the information to generate a written narrative. The examiner, using the writing rubric, graded this response at a Level 1: Entering because the text produced by the test taker did not demonstrate the ability to write full sentences and the syntactic errors contained in the text obstructed comprehensibility. A score of 2 could have been obtained if the test taker had written a full, syntactically correct sentence.

Event	lisen mexico musica
Who	six friends
When	monday 8:00 PM
Where	is my house
Other Information	my cousin is they Mexico

My cousin is they mexico
is you come to house my lisen musica
it will be this monday 8:00 PM

Figure 6–2. Example of student response for assessing writing.

Currently, the W-APT is used by 26 states to measure the English language proficiency of students (Zehr, 2011). The W-APT, now in the process of revision, will also develop Spanish language development (SLD) standards for grades pre-K–12 and a Spanish language proficiency assessment, PODER, for grades K–2.

The federal No Child Left Behind Act (NCLB) of 2001 (USDOE, 2002) and corresponding state statutes mandate that states annually administer a standards-based English language proficiency test to all ELs in kindergarten through grade 12 in public schools. Further, state educational agencies (SEAs) are responsible for reporting student English language proficiency levels to the US Department of Education. In some states SEAs must report results of English language proficiency tests to their respective governors, legislatures, and school districts.

Ongoing Language Proficiency Assessment

Why is ongoing assessment of EL language proficiency important and consequential? One answer to this question is because it is required by law. The No Child Left Behind (NCLB) Act of 2001, and, more specifically, Title III of that act, requires that language proficiency be continuously monitored to ensure that ELs attain English proficiency. Title III of the NCLB Act provides additional funding for school districts to assist with the implementation of programs designed to help ELs and immigrant students attain English proficiency and meet state-defined academic and content standards. As a result, Title III requires school districts to: (a) meet the English language proficiency standards that have been established by states; (b) conduct an annual assessment of English language proficiency; and (c) meet the annual measurable achievement objectives (AMAOs) for increasing the percentage of EL students developing and attaining English proficiency, which are set forth by individual states.

Why Are Annual Measurable Achievement Objectives Important?

The No Child Left Behind Act of 2001 requires all states to measure each public schools and district's achievement and establish annual achievement targets for the state. Specifically, Title III, Section 3122 of the NCLB Act requires states to develop annual measurable achievement objectives (AMAOs) for students identified as limited English proficient (LEP) with respect to: (1) making annual progress in English (AMAO 1); (2) attaining English proficiency on the state-identified English language proficiency (ELP) assessment (AMAO 2); and (3) making adequate yearly progress (AYP) in attaining academic proficiency in reading and mathematics (AMAO 3).

What happens if the three AMAOs are not met by schools? The NCLB Act stipulates that if a Title III school has failed to make progress toward meeting the same AMAOs for two consecutive years, the state's Board of Education will require the school to develop an improvement plan targeting the specific AMAO. If a Title III school has failed to meet the same AMAO for four consecutive years, the state's Board of Education will require the modification of the curriculum, program, or method of instruction.

Because of the NCLB Act, and Title III requirements, ongoing language proficiency assessment is "required" for all states. However, we cannot have valid and reliable assessment instruments without a well-defined set of language proficiency standards. Thus, as a response to the NCLB Act, TESOL has developed a set of proficiency standards (TESOL, 2006):

> *Standard 1:* ELs communicate for **social**, **intercultural**, and **instructional** purposes within the school setting.

> *Standards 2–5:* ELs communicate information, ideas, and concepts necessary for academic success in the area of **language arts (S2)**, **mathematics (S3)**, **science (S4)**, and **social studies (S5)**.

Additionally, TESOL (2006) has developed a set of language proficiency levels applicable for grades PreK through 12 that focus on listening, speaking, reading and writing and parallel, to some extent, the WIDA levels of proficiency.

WIDA and TESOL Levels of Proficiency

The new pre-K–12 English language levels of proficiency developed by TESOL (TESOL, 2006) are an extension of the levels of proficiency initially created in 2004 by the WIDA consortium (Gottlieb, Cranley, & Cammilleri, 2007). Although there are some minor changes in the general nomenclature of the two sets of proficiency levels, TESOL's five levels of English proficiency look very similar to the WIDA levels of language proficiency (WIDA, 2007b). The TESOL levels of English proficiency are noted below:

At **Level 1: Starting**, ELs have little or no understanding of English, and most of the time they respond nonverbally to simple commands or questions. It is important to remember that ELs at Level 1 build meaning from text from nonprint elements such as illustrations, graphs, or tables. Therefore, for EL students at Level 1, teachers should select texts that are rich in illustrations, or, if such texts are not available, make illustrations, graphs, or charts available to ELs as supplementary materials.

At **Level 2: Emerging**, ELs are beginning to understand phrases and short sentences. They can communicate limited information in routine situations by using memorized chunks of language. ELs at Level 2 begin to use general academic vocabulary and familiar expressions used in everyday communication.

At **Level 3: Developing**, ELs have a more developed vocabulary and start to understand more complex speech. They use English spontaneously, using simple sentences that are both comprehensible and appropriate but frequently marked by grammatical errors. They understand not only general academic vocabulary, but also specialized vocabulary. However, they still have some problems understanding and producing complex structures and academic language.

At **Level 4: Expanding**, ELs have language skills that are adequate for everyday communication demands, but they still make occasional structural and lexical errors. At this level, ELs are proficient in communicating in new or unfamiliar settings but have some difficulty with complex language structures and abstract academic concepts.

ELs at **Level 5: Bridging** are not fully proficient in English, but can express themselves fluently and accurately on a wide range of social and academic topics in a variety of contexts. ELs at this level of proficiency need very minimal language support to function in English-based instructional environments.

In addition to defining language proficiency levels for ELs, both WIDA and TESOL went a step further by clearly outlining and assigning performance indicators for each level of proficiency and standard. These performance indicators are examples of measurable language behaviors ELs are expected to demonstrate as they engage in classroom activities. Sample performance indicators consist of three elements: content, language function, and support/strategy. An example of a performance indicator for math (TESOL, 2005) is: "*State and confirm* (language function) *operation* (content) *represented visually* (support)."

For accountability purposes, many states have developed English language proficiency standards (i.e., the WIDA consortium) and designed instruments based on these new language proficiency standards. Two multistate language proficiency assessments, the WIDA ACCESS and the CELLA (Comprehensive English Language Learning Assessment) have been developed to measure language progress in ELs.

Consortium (Multistate) Instruments for Assessing English Language Proficiency

WIDA ACCESS for ELLs Test

After completing the English language proficiency standards in 2004 (revised in 2007), WIDA developed several assessment instruments for ELs based on the WIDA/TESOL language proficiency standards. Two instruments that were developed were the WIDA Assessing Comprehension and Communication in English State-to-State for English Language Learners for ELLs (ACCESS for ELLs) and the W-APT. These two instruments allow teachers and administrators to separate the purpose of language proficiency assessment from progress and placement. The placement of ELs is addressed by using the WIDA Access Placement Test (W-APT), a test previously discussed in detail, whereas the question of ongoing language proficiency assessment is addressed by ACCESS for ELLs. Table 6–4 provides a comparison of the two tests and highlights their differences and similarities (WIDA, n.d.).

ACCESS for ELLs is a large-scale assessment. Summative in nature, it is used to measure the annual language proficiency development of ELs. ACCESS for ELLs consists of the following grade level clusters: pre-K–K, 1–2, 3–5, 6–8, and 9–12. Each cluster addresses the five WIDA/TESOL standards: social and instructional language, English language arts, math, science, and social studies. For each grade level, the standards further specify one or more performance indicators for each of the four language domains: listening, speaking, reading, and writing.

ACCESS for ELLs has three tiers (A, B, and C) that correspond to the proficiency level of each EL taking the test. The tiers overlap in an effort to have a test designed for ELs within a particular grade level cluster and range of proficiency level.

- ◆ Tier A covers Level 1 (WIDA Entering/TESOL Starting) to Level 3 (WIDA/TESOL Developing)
- ◆ Tier B covers Level 2 (WIDA Beginning/TESOL Emerging) to Level 4 (WIDA/TESOL Expanding)
- ◆ Tier C covers Level 3 (WIDA/TESOL Developing) to Level 5 (WIDA/TESOL Bridging).

Table 6–4. A Comparison Between ACCESS for ELLs and W-APT

	ACCESS for ELLs	W-APT
Purpose	Annual evaluation of ELs language proficiency progress	Program placement
Assessment Domains	All four: listening, speaking, reading, and writing	All four: listening, speaking, reading, and writing
Standards Assessed	All five TESOL/WIDA standards	All five TESOL/WIDA standards
Time	2.5 hours	45–90 minutes
Format	Three tiers, each covering three levels	Single form measuring English language proficiency for all five levels
Language Domains	Speaking: 3 parts, 13 tasks, 15 minutes	Speaking: 2 parts, 8 tasks, up to 15 minutes
	Listening: 6–7 parts, 19–22 items, 30 minutes	Listening: 5 parts, 15–17 items, up to 20 minutes
	Reading: 6–8 parts, 23–30 items, 40 minutes	Reading: 5 parts, 15–17 items, up to 20 minutes
	Writing: 3–4 parts, 60 minutes	Writing: 2 parts, up to 30 minutes

Source: Adapted from "Comparing WIDA MODEL™, ACCESS for ELLs®, and W-APT™," by World-Class Instructional Design and Assessment (WIDA, n.d.). Retrieved from http://www.wida.us/assessment/comparing.aspx

As research in second language acquisition suggests, ELs are rarely fully at one level or the other. Quite often they are in the process of moving from one level (tier) to the next. Attaining a certain level of English proficiency is not similar to leaving a room, closing the door, and never looking back. Rather, it is more like being in constant transition, at times fully comfortable at one level with certain skills but not with others. For example, an EL can be at Level 3 in speaking, but at Level 1 or 2 in reading.

The decision as to which tier version of the test an EL should take is made by their teachers based on information generated by other language tests, for example, the W-APT.

An example of an ACCESS for ELLs test item for the reading domain in Tier B of the grade cluster 1–2, addressing social and instructional language (WIDA/TESOL Standard 3), is provided in Figure 6–3. Given a picture of a bulletin board, the EL is required to extract information from environmental print (such as signs, bulletin boards, or menus). The EL then reads a scenario and responds to corresponding questions. In the example provided in Figure 6–3, three test items associated with this particular scenario are provided below.

The first test item covers Level 2, which has the following model performance indicator (MPI), very similar to TESOL's sample performance indicators previously discussed.

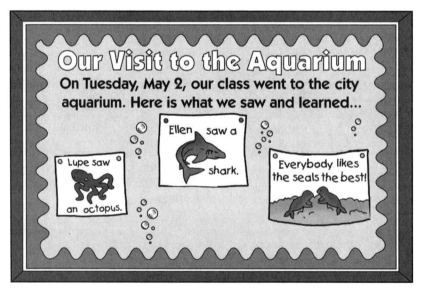

Figure 6–3. *ACCESS for ELLs test sample for the reading domain (bulletin board). Source: From ACCESS for ELLs®. Listening, Reading, Writing, and Speaking sample items, grades 1–12, by World-Class Instructional Design and Assessment (WIDA), 2008. Retrieved from http://www.wida.us/assessment/ACCESS/ACCESS_Sample_Items.pdf. Reprinted with permission.*

When did the class visit the aquarium?

A. March
B. May
C. September

The second test item listed below measures the following MPI, associated with Level 3 of language proficiency: "Restate information found in visually supported print such as school schedules, field trips, or celebrations."

What was everybody's favorite animal?

A. octopus
B. shark
C. seal

The third test item, designed for ELs at Level 4, is based on the following MPI: "Summarize information found in visually supported print on classroom or school activities."

What kind of animals are in the aquarium?

A. animals that live on land
B. animals that live in water
C. animals that live in the air

The Comprehensive English Language Learning Assessment (CELLA)

The Comprehensive English Language Learning Assessment (CELLA) test was developed by Accountability Works (AW), Educational Testing Service (ETS), and a consortium of five states: Florida, Maryland, Michigan, Pennsylvania, and Tennessee (CELLA, 2010). The emphasis of the CELLA is on academic English. The test was developed after a review of English language proficiency standards in multiple states. The purpose of the CELLA is to measure the progress of ELs in mastering the English language skills they need to succeed in school, as stipulated in Title III of the NCLB Act (2001). The CELLA measures four language domains: listening, speaking, reading, and writing. Additionally, the test has four grade level clusters for each language domain: Level A (grades K–2), Level B (grades 3–5), Level C (grades 6–8), and Level D (grades 9–12). The CELLA has a Locator Test which consists of 18 multiple choice questions used to determine which level of reading and writing assessment is most appropriate for each EL. It is important to note that when the CELLA test was developed it did not incorporate either the WIDA or the TESOL language proficiency levels, but preferred to create its own taxonomy, as shown in Table 6–5. This taxonomy is not as detailed as we have seen in the case of the WIDA/TESOL levels of language proficiency.

Compared to the examples easily obtained by the public for the WIDA's ACCESS for ELLs test, few examples of the CELLA are available for the public to view. In the demonstration section of the AW School Test website, a limited number of samples for the writing section of CELLA are available (Accountability Works, n.d, n.d.a, n.d.b). To assess writing ability in English, the writing construct has been divided into several subskills: grammar and writing, editing, and paragraph composition. Examples of these four subskills for the CELLA writing Level C are available on the AW School Test website (http://www.awschooltest.com/photos/CarmenTakesTEST.5.mov).

State-Developed Instruments for Assessing English Language Proficiency

Although some states have decided to use language proficiency instruments developed either by multistate consortia or by national test development companies, others have decided to develop their own assessment of EL language proficiency. Two states fall into this category: Texas (with its TELPAS test) and Colorado (with the CELApro).

Texas English Language Proficiency Assessment System (TELPAS)

Just like many of the other tests discussed previously, the Texas English Language Proficiency Assessment System (TELPAS) was developed in response to the NCLB Act's requirement of assessing

Table 6–5. CELLA Proficiency Level Descriptors

Level of Proficiency	Listening/ Speaking Proficiency Level Descriptors	Reading Proficiency Level Descriptors	Writing Proficiency Level Descriptors
Beginning	ELs speak in English and understand spoken English that is below grade level and require continuous support.	ELs read below grade level and require continuous support.	ELs write below grade level and require continuous support.
Low Intermediate	ELs speak in English and understand spoken English that is at or below grade level and require some support.	ELs read at or below grade level and require some support.	ELs write at or below grade level and require some support.
High Intermediate	ELs speak in English and understand spoken English that is at grade level, with minimal support.	ELs read at grade level with minimal support.	ELs write at grade level with minimal support.
Proficient	ELs speak in English and understand spoken English at grade level in a manner similar to non-English learners.	ELs read at grade level in a manner similar to non-English learners.	ELs write at grade level in a manner similar to non-English learners.

Source: Adapted from Florida CELLA Interpretive Guide, by Florida Department of Education, n.d. Retrieved from www.fldoe.org/aala/pdf/CELLA-Interpretive-Guide .pdf

ELs' progress in learning English (TELPAS, 2011). Structurally, the TELPAS is organized in two major sections. For ELs in grades K and 1, TELPAS is composed of listening, speaking, reading, and writing assessments rated holistically. For ELs in grades 2–12, TELPAS consists of multiple choice reading tests, holistically rated student writing collections, and speaking and listening assessments.

Similar to other English language proficiency tests, the TELPAS measures English learning based on identifiable stages of second language development. There are four proficiency levels assessed through TELPAS: beginning, intermediate, advanced, and advanced high (Telpas,2011). For example, for reading, descriptors are provided for each proficiency level, as seen in Table 6–6).

The majority of the test items in the TELPAS reading section of the test are organized under three TELPAS reading assessment objectives: (1) understanding of words and language structures, (2) basic understanding of a variety of texts, and (3) analyzing and evaluating information and ideas in a variety of texts. One example for understanding words and language structures is as follows.

Miguel uses a ruler to _____ the length of a pencil.

 A. line
 B. ask
 C. measure
 D. add

Table 6–6. TELPAS Proficiency Levels

Beginning:

Students at this level are typically new to the English language. They have little or no ability to derive meaning from English text. They generally understand very little English and tend to read very slowly and word by word. In order to figure out the meaning of what they read, they rely heavily on previous knowledge of the topic, the small bank of English words and phrases they have learned, and information from pictures. Because their English is so limited, their comprehension quickly breaks down when they try to read English in authentic social and academic contexts.

Table 6–6. *continued*

Intermediate:

Students at this level have a somewhat larger English vocabulary and a basic sense of simple English language structures. However, they tend to interpret English very literally and have difficulty following story lines that have a surprise twist or nonstandard format. They still rely heavily on what they already know about a topic to confirm meaning and increase comprehension, and pictures that illustrate meaning are still a needed support. Students at this level can read and understand short connected texts on familiar topics when high-frequency English is used. They have difficulty reading and understanding materials written for their grade level.

Advanced:

Students at this level have an emerging grade appropriate reading vocabulary and a grasp of the structure and grammatical features of the English language. They have the ability to read grade-level texts with some success, although second language acquisition support is still needed to help them understand language that is typically familiar to native English-speaking peers. With linguistic support these students can often demonstrate comprehension of main and supporting ideas on topics they know little about. Additionally, they can often understand English beyond its literal meaning, and they have an emerging ability to think analytically to build conceptual understanding as they read grade-level materials in English.

Advanced High:

Students at this level have the ability to read and understand, with minimal support related to second language acquisition, grade appropriate English used in academic and social contexts, with some exceptions when low-frequency or specialized vocabulary is used. With minimal visual and textual support and at a level nearly comparable to their native English-speaking peers, they are able to understand both explicit and implicit ideas, think analytically, and build conceptual understanding as they read grade-level materials in English.

Source: Adapted from *Educator Guide to TELPAS. Grades K–12,* by TELPAS, 2011. Retrieved from http://www.tea.state.tx.us/WorkArea/linkit.aspx ?LinkIdentifier = id&ItemID = 2147501849&libID = 2147501843

The TELPAS also assesses advanced and advanced high levels of language proficiency using cloze procedures. Content area cloze selections require students to fill in blanks with words that appropriately complete the surrounding academic context. This test format provides evidence of the extent to which ELs are developing the academic literacy in English necessary for understanding language and constructing meaning in subject area instructional materials. This type of test item is designed to assess general comprehension of content-based instructional materials, not mastery of the subject area academic content, skills, or terminology. For example, the student reads a paragraph that has several sentences with missing words:

Matteo was very happy. His math teacher showed the students many different _____ of maps.

  A. types
  B. places
  C. students
  D. teachers

This test item is a possible example of a mathematics cloze selection designed to assess understanding of words and language structures for grade 2.

Colorado English Language Acquisition Proficiency Test (CELApro)

The CELApro represents Colorado's standardized language proficiency assessment for ELs. The CELApro is an annual measure of a student's content knowledge relative to the Colorado English Language Development Standards (Colorado Department of Education, 2010). The standards and their corresponding indicators are organized by language domains, grade clusters, and proficiency levels. Table 6–7 provides an example of Standard 2 for K–2 (Colorado Department of Education, 2005).

The CELApro is an untimed test; however, estimated administration times are provided. The test is composed of four separately administered sections and assesses speaking, listening, reading, and writing proficiency. To assess speaking, the

Table 6–7. CELApro—*Example of Standard 2 Corresponding Indicators Organized by Language Domains, Grade Clusters, and Proficiency Levels for K–12*

Standard 2: English learners speak to convey information and understanding, using a variety of sources, for academic and social purposes.

I. Kindergarten to Second Grade

A. Beginning Level

1. Use gestures, single words, and simple phrases in greetings, routine conversations and to communicate needs.

2. Use both social and academic learned vocabulary in context.

3. State basic personal information, e.g., age, name, family members.

4. Participate in classroom group activities, e.g., chants, songs, choral readings.

5. Retell simple stories and personal experiences using key words and phrases.

6. Respond to simple questions related to immediate context with single words, e.g., yes/no, either/or, basic personal information.

7. Approximate pronunciation of a number of phonemes representing sounds particular to the English language and single words.

B. Intermediate Level

1. Imitate appropriate language in formal and informal settings.

2. Use vocabulary learned in content area lessons.

3. Use simple sentences to express needs and ideas about familiar topics in social and academic contexts.

4. Retell familiar stories and experiences using simple sentences.

5. Initiate conversation in social and academic settings using simple sentences.

6. Contribute to classroom and small group discussions by responding to and asking simple questions.

7. Approximate pronunciation, rhythm, stress, and intonation of English.

continues

Table 6–7. *continued*

C. Advanced Level

1. Communicate information and feelings clearly in conversations.

2. Contribute to classroom discussions by asking/answering questions, giving opinions, disagreeing, and sharing experiences.

3. Retell, narrates and paraphrases stories with descriptive detail including characters and setting.

4. Use both formal and informal language, e.g., interviewing, persuasive speech, with attention to grammar, vocabulary, intonation, and pronunciation.

5. Use expanded and descriptive vocabulary related to content areas.

Source: Adapted from *English Language Development Standards for the State of Colorado*, by Colorado Department of Education, 2005. Retrieved from http://www.aps.k12 .co.us/ela/Resources/ELD%20Standards%20April%202005.pdf

students are shown different pictures. They are required to identify the object(s) and describe its use. The rater marks students' responses as correct, incorrect, or no response. For example, if the student is shown the picture of a chair, it is anticipated that the child will say "chair." However, if the child responds with the word "silla," which is the Spanish word for chair, then the response will be marked as incorrect. More information regarding the structure and the grading of the CELApro can be found at the Colorado Department of Education's website (http://www.cde.state.co.us/cdeassess/training_ info.html).

Exiting Procedures for ELs

When ELs are identified as not being fully proficient in English, they are placed in educational programs that, regardless of format, have as their main goal the improvement of their English language proficiency. As the student becomes more proficient in English a decision must be made, should the EL remain in a program for ELs or exit the program?

The procedures used in three states (i.e., Michigan, Washington, and Massachusetts) provide examples of exiting procedures for ELs.

In Michigan, once EL students have been placed in the LEP (limited English proficient) program, they are evaluated on an annual basis to determine how well they are learning English and if they are becoming more proficient in the areas of listening, speaking, reading, and writing of the English language. ELs are also tested in the academic content areas of reading/language arts, math, and other core academic subjects. The purpose of this evaluation is to determine whether their level of proficiency is adequate to meaningfully participate in regular educational programs.

Teacher recommendation initiates the process for the student to exit the LEP program. In determining whether a student is able to participate in the regular educational program, the school district evaluates factors including the results of the assessment, the teacher recommendation that the student is ready to be exited from the program, whether the student is able to keep up with non-EL peers in the regular educational program, and whether the student is able to participate successfully in essentially all aspects of the instruction without the use of simplified or modified English language materials. Upon exit from the LEP program, ELs are monitored for a period of up to 2 years in order to determine whether they are achieving academically and continuing to achieve English language proficiency.

In Washington, students may be exited from EL services for various reasons, which include moving out of the district, parent waiver of services, LEP factors attributed primarily to special education, and transitioned or redesignated to general education classes. The transition/redesignation occurs when students test out of EL according to results of the Washington Language Proficiency Test-II (WLPT-II). The test annually assesses the growth of the state's K–12 English learners in reading, writing, listening and speaking.

In Massachusetts, an EL student exits the English language development program when it is determined, in consultation with the classroom teacher and/or a guidance counselor, that English language development instruction is no longer necessary. In making this determination, the school district uses multiple means of assessment, which include student grades, reports of teacher observation, and standardized test scores. Once a student has exited the program, the student is designated as FLEP (formerly limited English proficient) and school records are updated to reflect the student's redesignation.

Redesignated students are monitored for academic progress for 2 years after the reclassification. The monitoring is done by the classroom teacher/guidance counselor in consultation with the EL teacher. It is based on classroom participation, assignments, grades, and assessments, including performance on standardized state assessments. During this time, FLEP students receive language development support if and as needed. If a FLEP student fails to make academic progress, as measured by grades and assessments, during the first 3 to 6 months after the reclassification, and if a school-based team familiar with the student determines that this failure is due to lack of English proficiency, the student's instructional program will be redesigned and the student may be reclassified as LEP.

Accountability: Measuring Academic Knowledge Through Large-Scale Assessments

Large-Scale Assessment Accommodations for ELs: Defining the Issues

Under Title III of the NCLB Act (2001), states are required to measure whether or not ELs are making progress in attaining full English language proficiency. The same requirement applies to measuring academic knowledge. Currently, as a direct consequence of the NCLB Act, all public school districts must include ELs when reporting student progress in academic achievement goals. Title I of the NCLB Act strengthens the idea of accountability by requiring that all states develop annual assessments for grades 3 through 8 and one assessment in high school that are aligned with state standards.

The NCLB Act requires that all students demonstrate a high level of proficiency in English language arts and mathematics. Title I states that annual yearly progress for students in K–12 be answered by considering only the results obtained on statewide tests in reading and content area; performance on classroom-based assessments is not to be considered. In many cases, this level of proficiency in these two core areas presents quite a challenge for all students in schools, but even more so for ELs who are struggling to learn academic content and English. Thus, there is a common goal of Title I and Title III for ELs: these students must demonstrate a quick progress in English and content areas (e.g., math). The US educational system allows for a "catch-up" period that is generally limited to 2 years.

This increased level of accountability is bringing an increased focus on the academic needs of ELs from educators and school administrators. There have been many concerns regarding the quality of standardized assessments applied to ELs, especially whether the results from such large-scale tests are valid and reliable (Abella, Urritia, & Shneyderman, 2005). To address these critical issues, all states have developed and implemented accommodation policies for ELs when taking standardized large-scale tests that focus on content areas.

Test accommodation for ELs can be defined as the support provided to ELs to access the English content of the assessment in order to demonstrate what they know academically. Accommodations can be either modifications of the test itself or modifications of the test procedure (Butler & Stevens, 1997). In the category of modifications of the test, the following may be included: bilingual translations and glossaries (either in English or the student's native language). Accommodations such as flexible time limits, flexible setting, and/or the reading and explanation of directions belong to the category of modifications of the test procedures.

Abedi, Hofstetter, and Lord (2004) focus their attention on the effectiveness of EL accommodations. Effective accommodations should level the playing field for the ELs and test modifications should help ELs overcome the language barrier. If the language barrier is reduced, the test becomes a measure of ELs' academic content knowledge and not of their language proficiency.

An example of this would be using a specialized glossary (defined as a list of definitions for selected words, terms, or phrases in a text) as opposed to a standard dictionary. For example, in English there are several definitions for the word "view."

Let us suppose that a test prompt asks students to "give their own view." If an EL looks in the regular dictionary they will note that the word "view" is defined as a noun and has at least six separate definitions for the word. Non-ELs would probably identify the correct meaning of the word without any linguistic support. However, ELs may be easily confused and overwhelmed by the number of possibilities. This might potentially affect test validity because it measures language proficiency and not content knowledge.

To address this potential validity concern, a specialized glossary that supplies only the definition appropriate to that context should be used instead of a general dictionary. Using a glossary can help ELs understand what the test questions require and will not give them an unfair advantage over their non-EL peers.

Modifications and Accommodations for ELs: Examples and Effectiveness

Testing accommodations have been separated into test modifications and modifications of test procedures. This two-category structure is very broad; therefore, it is more useful to further separate EL accommodation in order to eliminate ambiguity. Mihai (2010) proposed a six-category system, to include

1. Accommodation related to time/scheduling (schedule changes, additional time, etc.),
2. Location (preferential seating, private setting, etc.),
3. Directions (in native language, read aloud),
4. Presentation (bilingual version, audio/video recorded),
5. Support (dictionaries, computers, etc.), and
6. Response format (in native language, point to responses in English).

Table 6–8 lists the top five most allowed EL test modifications. Most of the elements comprising Mihai's (2010) six-category system are represented; these most popular accommodations also require the least administrative costs. Unquestionably, they are very practical, but are they effective?

Research in the area of accommodations has compared scores of ELs from accommodated and nonaccommodated test

Table 6–8. *The Top Five EL accommodations*

Accommodation	Category	Number of States
Additional Time	Time/Scheduling	39
Use of Dictionaries	Support	38
Individual/Small-Group Administration	Location	34
Flexible Scheduling	Time/Scheduling	28
Read Aloud of Test in English	Presentation	25

Source: From *Assessing English Language Learners in the Content Areas: A Research-into-Practice Guide for Educators,* by F. Mihai, 2010, p. 72, Table 12, Ann Arbor: University of Michigan Press. Copyright 2010 by University of Michigan Press. Reprinted with permission.

administrations in an effort to make sure the validity of the test has been preserved. According to Sireci, Li, and Scarpati (2003), more studies are needed on the effects of accommodations on the actual test performance of nonnative English speakers. For example, many studies have analyzed the adequacy of translation of tests in the native language of the ELs, or whether the constructs that needed to be tested in accommodated tests are similar with the ones found in nonaccommodated versions of the tests.

There have been several studies that looked at the effectiveness of ELs using accommodations in large-scale assessments. For example, in one study investigating the extra time modification, Abedi, Courtney, and Leon (2003) found that ELs who received extra time had significantly higher scores than the students who were not given this accommodation. However, findings from a different study revealed that gains in scores were very small (Abedi, Hofstetter, Baker, & Lord, 2001). Hafner (2000) conducted another study that looked at the effectiveness of additional time for ELs in combination with another modification, extended oral presentations. The findings showed that giving students more time did increase ELs' and non-ELs' scores significantly, compared to the scores of the students who received only extended oral presentation of directions and test items.

Abedi, Courtney, and Leon (2003) looked at the effectiveness of several accommodations, such as a customized English dictionary, a computer test with pop-up glossaries (an option to pop up the glossary definition in a new window when the user clicks on a glossary term), additional time, and small-group administration with ELs in the fourth and eighth grade. Their findings revealed that the ELs in the fourth grade who had access to the computer test and additional time received significantly higher scores than the ELs who took the nonaccommodated version of the math test. ELs in the eighth grade who took the computer test with pop-up glosses scored significantly higher than the EL students who were provided with the customized dictionary or the ELs who took the test under standard conditions. One other important finding of the study revealed that at both grade levels, native English speakers did not perform significantly better when provided with any of the four accommodations. This is very strong evidence for the validity of such accommodations, which are supposed to level the playing field for ELs and not give them an unfair advantage over their non-EL peers.

In a study exploring the effectiveness of using an English glossary containing definitions of nontechnical words, Kiplinger, Haug, and Abedi (2000) administered items selected from the National Assessment of Educational Progress (NAEP) to fourth graders in Colorado. The study found that, after using this accommodation, the scores of ELs did not improve significantly compared to non-ELs. In fact, all students scored better when they took the test under accommodated conditions. The glossary accommodation generated the most gain in scores for ELs, although insignificant from a statistical point of view.

The research on EL accommodations for large-scale literacy assessment is still in beginning stages and more examination is needed to ensure that the existing accommodations do level the playing field for ELs. Anderson, Liu, Swierzbin, Thurlow, and Bielinski (2000) looked at whether bilingual accommodations provided to ELs during a reading test had an effect on student scores. The bilingual accommodations for the experimental group focused on providing ELs with the questions for the reading test in both English and Spanish. The experimental group ELs had access to test directions and test questions read aloud in Spanish, as well as test questions presented in both languages in writing side by side. The findings revealed that the accommodated EL group had a higher mean score than the unaccommodated group, but the mean scores of the two groups were not significantly different from a statistical point of view. The data from the study also revealed that the accommodations in focus did not give ELs a significant advantage over the native English speakers who participated in the study.

Albus, Bielinski, Thurlow, and Liu (2001) studied whether using a monolingual English dictionary with ELs taking a reading test improved their test performance. The results of their study indicated that there were no significant differences in scores between ELs who received the accommodation and ELs who did not. However, there was a slight gain between the ELs who used the dictionary accommodation and the ELs who were part of the control group and had no access to a dictionary while taking the reading test.

The research on the effectiveness of accommodations for ELs bring to light several important points. First, research findings are mixed and present conflicting results. For some accommodations, some studies found significant gains in scores for ELs taking standardized math assessments, whereas others identified gains in EL scores but without registering a statistical significance. A second point is that accommodations need to be studied in isolation, and not combined in clusters of accommodation. One example is additional time, where the effects on EL scores (not only for math, but for other content areas as well) are not very clear, mostly because this accommodation was clustered with other accommodations. Finally, one accommodation does not fit all. The research of Abedi, Courtney, Mirocha, Leon, and Goldberg (2005) has revealed that an accommodation that resulted in significant score gains for ELs at one grade level did not work for ELs at a different grade level.

Undoubtedly, there is need for more research not only on the accommodations that have been previously researched, but also on the entire range of available and state-sanctioned EL accommodations. Educators and researchers need to identify what works best for ELs. One example where research has informed the practice of EL accommodations is the language support provided to ELs. Dictionaries and glossaries seem to have a much more positive impact on EL student scores compared to when the test is translated, and research shows there is very little evidence for the effectiveness of dual language test booklets.

Modifications and Accommodations for ELs with Special Needs: Examples and Effectiveness

Because of current legislation, there has been an increased need to ensure academic achievement for all students. The NCLB Act requires that at least 95% of every subgroup of students, for example, ELs and special education students, must participate in statewide assessment for a district to demonstrate that enrolled students make adequate yearly progress. As a consequence, many special education students, ELs with communication disorders included, have access to testing accommodations so they can participate in large-scale tests designed to measure student progress. Because of the serious consequences of the NCLB Act, effective accommodations for ELs with communication disorders are very important in documenting student proficiency in core content areas.

Similar to accommodations for ELs, accommodations for students with disabilities permit changes in the administration of the assessments, allowing students to show what they know academically without negatively affecting the validity of the assessment. Many special education students have difficulty with the nonaccommodated format of standardized assessment. Access to accommodations can potentially improve the test participation and accuracy of students with disabilities (McDonnell, McLaughlin, & Morison, 1997).

Specific accommodations for students with special needs have been recommended. For example, Thurlow, Lazarus, Thompson, and Robey (2002) have proposed a five-category accommodation system, which consists of the following: presentation (large print, Braille, etc.), scheduling/timing (extended time, breaks, etc.), response (proctor/scribe, tape recorder, etc.), equipment/materials (calculator, abacus, etc.), and setting (carrel, separate room, etc.). Table 6–9 specifies in more detail this five-category accommodation system for students with disabilities.

However, what are some specific accommodations for ELs with special needs? Previously, we analyzed two tests that mea-

Table 6–9. *State-Sanctioned Accommodations for Students with Special Needs*

Category	Accommodations
Presentation	Large Print
	Braille
	Read Aloud
	Sign Interpretation
	Read/Reread/Clarify
	Visual Cues
	Administration by Other
	Additional Examples
Scheduling/Timing	Extended Time
	With Breaks
	Multiple Sessions
	Time Beneficial to Student
	Over Multiple Days
Response	Proctor/Scribe
	Computer or Machine
	Write in Test Booklets
	Tape Recorder
	Communication Device
	Spell Checker/Assistance
	Braille
	Pointing
Equipment/Materials	Amplification Equipment
	Light/Acoustics
	Calculator
	Templates/Graph Paper
	Audio/Video Cassette
	Noise Buffer
	Adaptive or Special Furniture
	Abacus

continues

Table 6–9. *continued*

Category	Accommodations
Setting	Individual
	Small Group
	Carrel
	Separate Room
	Seat Location/Proximity
	Minimize Distractions/Reduced Noise
	Student's Home
	Special Education Classroom

Source: Adapted from *2001 State Policies on Assessment Participation and Accommodations* (Synthesis Report 46), by M. L. Thurlow, S. Lazarus, S. Thompson, & J. Robey, 2002, Minneapolis: University of Minnesota, National Center for Educational Outcomes.

sured English language and literacy proficiency for ELs: the ACCESS for ELLs and the CELLA. It is very encouraging to note that these tests provide accommodations for students with special needs, and specifically students who are deaf or hard of hearing (DHH) or ELs with communication disorders. For example, the ACCESS for ELLs has specific guidelines for students who are deaf or hard of hearing (DHH), including those for whom American Sign Language (ASL) is their first language. Generally these students can participate in the reading and writing sections of the test with few or no accommodations necessary. For the listening and speaking parts of the test, speech-reading with spoken responses for those students who possess these abilities is allowed. This accommodation is determined on a case-by-case basis as determined by the Individual Education Program (IEP) team. Because translating the listening and speaking prompts into sign language is viewed as similar to translating into another spoken language, this accommodation is prohibited, as it changes the construct and has a negative impact on the validity of the test. Table 6–10 lists ACCESS for ELLs accommodations for ELs with special needs.

Table 6–10. ACCESS for ELLs Accommodations for ELs with Special Needs

Category	Recommended Accommodations	Non-Recommended Accommodations
Presentation Format/Test Directions	Explanation of directions (English)	Translation of test into native language
	Repeat directions	
	Use directions that have been marked by teacher	Translation of test into sign language
	Sign directions to students	
	Translation of directions into native language	Oral reading in native language
	Oral reading in English (Writing only)	Bilingual dictionaries
	Use of highlighters (yellow only) by student	
	Use of marker to maintain place	
	Large Print or visual magnification device	
	Audio amplification device or noise buffer	
	Student reads questions or responses aloud to self	
Setting Format	Test administered by school personnel familiar to student	
	Alone in study carrel	
	Administer test in separate room	
	With small groups	
	Preferential seating	
	Individually	
	By special education personnel	
	Special lighting/acoustics/furniture	
	Administer test with school personnel in nonschool setting (e.g., home or hospital)	

continues

Table 6–10. *continued*

Category	Recommended Accommodations	Non-Recommended Accommodations
Timing/ Scheduling	Extended testing time (same day) More breaks Extending sessions over multiple days (except Speaking)	
Response Format	Word processors or similar assistive device (writing only; spelling and grammar check and dictionary/thesaurus must be turned off) Write directly in test booklet Scribes Answer orally, point to answer (except writing)	Braille writers Responses in native primary language Tape recorders
Other	Provide verbal praise or tangible reinforcement to increase motivation Administer practice test or examples before the administration date of the assessment Allow use of equipment or technology that the student uses for other tests and school work (e.g., pencils adapted in size or grip, slant board or wedge)	Signing questions or answers

Source: Adapted from World-Class Instructional Design and Assessment (WIDA) ACCESS Placement Test (W-APT), 2007a. Retrieved from http://wida.us/assessment/w-apt/#about

The CELLA, similar to the ACCESS for ELLs, recognizes that there are ELs with special needs that require accommodations (Florida Department of Education, n.d.a.). Because this test measures language and literacy in English, there are several accommodations that are not allowed for all ELs with special needs because they will make the test invalid. These accommodations include: (a) the use of English to Heritage or Heritage to English dictionaries; (b) getting help in ELs' heritage language on specific test questions; (c) the translation of any part of the test other than the directions; and (d) the translation of the directions for the entire class. Table 6–11 presents the CELLA accommodations for ELs with special needs.

A brief overview of the types of accommodations for ELs with special needs have been discussed. However, these accommodations raise a critical question: are these accommodations successful in leveling the playing field for ELs with special needs?

To address this question we look to the research on the accommodations for ELs and non-ELs with special needs. Bolt and Thurlow (2004) surveyed the most allowed large-scale test accommodations for special education students, as well as their effectiveness. Table 6–12 lists the top five most frequent special needs accommodations.

Table 6–11. *CELLA Accommodations for ELs with Special Needs*

Category	Inventory
Schedule	Brief sessions with frequent breaks
	Specific time of day to test
	Additional time (however must complete one session before going to next)
	Tested over several days: not permitted to change responses from previous day and closely monitored on an individual basis

continues

Table 6–11. continued

Category	Inventory
Setting	Individual/small group administration
	Special lighting
	Adaptive furniture
	Special acoustics to enhance sound or rooms to decrease auditory distractions
	Opportunities for movement
	Stimuli reduced
	Test in familiar place
Presentation	May use magnification devices
	May use available means to maintain visual attention to test items
	Portions of the test may be masked
	Colored transparencies/overlays may be used
	Papers may be secured to work area
	Positioning tools (reading stand) may be used
	Student may highlight key words or phrases
	Test directions repeated, clarified, or summarized
	White noise
Responding	On multiple choice: written, signed, and verbal responses.
	A scribe may transcribe the student's responses directly onto an answer sheet
	For writing: can use writing guides, special paper (transcribed after), dictating responses into tape recorder (transcribed after)
Other	Visual magnification
	Assistive technology for writing without spelling or grammar check applications
	Braille and large print versions available

Source: Adapted from *CELLA Accommodations*, by Florida Department of Education, n.d.a. Retrieved from http://www.fldoe.org/aala/pdf/CELLA-TestAccommodations.pdf

Table 6–12. Most Frequent Special Education Student Accommodations

Accommodation	Category	Number of States
Individual Administration	Setting	44
Dictated Response to Scribe	Response	43
Small Group Administration	Setting	41
Large Print	Presentation	40
Braille	Presentation	38

Source: Adapted from "Five of the Most Frequently Allowed Testing Accommodations in State Policy," by S. E. Bolt & M. L. Thurlow, 2004, *Remedial and Special Education, 25*(3), 141–152.

In their analysis of accommodation effectiveness, Bolt and Thurlow (2004) focused on three accommodations: (1) dictated response to scribe, (2) access to large-print test materials, and (3) usage of Braille. These three accommodations have generated a lot controversy in terms of effectiveness (Thurlow, House, Boys, Scott, & Ysseldyke, 2000). The results of their meta-analysis are summarized in Table 6–13.

There has been very limited research done on the effectiveness of large-scale test accommodations for ELs with communication disorders. In general, studies focus on either EL accommodations for students who have no disabilities or on special education accommodations for students who are not ELs. Table 6–14 briefly summarizes the research done on assessing literacy for students with special needs, with an emphasis on students with communication disorders.

One important study conducted by Steinberg, Cline, Ling, Cook, and Tognatta (2009) does not directly address the issue of accommodations for ELs but emphasizes the achievement gap of ELs with communication disorders. The researchers looked at the validity and fairness of a state English language arts assessment for students who were DHH and analyzed score performance of four categories of students: nondisabled/non-EL, nondisabled/ELs, DHH/non-ELs, and DHH/ELs. Their analysis considered the internal structure of the English language arts assessments

Table 6–13. Research on the Effectiveness of Commonly Allowed Special Needs

Type of Accommodation	Studies
Dictated Response to Scribe	*Fuchs, Fuchs, Eaton, Hamlett, and Karns (2000):* On math problem-solving items, students with learning disabilities benefited from this accommodation more than the students without disabilities.
	Johnson, Kimball, Brown, and Anderson (2001): Students with disabilities who received this accommodation received significantly higher scores.
	Schulte, Elliott, and Kratochwill (2001): On math assessments, students with disabilities found significant differences between their scores and the scores of students without disabilities on several accommodation clusters that included dictated response.
	De La Paz and Graham (1997): Only small differences between dictated response and written essays.
	Graham (1990): When using a scribe, students with learning disabilities produced longer and higher quality essays.
Large Print	*Fuchs (2000):* No significant difference in scores for students with disabilities.
	Fuchs, Fuchs, Eaton, Hamlett, Binkley, and Crouch (2000): No significant difference in scores for students with disabilities.
	Burk (1999): No significant increase in the scores of students with or without disabilities when using this accommodation on computerized assessments.
	Brown (1998): Significant gains for third grade students with learning disabilities.

Table 6–13. *continued*

Type of Accommodation	Studies
Braille	*Bennett, Rock, and Novatkoski (1989):* Certain math items, such as the ones that depict certain figures or graphs or the ones that require knowledge of the tally system might be more difficult for students taking the Braille edition of the SAT.
	Bennett, Rock, and Kaplan (1987): Some items on the math portion of the SAT were significantly difficult for visually impaired students taking the Braille edition of the test.

Source: Adapted from *State Participation and Accommodation Policies for Students with Disabilities: 1999 Update* (Synthesis Report 33), by M. L. Thurlow, A. House, C. Boys, D. Scott, & J. Ysseldyke, 2000, Minneapolis: University of Minnesota, National Center for Educational Outcomes.

for consistency across the above-mentioned nondisabled and disabled groups for the fourth and eighth grade students. The findings revealed that the performance of students with disabilities was significantly below that of nondisabled students, with a difference of nearly one standard deviation between the mean performances of the two groups. On average, nondisabled ELs had scores slightly below those of non-EL DHH students, but significantly below nondisabled non-EL students. A very important finding of the study showed that DHH ELs performed more than 1.5 standard deviations below nondisabled, non-EL students and significantly below the non-EL DHH students. Clearly, there is a very urgent need to reduce this critical achievement gap between ELs with communication disorders and non-ELs.

A step in the right direction is to provide ELs with communication disorders with appropriate and effective accommodations that can have a positive impact on their academic performance. Based on available research done on EL accommodations, Abedi (2009) outlines a set of recommendations that should be used in the classification, instruction, and assessment

Table 6–14. *Literacy Assessment for Students with Special Needs*

Study	Summary
Lollis and LaSasso (2008)	The study analyzed the appropriateness of the North Carolina state-mandated Reading Competency Test when administered to students who are DHH. Eight reviewers, of which four were DHH, rated the reading passages of the exam for difficulty, appropriateness, interest, and structure. Their analysis took into account factors that might influence test performance due to the student's hearing loss, such as cultural bias or disability related stereotyping, content that would be less familiar to students who are DHH.
	50% of the reviewers rated six of the ten passages as being difficult for DHH students. Moreover, five items from the content passages and two items from the literary passages received negative comments from half the reviewers. The conclusion of the study was that a valid test for DHH students requires proactive input on test construction from teachers of DHH students.
Martin (2005)	The study examined the appropriateness of the New York State (NYS) English Language Arts Grade 8 Test for DHH students. For the first part of the study, eight experts (three of whom were deaf), who were teachers of DHH students evaluated the appropriateness of the ELA Grade 8 Test passages. In the second part of the study, the researcher analyzed the test responses of the 44 DHH student participants on the 2004 ELA Grade 8 Test. More than 60% of the reviewers rated the overall difficulty of the eight passages as being hard for students who are DHH and found that 18% of the multiple choice items and 28% of the constructed response ones did not pass the item quality indicators. Specifically, the reviewers identified three skills as not being taught to students prior to test administration: literary device, author point of view and author technique. The test results of 44 DHH students who had taken the exam revealed congruence between the expert opinions on the test items and the students' performances on the test. Only 6 of 25 multiple choice items were correctly answered by 50% of students.

Table 6–14. *continued*

Study	Summary
Cahalan-Laitusis, Cook, and Aicher (2004)	The study investigated test results on third and seventh grade assessments of English/language arts. The analysis employed differential item functioning (DIF), which identifies items that are much harder or easier for group if test takers when compare to a reference group of test takers of the same ability. The researchers compared students with learning disabilities that received a read-aloud accommodation or extra time to two separate reference groups: students with and without disabilities who received no accommodations. The research results indicated that 7–12% of the test items functioned differently for students with learning disabilities that received read-aloud accommodations when compared to either of the reference groups. However, providing the students with learning disabilities with extra time resulted in only 0–1% of the items showing DIF.
LaSasso (1999)	The study looked at the limitations of tests and other assessment instruments that are administered to students during or after reading to measure reading comprehension. The author stated that conclusions about what deaf students learned were based on standardized tests, informal tests, and portfolios The study reviewed documented differences in test-taking abilities of deaf and hearing students, and listed specific compensatory test-taking strategies used by deaf readers. The author suggested instruction needed to include specific test-taking abilities in order to demonstrate mastery of subject matter. Therefore, the author recommended that deaf students needed to be exposed to instruction in multipurpose reading and to different test formats.

of ELs with special needs in general, and ELs with communication disorders in particular:

1. Assessment instruments for ELs with communication disorders should be made as accessible as possible to

control for cultural, linguistic, etc., biases. It is important to remember that instruments constructed for the general English-speaking population might not be valid for ELs with communication disorders.

2. Accommodations should level the playing field. For example, for ELs with communication disorders, selected accommodations should directly address either their communication disorder or their language needs.

3. Accommodations should not affect the construct being tested negatively. The validity of accommodations must be established so that the results obtained can be aggregated with the results of non-ELs.

4. Accommodations should be practical and easy to implement.

Summary

We have highlighted several protocols and instruments used nationally to assess language proficiency in ELs; however, this list is not exhaustive. Assessments used to identify ELs that have a disability are not included in this chapter, because the routine procedure usually followed is to identify struggling ELs as ELs first, before they are identified as students with disabilities. Although the ESOL or bilingual professional use the above measures to identify and place ELs in accordance to their language proficiency, it is the SLP, as a key member of an interdisciplinary team that determines if an EL has a communication disorder by making use of the information provided by the selected measures of language proficiency. The next chapter discusses the procedures used by the SLP to identify and determine appropriate services for ELs with communication disorders.

References

Abedi, J. (2009). English language learners with disabilities: Classification, assessment, and accommodation issues. *Journal of Applied Testing Technology, 10*(2).

Abedi, J., Courtney, M., & Leon, S. (2003). *Research-supported accommodations for English language learners in the NAEP* (CSE Tech.

Rep. No. 586). Los Angeles: University of California's National Center for Research on Evaluation, Standards, and Student Testing.

Abedi, J., Courtney, M., Mirocha, J., Leon, S., & Goldberg, J. (2005). *Language accommodations for English language learners in large-scale assessments: Bilingual dictionaries and linguistic modification* (CSE Tech. Rep. No. 666). Los Angeles: University of California's National Center for Research on Evaluation, Standards, and Student Testing.

Abedi, J., Hofstetter, C. H., Baker, E., & Lord, C. (2001). *NAEP math performance and test accommodations: Interactions with student language background* (CSE Tech. Rep. No. 536). Los Angeles: University of California's National Center for Research on Evaluation, Standards, and Student Testing.

Abedi, J., Hofstetter, C. H., & Lord, C. (2004). Assessment accommodations for English language learners: Implications for policy-based empirical research. *Review of Education Research, 74*(1), 1–28.

Abella, R., Urritia, J., & Shneyderman, A. (2005). An examination of the validity of English-language achievement test scores in an English language learner population. *Bilingual Research Journal, 29*(1), 127–144.

Accountability Works. (n.d.). Demonstrations of CELLA Online. Retrieved from http://www.awschooltest.com/news.php?viewStory=78

Albus, A., Bielinski, J., Thurlow, M., & Liu K. (2001). *The effect of simplified English language dictionary on a reading test* (LEP Projects Report 1). Minneapolis: University of Minnesota, National Center on Educational Outcomes.

Academic Language Programs Department—LAS Links. Retrieved from http://www2.yisd.net/education/components/docmgr/default.php?sectionetailid=162164&catfilter=10502#showdoc

American Speech-Language-Hearing Association. (2010). *Roles and responsibilities of speech-language pathologists in schools* [Professional issues statement]. Retrieved from www.asha.org/policy

Anderson, M., Liu, K., Swierzbin, B., Thurlow, M., & Bielinski, J. (2000). *Bilingual accommodations for limited English proficient students on statewide reading rests: Phase 2* (Minnesota Rep. No. 31). Minneapolis, MN: National Center for Educational Outcomes.

Bennett, R. E., Rock, D. A., & Kaplan, B. A. (1987). SAT differential item performance for nine handicapped groups. *Journal of Educational Measurement, 24*(1), 41–55.

Bennett, R. E., Rock, D. A., & Novatkoski, I. (1989). Differential item functioning on the SAT-M braille edition. *Journal of Eductional Measurement, 26*(1), 67–79.

Bolt, S. E., & Thurlow, M. L. (2004). Five of the most frequently allowed testing accommodations in state policy. *Remedial and Special Education, 25*(3), 141–152.

Briggs, M. (1991). Team development: Decision-making for early intervention. *Infant-Toddler Intervention, 1*(1), 1–9.

Brown, P. J. (1998). *Findings of 1997 Spring Field Test.* Delaware Department of Education.

Burk, M. (1999). *Computerized test accommodations.* Washington, DC: A.U. Software.

Butler, F. A., & Stevens, R. (1997). *Accommodation strategies for English language learners on large-scale assessments: Student characteristics and other considerations* (CSE Tech. Rep. No. 448*).* Los Angeles: University of California's National Center for Research on Evaluation, Standards, and Student Testing.

Cahalan-Laitusis, C., Cook, L. L., & Aicher, C. (2004). *Examining test items for students with disabilities by testing accommodation.* Paper presented at the Annual Meeting of the National Council on Measurement in Education, San Diego, CA.

Calderón, M. E. (2007). *Teaching reading to English language learners, Grades 6–12: A framework for improving achievement in the content areas.* Thousand Oaks, CA: Corwin Press.

California Department of Education. (n.d.). *California English language development.* Retrieved from http://www.cde.ca.gov/ta/tg/el/cefceldt.asp

California Department of Education. (n.d.a). *Home Language Survey form.* Retrieved from http://www.cde.ca.gov/ta/cr/documents/hls form.doc

Colorado Department of Education. (2005). *English Language Development Standards for the State of Colorado.* Retrieved from http://www.aps.k12.co.us/ela/Resources/ELD%20Standards%20April%20 2005.pdf

Colorado Department of Education. (2010). *Colorado Student Assessment System. 2010–2011 Procedures Manual for CSAP, CSAPA, CEL-Apro.* Retrieved from http://bvsd.org/assessment/accommodations/Documents/2011_Procedures_Manual.pdf

Comprehensive English Language Learning Assessment (CELLA). (2010). Bethesda, MD: Accountability Works. Retrieved from http://www.awschooltest.com/photos/Revised_CELLA_Technical_Summary_ Report.2010.pdf

De La Paz, S., & Graham, S. (1997). Strategy instruction in planning: Effects on the writing performance and behavior of students with learning difficulties. *Exceptional Children, 63,* 167–181.

Florida Department of Education. (2001). *Preparing Florida teachers to work with limited English proficient students.* Retrieved from http://www.fldoe.org/profdev/pdf/final_esol.pdf

Florida Department of Education. (2011). *Consent Decree.* Retrieved from http://www.fldoe.org/aala/cdpage2.asp

Florida Department of Education. (n.d.). *Florida CELLA Interpretive Guide*. Retrieved from www.fldoe.org/aala/pdf/CELLA-Interpretive-Guide.pdf

Florida Department of Education. (n.d.a.). *The CELLA Test accommodations*. Retrieved from http://search.fldoe.org/default.asp?cx=012683 245092260330905%3Aalo4lmikgz4&cof=FORID%3A11&q=CELLA+test+accomodations

Friend, M., & Cook, L. (2009). *Interactions: Collaboration skills for school professionals*. Boston, MA: Pearson.

Fuchs, L. S. (2000). *The validity of test accommodations for students with learning disabilities: Differential item performance on mathematics tests as function of test accommodations and disability status*. Delaware Department of Education.

Fuchs, L. S., Fuchs, D., Eaton, S. B., Hamlett, C., Binkley, E., & Crouch, R. (2000). Using objective data sources to enhance teacher judgments about test accommodations. *Exceptional Children, 67*, 67–81.

Fuchs, L. S., Fuchs, D., Eaton, S. B., & Karns, K. (2000). Supplementing teacher judgments of mathematics test accommodations with objective data sources. *School Psychology Review, 29*, 65–85.

Gottlieb, M., Cranley, M.E., & Cammilleri, A. (2007). *Understanding the WIDAEnglish language proficiency stgandards. A resource guide*. WI: Board of Regents of the University of Wisconsin System, on behalf of the WIDA Consortium. Retrieved from http://www.wida.us/standards/Resource_Guide_web.pdf

Graham, S. (1990). The role of production factors in learning disabled students' compositions. *Journal of Educational Psychology, 82*, 781–791.

Hafner, A. L. (2000). *Evaluating the impact of test accommodations on test scores of LEP students and non-LEP students*. Dover, DE: Delaware Department of Education.

IDEA Language Proficiency Tests (IPT). (2005). Brea, CA: Ballard & Tighe. Retrieved from http://www.ballard-tighe.com/products/la/iptFamilyTests.asp

Indiana Department of Education. (2006). *Language Assessment Scales-Links (LAS Links)*. Monterey, CA: CB/McGraw-Hill. Retrieved from http://www.doe.in.gov/lmmp/las-links.html

Johnson, E. S., Kimball, K., Brown, S. O., & Anderson, D. (2001). A statewide review of the use of accommodations in large-scale, high-stakes assessments. *Exceptional Children, 67*, 251–264.

Kiplinger, V. L., Haug, C. A., & Abedi, J. (2000, June). *A math assessment should test math, not reading: One state's approach to the problem*. Paper presented at the 30th annual National Conference on Large-Scale Assessment, Snowbird, UT.

LaSasso C. (1999). Test-taking abilities: A missing component of the curriculum for deaf students. *American Annals of the Deaf, 144,* 35–43.

Lollis, J., & LaSasso, C. (2008). The appropriateness of the NC state-mandated reading competency test for deaf students as a criterion for high school graduation. *Journal of Deaf Studies and Deaf Education Advance.* doi: 10.1093/deafed/enn017

Loop, C. (2002). Which tests are commonly used to determine English and/or Spanish language proficiency? *AskNCELA,* (25). Washington, DC: National Clearinghouse for English Language Acquisition.

Martin P. *(2005) An examination of the appropriateness of the New York State English language arts: Grade 8 test for deaf students.* Unpublished doctoral dissertation, Gallaudet University, Washington, DC.

McDonnell, L. M., McLaughlin, M. J., & Morison, P. (Eds.). (1997). *Educating one and all: Students with disabilities and standards-based reform.* Washington, DC: National Academy Press.

Mihai, F. M. (2010). *Assessing English language learners in the content areas: A research into practice guide for educators.* Ann Arbor: University of Michigan Press.

Minnesota Department of Education. (2011). *English learner education program guidelines. Identification and program basics.* Retrieved from http://search.education.state.mn.us/search?q=identification+and+placement+procedures+for+ELs+&searchbutton=Go&output=xml_no_dtd&oe=UTF-8&ie=UTF-8&client=New_frontend&proxystylesheet=New_frontend&site=default_collection

No Child Left Behind Act. (2001). Pub. L. No. 107-110, 115 Stat. 1446. Retrieved from http://www2.ed.gov/policy/elsec/leg/esea02/index.html

Ortiz, A., & Yates, J. R. (2002). Considerations in the assessment of English language learners referred to special education. In A. J. Artiles & A. Ortiz (Eds). *English language learners with special education needs* (pp. 65–85). McHenry, IL: Center for Applied Linguistics and Delta Systems.

Pena, E., & Quinn, R. (2003). Developing effective collaboration teams in speech-language pathology: A case study. *Communication Disorders Quarterly, 24,* 53–63.

Rhodes, R. L., Ochoa, S. H., & Ortiz, S. O. (2005). *Assessing culturally and linguistically diverse students: A practical guide.* New York, NY: Guilford Press.

Rosa-Lugo, L. I., & Fradd, S. (2000). Preparing professionals to serve English-language learners with communication disorders. *Communication Disorders Quarterly, 22*(1), 29–42.

Schrank, F. A., Wendling, B., Alvarado, C., & Woodcock, R. (2010). *Woodcock-Muñoz Language Survey—Revised Normative Update (WMLS-R NU)*. Itasca, IL: Riverside.

Schulte, A. G., Elliot, S. N., & Kratochwill, T. R. (2001). Experimental analysis of the effects of testing accommodations on students' standardized achievement test scores. *School Psychology Review, 30*(4), 527–547.

Sireci, S. G., Li, S. & Scarpati, S. (2003). *The effects of test accommodation on test performance: A review of the literature.* Center for Educational Assessment Research Report No. 485. Amherst, MA: School of Education, University of Massachusetts.

Spencer, S. (2005). Lynne Cook and June Downing: The practicalities of collaboration in special education service delivery. *Intervention in School and Clinic, 40*(5), 296–300.

Steinberg, J., Cline, F., Ling, G., Cook, L., & Tognatta, N. (2009). Examining the validity and fairness of a state standards-based assessment of English-language arts for deaf or hard of hearing students. *Journal of Applied Testing Technology, 10*(2).

Teachers of English to Speakers of Other Languages (TESOL). (2005). *PreK–12 English Language Proficiency Standards in the Core Content Areas.* Retrieved from http://www.projectshine.org/sites/default/files/English%20Language%20Proficiency%20Standards%20in%20the%20Core%20Content%20Areas.pdf

Teachers of English to Speakers of Other Languages (TESOL). (2006). *PreK–12 English language proficiency standards.* Alexandria, VA: Author.

Teachers of English to Speakers of Other Languages (TESOL). (2007). *TESOL position statement on the identification of English language learners with special educational needs.* Retrieved from http://www.tesol.org/s_tesol/bin.asp?CID=32&DID=8283&DOC=FILE.PDF

TELPAS. (2011). *Educator guide to TELPAS. Grades K–12.* Retrieved from http://www.tea.state.tx.us/WorkArea/linkit.aspx?LinkIdentifier=id&ItemID=2147501849&libID=2147501843

Thurlow, M. L., House, A., Boys, C., Scott, D., & Ysseldyke, J. (2000). *State participation and accommodation policies for students with disabilities: 1999 Update* (Synthesis Report 33). Minneapolis: University of Minnesota, National Center for Educational Outcomes.

Thurlow, M. L., Lazarus, S., Thompson, S., & Robey, J. (2002). *2001 state policies on assessment participation and accommodations* (Synthesis Report 46). Minneapolis: University of Minnesota, National Center for Educational Outcomes.

US Department of Education. (2002). Office of Elementary and Secondary Education. *No Child Left Behind: A desktop reference.* Washington, DC.

Woodcock, R. W., Muñoz-Sandoval, A. F., Ruef, M. L., & Alvarado, C. G. (2005). *Woodcock-Muñoz Language Survey—Revised*. Rolling Meadows, IL: Riverside.

World-Class Instructional Design and Assessment (WIDA) ACCESS Placement Test (W-APT). (2007a). Retrieved from http://wida.us/assessment/w-apt/#about

World-Class Instructional Design and Assessment (WIDA). (2007b). *The WIDA English Language Proficiency Standards, 2007 Edition, Pre-Kindergarten through grade 12*. Madison: University of Wisconsin.

World-Class Instructional Design and Assessment (WIDA). (2007c). *Writing rubric of the WIDA Consortium*. Retrieved from http://title-iii.pbworks.com/f/Writing+Rubric.pdf

World-Class Instructional Design and Assessment (WIDA). (2008). *ACCESS for ELLs®. Listening, Reading, Writing, and Speaking sample items, grades 1–12*. Retrieved from http://www.wida.us/assessment/ACCESS/ACCESS_Sample_Items.pdf

World-Class Instructional Design and Assessment (WIDA) (n.d.). *Comparing WIDA MODEL™, ACCESS for ELLs®, and W-APT™*. Retrieved from http://www.wida.us/assessment/comparing.aspx

World-Class Instructional Design and Assessment (WIDA). (n.d.a). *English language proficiency standards. WIDA's ELD Standards, 2012 Edition*. Retrieved from http://www.wida.us/standards/elp.aspx

Zehr, M. A. (2011, May). *WIDA tally: Half of states are now members of consortium*. Education Week, Bethesda, MD. Retrieved December 26, 2011, from http://blogs.edweek.org/edweek/learning-the-language/2011/01/wida_tally_consortium_now_has.html

7

An Interdisciplinary Approach to the Assessment of English Learners with Communication Disorders

Introduction

States often diverge on policies and procedures to identify ELs who need special services. They are challenged to a varying degree to determine whether a student's academic difficulties stem from learning a second language or from the presence of a communication disorder, or from both. The framework in which states must identify, evaluate, and provide evidenced-based intervention for ELs with communication disorders are couched in IDEA (2004) and NCLB (2001). This chapter focuses on the identification practices and protocols used by SLPs to identify ELs with a communication disorder and to determine eligibility for speech-language services and/or programs.

Identification Practices and Protocols for ELs with a Communication Disorder: Disability Determination, Eligibility, and Intervention

Different states have developed their own criteria or relied on the skilled judgment of professionals responsible for conducting special education assessments to guide the assessment and identification process (ASHA, n.d.). According to parents and school personnel, variations in these criteria and how they are applied have contributed to confusion when children move within and across school districts. In addition, as school administrators and boards of education have examined state special education prevalence data, increasing attention has been given to discrepancies among districts in the numbers of children identified as having speech-language disabilities, particularly in ELs. In a study conducted by Klingner and Harry (2006), researchers examined the special education referral and decision-making process for ELs in an urban school district in a southern state. Specifically, the researchers focused on the Child Study Team (CST) meetings, placement conferences/multidisciplinary team meetings, and the process that was used to determine if ELs who were struggling had disabilities. The researchers posed the following questions: (1) How is it determined whether ELs who struggle academically have a disability? (2) What is the decision-making process? (3) To what extent do the professionals involved understand second language acquisition? And (4) what considerations are given to language issues?

The researchers found that professionals were confused about when to refer an EL, were not always able to differentiate between English language acquisition and a disability, depended to a greater extent on test scores, misinterpreted the child's lack of full language proficiency as having a disability, and did not fully consider other factors that might affect a student's performance. In general, the findings of this study revealed that in practice, only cursory attention was given to prereferral strategies and/or response to intervention models (RtI) with ELs. Most importantly, there was a great deal of variability across schools in how district policies were carried out, how assessments were conducted, and how decisions were made (Spaulding, Plante, & Farinella, 2006).

The steady increase in the number of students whose primary language spoken in the home is a language other than English has created a need for the development of consistent state policies and procedures to appropriately identify and provide educational interventions for ELs and bilingual students with disabilities. There is widespread anecdotal evidence suggesting that ELs may be either bypassed for consideration as a child with a disability because professionals assume the child is not achieving solely because of his or her language difference, *or* overrepresented on special education rosters due to inappropriate placement based on inaccurate measures and ill-conceived procedures.

Roseberry-McKibben (2008) outlines the procedure commonly used to determine a student's eligibility for special education and/or related services (Figure 7–1). The process routinely begins with a teacher referral. If an EL student is suspected of a speech or language disorder, an interdisciplinary team (also often termed a "child study committee") convenes to review existing data and discuss possible interventions prior to referral for an evaluation. In an effort to reduce inappropriate identification and placement of ELs in special education, prereferral strategies are often implemented (Fuchs, Mock, Morgan, & Young, 2003). During this time it is important that a team of professionals

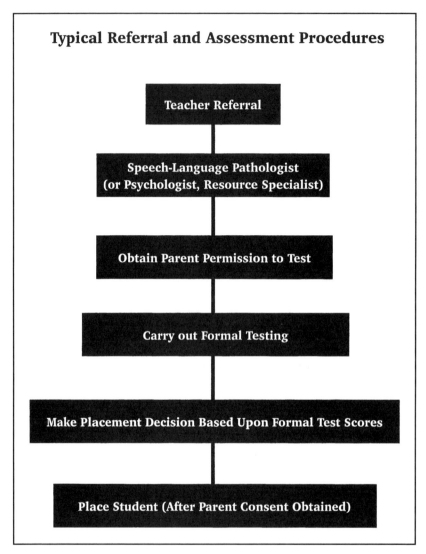

Figure 7–1. *Typical referral and assessment procedures.* Source: *From* Multi-cultural Students with Special Language Needs *(3rd ed.), by C. Roseberry-McKibben, 2008, Oceanside, CA: Academic Communication Associates.*

gather information about the student using a variety of strategies to determine whether a formal evaluation is warranted. A model, such as the one shown in Figure 7–2, can be used to guide the process of data collection. The purpose of these strategies is to

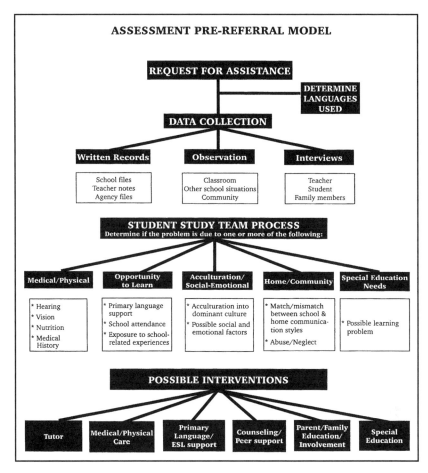

Figure 7–2. *Assessment prereferral model.* Source: *From* Multicultural Students with Special Language Needs *(3rd ed.), by C. Roseberry-McKibben, 2008, Oceanside, CA: Academic Communication Associates.*

provide students with assistance within the general education environment prior to conducting a formal evaluation to determine whether the student has a communication disorder.

With the reauthorization of IDEA (2004), response to intervention (RtI) multitiered models have been established as a vehicle for supporting monolingual English students and ELs with meaningful prereferral strategies. RtI has been recognized as a promising alternative for use with ELs (Burns, Griffiths, Parson, Tilly, & VanDerHeyden, 2007; Collier, 2010; Echevarria & Vogt,

2011; Ehren, 2005; Fuchs & Deshler, 2007; Klingner & Edwards, 2006; Mellard & Johnson, 2007; Moore & Montgomery, 2008; Schraeder, 2008), and the SLP can collaborate with school professionals and specialized instructional support personnel in the implementation of RtI models.

Several RtI models, flow charts, guiding questions, and recommendations have been offered to guide assessment professionals in the collection of critical student information. These resources can be used to facilitate decision making regarding the need for a more extensive formal evaluation of EL students (Batsche, Elliott, Graden, Grimes, Kovaleski, Prasse, et al., 2005; Leung, 1993; Linan-Thompson & Ortiz, 2009; Rinaldi & Samson, 2008; Rosa-Lugo, Rivera, & Rierson, 2010). Specifically, RtI models that focus on the use of screening and progress-monitoring tools and effective, high-quality, and linguistically and culturally responsive core curricula as a precursor to the identification of ELs with communication disorders have been recommended (Figures 7–3 and 7–4) (Esparza Brown, 2011, personal communication; Esparza Brown & Doolittle, 2008; Esparza Brown & Sanford, 2011).

To determine the presence of a disability, the normal behaviors of dual code learners and users must be identified, and differentiated from disabilities. Possible indicators of a language disorder have been described in the literature (Goldstein, 2004a; Goldstein, 2004b; Kayser, 1995; Kohnert, 2008; Ortiz, 1997; Paradis, 2005; Roseberry-McKibben, 2008). These indicators offer assessment professionals a framework to establish if the child: (a) meets the federal definition of a "child with a disability," (b) meets the criteria associated with one of the disability categories established in the law (e.g., speech-language impairment), and (c) if special education and/or related services are necessary to address the disability. For ELs the disability determination of "language disorder" is appropriate only for students with disabilities affecting their underlying ability to learn any language (Roseberry-McKibben, 2008). For example, the federal regulation at 34 CFR § 300.304 of IDEA (PL 108-146) (2004) requires that:

◆ assessments and other evaluation procedures are selected and administered to ensure that they measure the extent to which a child has a disability and needs special edu-

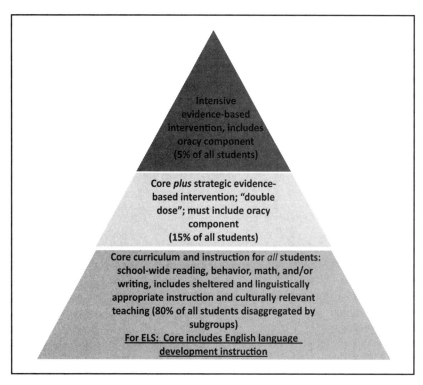

Figure 7–3. *Response to Intervention: Three-tier model for ELs.* Source: *From J. Esparza Brown, 2011, personal communication.*

cation, rather than measuring a child's English language skills;

◆ evaluators conduct assessments in the child's native/ dominant language;

◆ a variety of assessment tools and strategics are used to gather relevant functional and developmental information about the child;

◆ any standardized tests administered to a child are valid for the specific purpose for which they are used and are administered by trained and knowledgeable personnel in accordance with any instructions provided by the test publisher; and,

◆ no single procedure is used as the sole criterion for determining whether an EL child or student has a disability.

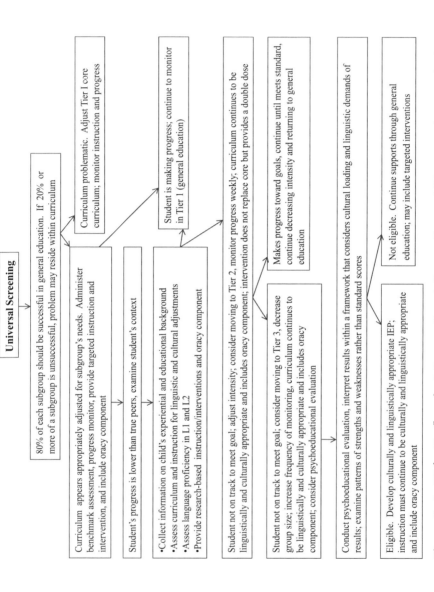

Universal Screening

80% of each subgroup should be successful in general education. If 20% or more of a subgroup is unsuccessful, problem may reside within curriculum

Curriculum appears appropriately adjusted for subgroup's needs. Administer benchmark assessment, progress monitor, provide targeted instruction and intervention, and include oracy component

Student's progress is lower than true peers, examine student's context

• Collect information on child's experiential and educational background
• Assess curriculum and instruction for linguistic and cultural adjustments
• Assess language proficiency in L1 and L2
• Provide research-based instruction/interventions and oracy component

Student not on track to meet goal; adjust intensity; consider moving to Tier 2, monitor progress weekly; curriculum continues to be linguistically and culturally appropriate and includes oracy component; intervention does not replace core but provides a double dose

Student not on track to meet goal; consider moving to Tier 3, decrease group size; increase frequency of monitoring, curriculum continues to be linguistically and culturally appropriate and includes oracy component; consider psychoeducational evaluation

Conduct psychoeducational evaluation, interpret results within a framework that considers cultural loading and linguistic demands of results; examine patterns of strengths and weaknesses rather than standard scores

Eligible. Develop culturally and linguistically appropriate IEP; instruction must continue to be culturally and linguistically appropriate and include oracy component

Curriculum problematic. Adjust Tier I core curriculum; monitor instruction and progress

Student is making progress; continue to monitor in Tier 1 (general education)

Makes progress toward goals, continue until meets standard, continue decreasing intensity and returning to general education

Not eligible. Continue supports through general education; may include targeted interventions

Figure 7–4. *RtI for ELs flow chart. Source: From J. Esparza Brown, 2011, personal communication.* ***Note:*** *When L1 instruction is not provided, expectations regarding rates of learning and grade-level benchmarks may not be met.*

286

When a speech-language disability is suspected in an EL, the SLP ideally must use a combination of assessment procedures and strategies that include:

- information obtained from the parents (medical, educational history; concerns regarding their child's communication);
- hearing screening;
- formal and informal assessment (e.g., standardized tests, language samples; alternative assessment strategies);
- review of classroom performance (e.g., work samples, journals, narratives, criterion-referenced tests);
- review of student record (e.g., performance on state or district assessments of prereading and reading abilities, attendance, discipline, health records, universal screening results);
- observation in the classroom, using checklists to quantify student behaviors, ideally during diverse instructional activities; and
- information obtained from teachers.

Roseberry-McKibben (2008) highlights a process that can be followed to determine if a language disorder is present (Figure 7–5). This assessment wheel highlights the various activities that SLPs use in the evaluation of ELs.

Practices Used by SLPs for EL Identification, Disability Determination, and Placement

Determining a Language Difference from a Disorder: The Role of Language Proficiency

Any student who has been identified as a student of limited English proficiency and is referred for an evaluation to determine if a disability is present is required to receive an assessment that considers the language or languages in which they can best demonstrate their cognitive, linguistic, and academic competence (Ortiz & Yates, 2002). This evaluation should be

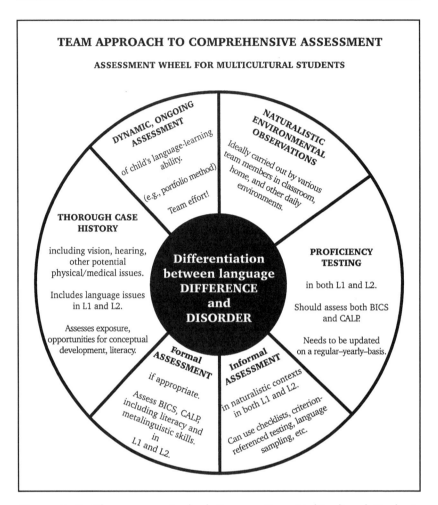

Figure 7–5. *The assessment wheel.* Source: *From* Multicultural Students with Special Language Needs *(3rd ed.), by C. Roseberry-McKibben, 2008, Oceanside, CA: Academic Communication Associates.*

conducted in the student's first acquired or home language, in English, or a combination of languages that the child brings to the assessment (Juarez, 1983; Langdon& Irvine Saenz, 1996).

The decision regarding the language selection for evaluation is often based on the results of the performance of the EL on a measure of language proficiency that has been previously determined by a designated professional in the school system (e.g., ESOL professional, general education teacher, bilingual teacher). In the absence of this information a designation of non-English speaker and limited English speaker (LES) requires an evaluation by a bilingual SLP or the use of an interpreter that is proficient in the language(s) being assessed. A designation of fluent English speaker (FES) allows students to be evaluated in English exclusively under the following circumstances: they have never spoken any language other than English, they are not proficient in their first language any longer, or they have been mainstreamed and no longer receive EL services. However, if the student understands the non-English language spoken in the home at a conversational level, but speaks only a few basic words or phrases, the evaluation should be done bilingually to determine the extent of the low functioning in the both languages. Often students who come from code-switching communities must also be provided with the opportunity to demonstrate their language use to determine if the code-switching behaviors are appropriate or indicative of a communication disorder.

Instruments and Assessment Practices Used by SLPs for EL Identification, Disability Determination, and Placement

IDEA (1997) requires that ELs be assessed in their native language(s) (L1) and English (L2) using appropriate test instruments and assessment practices. Despite the persistent shortage of norm-referenced assessment procedures in languages other than English (Langdon & Cheng, 2002; Peña, Iglesias, & Lidz, 2001), SLPs typically administer tests normed on monolingual English speakers and then use measures normed on a specific language group (e.g., monolingual Spanish speakers) to determine if the EL has a disorder.

Prior to determining if the child has a language difference or a language disorder, the SLP must first obtain information about a child's language proficiency and functioning in L1 and L2. Similar to the ESOL professional (see chapter 6), the SLP often uses the Woodcock-Muñoz Language Survey—Revised Normative Update (WMLS-R NU) (Shrank, Wendling, Alvarado,

& Woodcock, 2010) to assess the level of English language proficiency (ELP) in ELs. The SLP also uses the WMLS-R NU to help them decide whether or not a bilingual speech-language assessment is warranted. This practice can be problematic. In the WMLS-R NU cluster scores provide the primary basis for interpretation. SLPs generally administer selected subtests (e.g., subtest 1—Picture Vocabulary, subtest 2—Verbal Analogies, subtest 5—Understanding Directions, and subtest 6—Story Recall) that contribute to related cluster scores to assess the level of oral English language proficiency (Table 7–1).

If the child obtains low CALP scores (levels 1 or 2) on the WMLS-R NU, the SLP might assume that the child does not need to be assessed further in that language. It is possible that the child may score limited Spanish (CALP level 3) on this measure and yet perform within normal limits on other measures of language tasks in Spanish. This is particularly likely to occur when the child is not being instructed in Spanish. Therefore, it is recommended that SLPs assess the child's functional language

Table 7–1. *WMLS-R NU (Oral Language Cluster—Total)*

Academic Language Cluster: Oral Language Cluster—Total WMLS-R Tests			
Picture Vocabulary	Verbal Analogies	Understanding Directions	Story Recall
Student is required to recognize an object and provide object name	Student is required to analyze relationship between words and then project that onto the second part of the analogy	Student is required to listen to a series of oral commands and apply the sequence to specified objects in a picture	Student is required to listen to a story and retell using own words

Source: Adapted from *Interpretive Supplement: Instructional Interventions for English Language Learners Related to the Woodcock-Muñoz Language Survey—Revised Normative Update,* by F. A. Schrank, C. G. Alvarado, & B. J. Wendling, 2010b, Rolling Meadows, IL: Riverside.

in Spanish and, as with all measures, careful interpretation of results is warranted.

Despite the limitations found with using static, standardized, quantitative, norm-referenced approaches to assess ELs, several standardized assessment instruments and practices are consistently used by bilingual and monolingual SLPs (with the assistance of a translator when warranted) to determine whether a student has a language delay, difference, or disorder (Caesar & Kohler, 2007; Langdon, 1989). Of the norm-referenced measures, the Clinical Evaluation of Language Fundamentals—Fourth Edition (CELF-4 English; Semel, Wiig, & Secord, 2003) is one of the most frequently used standardized test (Senaga & Inglebret, 2003).

This is often followed by the Expressive One-Word Picture Vocabulary Test: Spanish-Bilingual Edition (EOWPVT-SBE; Brownel, 2000a); the Receptive One-Word Picture Vocabulary Test: Spanish-Bilingual Edition (ROWPVT-SBE; Brownell, 2000b); the Preschool Language Scale (Zimmerman, Steiner, & Pond, 1992); and the Structured Photographic Expressive Language—Third Edition (SPELT-3) (Dawson, Stout, & Elyer, 2003).

To better understand these assessment measures, we provide a brief overview of each of the tests, their use, and their importance in determining a language difference or disorder.

Clinical Evaluation of Language Fundamentals—Fourth Edition (CELF-4 English)

The CELF-4 (Semel, Wiig, & Secord, 2003) is administered individually to determine whether a student (aged 5 through 21) has a language disorder or delay. This revised test measures four aspects of language (morphology and syntax, semantics, pragmatics, and phonological awareness) and can be administered in 30 to 60 minutes. The focus of this instrument is to evaluate a student's general language ability and to determine whether or not a language disorder is present. This is achieved by administering four subtests that yields a core language score. The CELF-4 (English) consists of 19 subtests that are exemplified in Table 7–2.

Table 7–2. CELF-4 English Subtests

Subtest	Subtest Task	Composite Score Formed Ages 5–8	Composite Score Formed Ages 9–21
Concepts and Following Directions	The student points to pictured objects in response to oral directions	Core	9–12 Core
Word Structure	The student completes sentences using the targeted structure(s)	Core	
Recalling Sentences	The student imitates sentences presented by the examiner	Core	Core
Formulated Sentences	The student formulates a sentence about visual stimuli using a targeted word or phrase	Core	Core
Word Classes 1 and 2	The student chooses two related words and describes their relationship	Receptive/ Content	Core
Sentence Structure	The student points to a picture that illustrates the given sentence	Receptive/ Structure	
Expressive Vocabulary	The student identifies a pictured object, person, or activity	Content	Content
Word Definitions	The student defines a word that is presented and used in a sentence		Core/Content

Table 7–2. continued

| Subtest | Subtest Task | Composite Score Formed | |
		Ages 5–8	Ages 9–21
Understanding Spoken Paragraphs	The student responds to questions about orally presented paragraphs; questions target main idea, details, sequence, inferential, and predictive information	Supplemental	Content/ Receptive
Sentence Assembly	The student produces two semantically/ grammatically correct sentences from visually and orally presented words/groups of words		Content
Semantic Relationships	The student listens to a sentence and selects the two choices that answer a target question		Receptive/ Language Memory
Number Repetition 1 and 2	The student repeats a series of numbers forward, then backward	Working Memory	Working Memory
Familiar Sequences 1 and 2	The student names days of the week, counts backward, orders other information while being timed	Working Memory	Working Memory

continues

Table 7–2. continued

Subtest	Subtest Task	Composite Score Formed	
		Ages 5–8	Ages 9–21
Rapid Automatic Naming	The student names colors, shapes, and color-shape combinations while being timed	Supplemental subtest	Supplemental subtest
Word Associations	The student names words in specific categories while being timed	Supplemental subtest	Supplemental subtest
Phonological Awareness	The student rhymes, segments, blends, identifies sounds and syllables in words and sentences	Supplemental subtest	Supplemental subtest
Pragmatics Profile	The examiner elicits information from a parent or teacher about the student's social language skills.	Supplemental subtest	Supplemental subtest
Observational Rating Scales	Parent, teacher, and student each rate the student's classroom interaction and communication skills.	Supplemental subtest	Supplemental subtest

Source: Adapted from CELF Technical Report, 2008. Retrieved from http://www
.pearsonassessments.com/NR/rdonlyres/F7DBBC32-B63E-4B8E-B1C4-59D
8358E5CA5/0/CELF_4_Tech_Report.pdf

The CELF-4 subtests provide a measure of specific aspects of language form, content, use, and working memory with resulting index scores that provide useful information regarding a student's strengths and weaknesses. These index scores are highlighted below:

Core—The Core Language Score

◆ The Core Language Score is a measure of general language ability that quantifies a student's overall language performance and is used to make decisions about the presence or absence of a language disorder. It is derived by summing the scaled scores from the subtests that best discriminate typical language performance from disordered language performance.

Receptive—The Receptive Language Index

◆ This is a measure of listening and auditory comprehension and is derived by summing the scaled scores from a combination of two or three receptive subtests.

Expressive—The Expressive Language Index

◆ The Expressive Language Index is an overall measure of expressive language skills. The subtests used to derive the receptive language and expressive language scores depend on the student's age.

Content—The Language Content Index

◆ This is a measure of various aspects of semantic development, including vocabulary, concept and category development, comprehension of associations and relationships among words, interpretation of factual and inferential information presented orally, and the ability to create meaningful, semantically and syntactically correct sentences.

Structure —The Language Structure Index

◆ This index is an overall measure of receptive and expressive components of interpreting and producing sentence structure. This index is used only for students aged 5 to 8.

Language Memory—The Language Memory Index

♦ This is a measure of the ability to recall spoken directions, formulate sentences with given words, and identify semantic relationships. It provides a measure of the ability to apply working memory to linguistic content and structure. This index is used for students aged 9 to 21 years.

Working Memory—The Working Memory Index

♦ This is a measure of attention, concentration, and recall. The complex manipulation of stimuli in short-term memory underlies the concept of working memory. All subtest scaled and composite standard scores of the test can be converted to percentile ranks and test-age equivalents.

Clinical Evaluation of Language Fundamentals—Fourth Edition, Spanish Edition (CELF-4 Spanish)

The Spanish edition of the CELF-4 (Semel, Wiig, & Secord, 2006) is an individually administered clinical tool for the identification, diagnosis, and follow-up evaluation of language and communication disorders in Spanish-speaking students aged 5 to 21. The CELF-4 Spanish is a norm-referenced standardized assessment developed specifically for Spanish speakers living in the United States as a parallel test to the CELF-4. It is not a translation of the English edition of the CELF-4. The test is normed on a current sample of Spanish speakers in the US, representing many countries of origin (25% from the Caribbean [Puerto Rico, Dominican Republic, and Cuba], 28% from Central and South America, and 46% from Mexico). This test evaluates interpersonal communication (BICS), elements of more advanced academic language (CALP), and includes a Pragmatics Profile and an Observational Rating Scale. It consists of 16 subtests, exemplified in Table 7–3.

Table 7-3. *CELF-4 Spanish Subtests*

Subtest	Subtest Task
Concepts and Following Directions (Conceptos y siguiendo direcciones)	The student points to pictured objects in response to oral directions
Word Structure (Estructura de palabras)	The student completes sentences using the targeted structure(s)
Recalling Sentences (Recordando oraciones)	Examiner presents sentence and student is required to imitate the sentence
Formulated Sentences (Formulación de oraciones)	The student formulates a sentence about visual stimuli using a targeted word or phrase
Word Classes—1 and 2 (Clases de palabras 1 y 2)	The student chooses two related words and describes their relationship
Sentence Structure (Estructura de oraciones)	The student points to a picture that illustrates the given sentence
Expressive Vocabulary (Vocabulario expresivo)	The student identifies a pictured object, person, or activity given a stimulus
Word Definitions (Definiciones de palabras)	The student defines a word that is presented and used in a sentence
Understanding Spoken Paragraphs (Entendiendo párrafos)	The student responds to questions about orally presented paragraphs; questions target main idea, details, sequence, inferential, and predictive information
Number Repetition 1 and 2 (Repetición de números 1 y 2)	The student repeats a series of numbers forward, then backward
Familiar Sequences 1 and 2 (Secuencias familiars 1 y 2)	The student names days of the week, counts backward, orders other information while being timed

continues

Table 7–3. *continued*

Subtest	Subtest Task
Rapid Automatic Naming (Enumeración rápida y automática)	The student names colors, shapes, and color-shape combinations while being timed
Word Associations (Asociación de palabras)	The student names words in specific categories while being timed
Phonological Awareness (Conocimiento fonológico)	The student rhymes, segments, blends, identifies sounds and syllables in words and sentences
Pragmatics Profile (Clasificación pragmática)	The examiner elicits information from a parent or teacher about the student's social language skills.
Observational Rating Scales Escala de valoración del lenguaje)	Parent, teacher, and student each rate the student's classroom interaction and communication skills.

Source: Adapted from *The Clinical Evaluation of Language Fundamentals—Fourth Edition, Spanish Edition (CELF-4 Spanish)*, by E. Semel, E. H. Wiig, & W. A. Secord, 2006, San Antonio, TX: Pearson.

Preschool Language Scale — Fourth Edition (PLS-4), English and Spanish Editions

The PLS-4, English Edition (Zimmerman, Steiner, & Pond, 2002a), is designed to identify young children from birth to 6 years, 11 months old who might have a language disorder or delay. Test administration varies between 20 and 45 minutes. PLS-4 English consists of two subscales, Auditory Comprehension and Expressive Communication. The Auditory Comprehension subscale measures a child's ability to understand spoken language; the Expressive communication subscale measures the ability of a child to self-express verbally. The test also provides three supplemental measures, which include an articulation screener, a language sample checklist, and a caregiver questionnaire.

In terms of test procedures, test items for infants and toddlers focus on skills that are considered important precursors of language development, such as attention to a speaker and object-specific play. For example, tasks for a 12-month-old include identifying familiar objects, playing appropriately with objects, following simple directions, babbling two syllables together, and having a vocabulary of at least one word.

Children aged 2 and 3 are engaged in interactive play activities with brightly colored objects and toys. Preschoolers are asked to respond to pictures, answer questions, and tell stories about the pictures. Many of these tasks assess comprehension of basic vocabulary, concepts such as big, little, long, and so forth, and grammatical markers.

For 5- and 6-year-old children, the test measures their ability to understand complex sentences, compare objects, and make inferences. Typical tasks in the PLS-4 English Edition for a 6-year-old child include identifying initial sounds in words, defining words such as "shirt," and recognizing and repairing grammatical errors in sentences.

To make sure that very young children are not penalized for failure to respond, some items for the youngest age can be scored as "passed" when the expected behavior is reported by the caregiver or seen during testing in spontaneous interactions with the examiner or caregiver. When the caregiver reports that the child has performed the behavior at home, the caregiver is required to provide specific examples.

Each of the 62 auditory comprehension tasks and 68 expressive communication tasks may include one or more subitems. For each task, pass criteria are listed on the PLS-4 Record Form, which simplifies test administration. For infant and toddler behaviors, the Record Form includes a description of the target behavior. For example, "Turns head or searches with eyes" is the pass criteria for the behavior for the "Actively searches to find a person who is talking" behavior. For older children, the pass criteria may be "3 correct" out of four or five questions that comprise one test item, such as naming objects or answering questions. Test items that are passed receive a score of "1" and those that are not passed receive a score of "0."

The PLS-4, Spanish Edition (Zimmerman, Steiner, & Pond, 2002b), follows the structure of PLS-4 English, although it is not a translation of the English version. There are several important differences. First, test items, the examiner's manual, the Record Form, and the picture manual are Spanish-edition specific. Then, test subitems are sometimes different to reflect the linguistic characteristics of the two languages. For example, in the English edition, "babies" and "horses" are examples of plurals. In the Spanish edition, based on data from Spanish speakers, "limones" and "ratones" are used as example of plurals. Last, but not least, separate norms have been developed for the Spanish edition based on 1,188 Spanish-speaking children living in the US.

The vocabulary used in PLS-4 Spanish test items is typical of vocabulary used in the Southwest. Dialectal variations are listed in the test and can be used to determine acceptable responses. Children who are from a different region may not use the vocabulary in PLS-4 Spanish; therefore, PLS-4 Spanish provides acceptable vocabulary items. The test manual suggests that the test examiner should interview the parent before the evaluation to determine if the words used by their children are acceptable substitutions. Additionally, bilingual children may respond in both English and Spanish or code-switch.

Receptive One-Word Picture Vocabulary Test and Expressive One Word Picture Vocabulary Test, English and Spanish Editions

The Expressive One-Word Picture Vocabulary Test, Fourth Edition (EOWPVT- 4) (Brownell, 2010a) and the Receptive One-Word Picture Vocabulary Test, Fourth Edition(ROWPVT- 4) (Brownell, 2010b) are administered to children aged 2 years to 18 years and 11 months. The EOWPVT is designed to assess expressive vocabulary, whereas the main purpose of ROWPVT is to measure receptive vocabulary. Test administration for each is approximately 20 minutes. To administer the EOWPVT, the examiner presents a series of illustrations showing objects, actions, or concepts. The child is asked to name each illustration. The test begins with an illustration the child is expected to name successfully. The examiner then presents items that become progressively more difficult. When the examinee is unable to correctly name a number of consecutive illustrations, testing discontinues.

To administer the ROWPVT, the examiner presents a series of test plates that each shows four illustrations. The examiner orally presents a stimulus word, and the child is expected to identify the illustration that depicts the meaning of the word. Like the EOWPVT, the test begins with a word the child should be able to identify. The examiner then presents items that become progressively more difficult. When the examinee is unable to correctly identify the meaning of a specified number of items, testing is stopped. EOWPVT was conormed with the ROWPVT, so accurate comparisons can be made between a student's receptive and expressive vocabulary skills.

Both the EOWPVT (Brownell, 2000a) and the ROWPVT (Brownel, 2000b) have bilingual versions assessing the expressive and receptive vocabulary of children who are bilingual in Spanish and English, aged 4 to 12. They are the Expressive One-Word Picture Vocabulary Test: Spanish-Bilingual Edition (EOWPVT-SBE) and the Receptive One-Word Picture Vocabulary Test: Spanish-Bilingual Edition (ROWPVT-SBE). These versions assess total acquired vocabulary by allowing children to respond in both languages, and the record forms include acceptable responses and stimulus words in both languages.

Structured Photographic Expressive Language Test— Third Edition (SPELT-3)

The Structured Photographic Expressive Language Test—Third Edition (SPELT-3) (Dawson, Stout, & Elyer, 2003) assesses morphosyntactic skills in children aged 4 years to 9 years and 11 months. It requires the child to look at color photographs of everyday situations and familiar objects and answer simple questions about each one. These questions, presented orally by the examiner, elicit specific morphological syntactic structures and are used nationally to assess children who experience language problems. The SPELT-3 is a revision of the SPELT-2 (Werner & Kresheck, 1983), which has been shown in the past to have high levels of discriminant accuracy in identifying preschoolers with language impairment (Perona, Plante, & Vance, 2005). Using 54 (4 by 6 inches) stimulus pictures the examiner elicits simple verbal questions and statements to elicit specific morphological and syntactic structures. This assessment tool allows for analysis of specific language structures that may not occur in spontaneous language samples. The manual includes explicit scoring guidelines, listing expected responses and typical errors. A separate chapter addresses African American vernacular response variations.

Spanish Structured Photographic Expressive Language Test—Third Edition (Spanish SPELT-3)

The importance of measuring language proficiency in the development of a second language resulted in the development of the Spanish version of the *Spanish SPELT-Preschool* and the *Spanish SPELT-2* (Werner & Krescheck, 1983). The Spanish *SPELT-3* (Langdon, 2011) assesses the expressive language of Spanish-speaking children. Although this test is not a direct translation of the English SPELT-3, it also assesses morphology and syntax skills in monolingual or bilingual children aged 4 years to 9 years and 6 months. It also samples the child's ability to use pragmatically appropriate language for various purposes.

The primary purpose of the Spanish SPELT-3 is to: (1) aid in identifying children who may be in need of language intervention; and (2) assist in targeting intervention that considers the child's strengths and weaknesses. This test utilizes actual photographs of children in contexts that are conducive to specific utilization of linguistic markers, particularly those related to noun, adjective, and verb morphology. This test allows analysis of a child's ability to express common grammatical form, as well as to perform rule-governed changes in sentence structure.

Important Considerations Regarding Language Assessment Instruments for ELs with Communication Disorders

SLPs have become increasingly aware of the inappropriateness of many standardized tests used with ELs; however, they continue to rely primarily on the use of norm-referenced tests to determine if an EL has a disorder (Crowley, 2003; Kriticos, 2003; Roseberry-McKibben, 2008). Reliance on these instruments often occurs because SLPs and other professionals believe that federal law (i.e., IDEA) requires their use to determine a disability and subsequently eligibility for special education intervention. According to federal law, however, standardized tests are not required. Yet, they are often used because they provide scores (i.e., percentile ranks, standard scores) that are used as guidelines to determine if a student is eligible for special education services. Furthermore, they are often used because they are perceived as more expedient and convenient to administer. Given the paucity of standardized tests for ELs in most languages and the continued use of standardized tests to assess the language development of ELs, several important considerations regarding their use are provided.

Standardized Testing and Bias

Selecting an appropriate standardized test is a challenging task. It is often recommended that professionals examine test items and consult test manuals to review the adequacy, reliability, and validity of tests used with ELs with different language profiles (Caesar & Kohler, 2007; Hutchinson, 1996). Many standardized tests, designed from a middle-class, literate Western framework, contain many potential sources of bias (Goldstein, 2000; Kayser, 1998; Roseberry-McKibben, 2008). These may include content bias (use of activities and items that are not familiar to the child), value bias (use of a test item that is inconsistent with the child's value system), format bias (using test procedures and/or materials that are unfamiliar to the child), an/or examiner bias (examiner may be unfamiliar with the cultural and/or linguistic characteristics of the child and/or have low expectations of the child and interpret results based on these assumptions). These tests are also designed with the assumption that a child will have the experiential background to perform optimally in a testing situation with test tasks that are administered by an unfamiliar adult using a language that the child might not yet have mastered.

Test Administration and Interpretation

Modifying how a test is administered, scored, and interpreted has been discussed as one way to minimize test bias (Bedore et al., 2005; Goldstein, 2002; Greenfield, 1997; Hamayan & Damico, 1991; Kayser, 1995, 1998; Roseberry-McKibben, 2003; Saenz & Huer, 2003). Although a variety of recommendations to modify standardized tests for ELs have been offered, these have not always resulted in eliminating test bias. Some of the modifications have included:

- Providing instructions to the child in L1 and English
- Rephrasing of instructions
- Providing the student with extra time
- Asking the child to clarify an "incorrect" response and score the response within the context of the child's cultural and linguistic background
- Using a dual scoring system
- Completing the assessment over a period of time

Some recommendations to reduce bias in test *interpretation* have included:

- Consulting the literature to determine if the errors demonstrated by the child are typical of other ELs from similar backgrounds
- Incorporating cautionary statements and disclaimers regarding deviations from standardized assessment procedures
- Avoiding the use of only standardized test results to determine disability and eligibility for special education services

Translated Tests

Determining which tests are most appropriate for a given purpose requires that the SLP be familiar with the theoretical framework of the test and the possible limitations of the test (Goldstein, 2000; McCauley & Swisher, 1984; Plante & Vance, 1994). Often, translated versions of speech-language tests have been used with ELs without considering the inherent problems in their use. For example, many translations provide word-for-word translations that do not account for a lack of equivalent linguistic form in the second language. Additionally, translated tests do not consider the effects of second language acquisition on a student's performance. As a precaution, scores from these translated versions should not be used to diagnose a communication disorder.

Tests in the Primary Language

To counteract the practice of using translated versions of English assessment instruments, many professionals use tests specifically developed for bilingual children, some of which were discussed above. These tests have been specifically developed in the primary language to assess the language skills of ELs. Although many tests have proven to be useful in the identification and diagnosis of language and communication disorders in children (i.e., Semel, Wiig, & Secord, 2006) the use of tests in the primary language has also been problematic (Pena & Kester, 2004; Perona, Plante, & Vance, 2005; Restrepo & Silverman, 2001). For example, several assessment instruments developed to accommodate a child's various proficiency levels in Spanish and English do not represent all the existing dialects of Spanish. Therefore, the SLP will need to be familiar with different dialects and what is acceptable across dialects to determine acceptable and unacceptable responses.

Another challenge is the availability of reliable phonological and language development norms. Although developmental norms have been developed for Spanish (e.g., Acevedo, 1993; Anderson, 1995; Fantini, 1985; Goldstein & Iglesias, 1996; Jimenez, 1987; Merino, 1992), developmental data on languages other than English continues to be limited.

Alternatives to Standardized Assessment

A critical question often asked by SLPs is: if standardized testing has such limitations and challenges, then what should we use to identify ELs with possible disabilities and to determine appropriate services? We have previously discussed that IDEA (2004) requires that ELs be assessed in their native language(s) (L1) and English (L2) using appropriate test instruments and assessment practices. We also noted that although IDEA allows for the use of norm-referenced standardized tests, it also allows for the use of subjective and qualitative measures. One option often recommended to SLPs is to use alternative assessment procedures (IDEA, 2004; Kohnert, 2008; Roseberry-McKibben, 2008; Saenz & Huer, 2003). Several alternative assessment procedures have been recommended. These include: (a) criterion-referenced testing, (b) language sampling, (c) dynamic assessment, (d) observation, and (e) use of interpreters. Each of these is briefly described.

Criterion-Referenced Testing

Criterion-referenced testing differs from norm-referenced testing. Criterion-referenced tests are administered to primarily gauge a child's skill level or capability, as opposed to determining a child's overall level as compared to others who are given the same test. The SLP often uses criterion-referenced measures to obtain a profile of a child's strengths and weaknesses. Criterion-referenced measures allow for reporting results using percentage of items passed, instead of normative standard scores (Battle, 2002; Laing & Kamhi, 2003).

Criterion-referenced tests are often used when norms that might be used to provide a norm-referenced interpretation of test performance are unavailable or inappropriate, or when information concerning specific skills or behaviors of a test taker is required by the clinical question being posed (McCauley, 1996). One drawback for using criterion-referenced measures is that their use still presumes a developmental framework that might not be appropriate or available for ELs (Goldstein, 2000). An example of a criterion-referenced measure is the Diagnostic Evaluation of Language Variation (DELV) (Seymour, Roeper, & de Villiers, 2005). This measure is appropriate for children who are mainstream American English (MAE) speakers and those who speak a variation of MAE (i.e., African American English [AAE]). The goal of this measure is to assist SLPs in distinguishing normal developmental language changes and patterns of variation from true markers of language disorder or delay.

Language Samples

Another alternative assessment technique used by SLPs is language sampling (Beck, 1995; Caesar & Kohler, 2007; Hux, 1993). Many experts (Gutierrez-Clellen, Restrepo, & Bedore, Pena & Anderson, 2000; Kayser & Restrepo, 1995) suggest that this approach allows the SLP to obtain language information about the conversational skills, syntactic structures, grammatical competency, and language use of ELs. They also note that language samples are useful in differentiating between a language disorder and a language difference.

Gathering a language sample in all languages used by the EL requires that the SLP have language proficiency in the child's language. If the child's primary language is not English, then the SLP should enlist the services of a bilingual SLP or use a properly trained interpreter to assist in the collection and analysis of the language sample. Additionally, the SLP should be familiar with a variety of elicitation techniques and analysis protocols and use these appropriately in analyzing the obtained sample (Retherford, 2000).

Although conversation followed by narration (i.e., giving a child a book to read) has been identified as the technique most often used by SLPs to elicit language samples, a number of alternate techniques have been recommended (Cornejo, Weinstein, & Najar, 1983; Hux, Morris-Friehe, & Sanger, 1993; Kayser, 1995, 1998; Langdon, 1992). These include: having a child describe an object; engage in a game or problem-solving activity in order to verbalize an answer to a problem; and narrating or describing a sequence of events. When storytelling is used in the context of a spontaneous language sample, the SLP should use procedures to analyze story structures in a narrative (see Bloome, Champion, Katz, Morton, & Muldrow, 2001; Champion & Mainess, 2003; Champion & Seymour, 1995; Gutierrez-Clellen & Quinn, 1993; Hester, 2010; Rollins, McCabe, & Bliss, 2000). It is also recommended that SLPs obtain language samples as the child engages in activities across settings (e.g., home and school) with a variety of conversational partners in order to yield a more representative and reliable measure of the child's language abilities.

A variety of strategies are available to analyze language samples (see Bliss, 2002; Gutierrez-Clellen et al., 2004; Linares,

1981; Long & Channell, 2001; Owens, 2004; Roseberry-McKibben, 2007). The main areas of language sample analysis are form (morphology, syntax, discourse structure), content (objects, actions), and use (semantics) (Swisher, 1994). Although many of these procedures require time, training, and skill in their application, they are valuable in assessing the language skills of ELs and capturing their strengths and weaknesses (Kemp & Klee, 1997; MacWhinney, 1996, 2000a, 2000b). The following are examples of analysis techniques used by SLPs to describe the child's language.

Mean Length of Response (MLR)

One of the frequently reported measures of linguistic skill in young children has been the mean length of response (MLR). MLR is a measure of expressive language development and has been defined as the average number of words used in 50 consecutive verbal utterances. Normative data are available and MLR measurement is known to be reliable (Webster & Shelton, 1964). MLR has also been recommended for languages that are highly inflected (i.e., Spanish) (Schnell de Acedo, 1994).

Mean Length of Utterance (MLU)

Mean length of utterance (MLU) is a measure of linguistic productivity in children. MLU is the average length of morphemes in the child's utterances and is traditionally calculated by collecting 100 utterances spoken by a child and dividing the number of morphemes by the number of utterances (MLU = number of morphemes/number of utterances). A higher MLU is taken to indicate a higher level of language proficiency (Owens, 2004). To measure morphological production in Spanish-speaking children, Linares (1981) recommended a procedure to calculate the mean length of utterance-morphemes (MLU-m) in Spanish.

The use of MLU has been challenged, specifically for counting verb inflections and the use of mean length of utterance-words (MLU-w) has been offered as an alternative (Schnell de Acedo, 1994). MLU-w is calculated by summing the number of words for each utterance and dividing by the number of utterances. Caution in using MLU as the only diagnostic measure of language proficiency in children is recommended.

Type-Token Ratio (TTR)

Language samples can also be analyzed using the Type-Token Ratio (TTR). TTR is a measure of vocabulary variation that a child uses expressively and measures the proportion of different words (types) to total words (tokens). The TTR is calculated by the ratio TTR = number of different words in a sample/total number of words in a sample, and reflects the diversity of words used by the client during a language sample.

Terminal Units (T-Units)

Another measure of analysis used in language sampling is the T-unit (minimal terminal unit). T-unit analysis, developed by Hunt (1965), has been used extensively to measure overall syntactic complexity, especially in older children. T-units are defined as any clause and its subordinate clauses that are attached to or embedded in the main clause. The application of this analysis technique to measure the syntactic language skills of school-age children (Klecan-Aker & Hedrick, 1985) and specifically bilingual Spanish children is offered as one way to quantify and analyze the language assessment of ELs with different levels of English proficiency (Gutiérrez-Clellen, Restrepo, Bedore, Peña, & Anderson, 2000; Kayser & Restrepo, 1995).

Computer-Aided Language Sample

Recent advances in computer technology have made analysis of language samples a realistic option (Long & Channell, 2001). Wider availability of software and hardware technologies has increased an SLP's potential for using Computer-Aided Language Sample Analysis protocols. Despite their availability, many SLPs continue to analyze their language samples based on nonstandardized, self-designed procedures (Hux, Morris-Friehe, & Sanger, 1993). Programs such as the CLAN program (Child Language Analysis) used in the CHILDES project (MacWhinney, 1996); the SALT (Systematic Analysis of Language Transcripts; Miller & Chapman, 2008); the PAL (Pye Analysis of Language; Pye, 1987); and the CP (Computerized Profiling) program (Long, Fey, & Channel, 2000) are some of the computer-aided language sample analysis protocols that are available to SLPs. Although some programs now include separate databases to compare Spanish-English bilinguals and African American English (AAE)–speaking children, overall tools or established protocols remain limited for other languages (Hammett Price, Hendricks, & Cook, 2010; Hux et al., 1993; Kemp & Klee, 1997; Kohnert, 2008; Miller & Iglesias, 2006; Miller, Freiberg, Rolland, & Reeves, 1992).

There are many ways the SLP can analyze language samples. In general, the use of this alternative assessment can provide the SLP with information on the language proficiency of the EL. Observation of the child with different language partners, across settings, using all languages, and including code-switching or use of dialects assists the SLP to obtain a more comprehensive view of the EL.

Dynamic Assessments

Static procedures to assess ELs are often used by SLPs to make disability determinations. One challenge with this practice is that judgments about the language proficiency of ELs are made using the results of testing that measure the student's skills at one point in time and do not consider the child's ability to learn. In recent years, dynamic assessment has been recommended as an alternative means of assessing ELs who are suspected of having language disabilities (Hux, 1993; Laing & Kamhi, 2003; Lidz & Pena, 1996; Pena, Quinn, & Iglesias, 1992). Initially described by Vygotsky (1986) as part of his model of cognitive development, dynamic assessment refers to approaches that evaluate a student's ability to learn when provided with instruction, such as the test-teach-retest paradigm. Studies (Butler, 1997; Gutierrez-Clellen, 2000; Lidz & Pena, 1996; Pena, Iglesias, & Lidz, 2001) have addressed the use and effectiveness of dynamic assessment with ELs and note its promise for distinguishing language differences from language learning disabilities (Gutierrez-Clellen & Peña, 2001).

Response to Intervention (RtI), discussed earlier in this chapter, uses the principles of dynamic assessment. The focus in RtI is on measuring the students' response to effective instruction. As appropriate and comprehensible instructional support is provided to ELs, a variety of informal assessment tools and observational protocols can be used to assess how ELs use language in the classroom and across social contexts (Collier, 2010). Their performance can be compared to their similar classmates rather than using national norms (Mattes & Saldana-Illingworth, 2009). Portfolio methods of assessment can also be used to evaluate samples of student work over time. It has been suggested that RtI, used as a form of dynamic assessment, can be helpful in discriminating language differences from language disorders in ELs (Rosa-Lugo, Rivera, & Rierson, 2010).

Observations

SLPs are often required to obtain information on the student's use of language in various academic and social contexts. By observing and examining the language strategies used by students to communicate with their peers and others, the SLP can obtain information about the child's language performance and identify observed behaviors that are characteristic of children in the normal process of acquiring a second language and children with a communication disorder.

The use of observation as an alternative assessment is highly recommended by many researchers (Collier, 2011; Kayser, 2008; Waxman, Padron, Franco-Fuenmayor, & Huang, 2009). Observation is a quantitative method of measuring specific behaviors observed in children and teachers as they interact in the classroom setting. Rating scales, interviews, and observational techniques and protocols have traditionally been used by SLPs to gather information about the child's language capabilities over multiple contexts with a variety of communication partners. Most observations require that the observer use a coding system to record what students and teachers do during learning activities within the classroom and often include the following (Stallings & Mohlman, 1988):

◆ A purpose for the observation
◆ Operational definitions of all the observed behaviors
◆ Training procedures for observers
◆ A specific observational focus
◆ A unit of time

◆ An observation schedule
◆ A method to record the data
◆ A method to process and analyze data

To determine whether a communication disorder exists in an EL it is important that all data obtained through rating scales, interviews, and observational techniques and protocols support the diagnosis of a language disorder. Observation protocols that have been used to observe teachers and EL students as they work in classrooms are the Sheltered Instruction Observation Protocol (SIOP; Short & Echevarria, 1999), used to observe and rate teachers in the classroom, and the Transitional Bilingual Pedagogical (TBP) Observation Protocol (Bruce et al, 1997), used to observe instructional practices in transitional bilingual classrooms. The Bilingual Classroom Communication Profile (BCCP; Roseberry-McKibben, 1993) is another protocol that is used in conjunction with other alternative measures to provide a comprehensive picture of the student's use of language. Mattes and Saldana-Illingworth (2008) have compiled a number of observational communication protocols and interview questionnaires that are useful for assessing the speech and language of ELs.

Use of Interpreters

As a supplement to the alternative assessments described above, the use of interpreters plays a critical role in assessing ELs. Interpreters convey information from one language to the other and facilitate communication between individuals that do not speak the same language, whereas translators translate written documents from one language to another (Kayser, 1995; Langdon & Cheng, 2002; Roseberry-McKibben, 2008). During a student evaluation, the interpreter usually takes a leading role. Langdon and Cheng (2002) and Matsuda and O'Connor (1993) have discussed the role and responsibilities of an interpreter/translator and the criteria that should be used in their selection (Hegde & Maul, 2006; Murphy & Dillon, 2008). Specifically, the SLP and the interpreter must work together to assess ELs in the absence of a bilingual SLP who speaks the client's language and adheres to legal requirements and professional ethics. The interpreter must have excellent communication skills in the language of the child and must be trained in the role of interpreter.

Langdon and Cheng (2002) outline a three-step process that can be used by the SLP as they work with interpreters. The three steps of the process are: (1) briefing, (2) interaction, and (3) debriefing (BID). During the *briefing* step, the SLP and the interpreter review the client's background information and outline the purpose of the assessment. The use and review of materials, seating arrangements, and type of interpreting is planned. During the *interaction* step, the interpreter and the SLP work as a team in test administration or use of alternate assessments. In this task, the interpreter acts as a bridge between the SLP and the client and attempts to engage and elicit responses from the student. The third step, *debriefing*, consists of reviewing the process as well as the outcome of the assessment process. The SLP and interpreter discuss the student's performance during tests, the interpreter's observations, test scoring, and the challenges encountered during the testing session. If the interpreter has been appropriately trained they can provide the SLP with valuable information that will shed light on the linguistic functioning of the child.

Final Thoughts Regarding Assessment

Alternative assessments are promising tools that should be included as part of an assessment battery. The use of these tools and strategies can contribute to the accurate identification of ELs with communication disorders. These measures can also be used by the SLP to plan intervention programs, document treatment effectiveness, and determine when services are no longer necessary.

The assessment process is incomplete without a final written report outlining the findings of the evaluation. Report formats vary from school district to school district; however, certain information should consistently be included in the diagnostic report. Information obtained through the case history should be included (i.e., client's language history, schooling history, and language proficiency) as well as all testing results (to include standardized and alternative assessments), modifications, and use of interpreters.

Ultimately, the written report should serve as a document that presents an accurate representation of the student written in a language understood by all professionals that will work with the student and the families of the child. SLPs are responsible for supporting the diagnosis of a communication disorder. Because this report is used to determine eligibility for speech and language services or programs, document progress, or determine if a child no longer needs services, it is extremely important that this report be detailed and precise (Burrus & Haynes, 2009; Goldfarb & Serpanos, 2009; Stein-Rubin & Fabus, 2011).

Eligibility and Dismissal Decisions

Eligibility Decisions

Determining whether a child has a communication disorder is a significant decision because of its educational consequences. The SLP is responsible for gathering all the critical information, obtained through formal testing and informal procedures, to determine whether the EL is experiencing challenges due to a true communication disorder or to something else, such as a communication difference. To determine the presence or absence of language impairment and if the student meets the eligibility criteria for speech-language services or programs in the schools, the SLP must address three questions:

1. Does the student have a communication difference or disorder? In other words, is there a disability that is manifested across all languages spoken by the child?
2. If so, does the disability have an adverse effect on educational performance resulting from the disability?
3. Are specially designed instruction and/or related services and supports needed to help the student make progress in the general education curriculum?

If it is determined, after supporting the student with meaningful RtI strategies, that the student demonstrates a language disorder in L1 and L2, then best practice is for the student to receive specially designed instruction and support for students with disabilities (Linan-Thompson & Ortiz, 2009; Restrepo-Gutierrez-Clellan, 2004). It is important to note that a child cannot be determined to have a disability if one of the determinant factors is limited English proficiency (IDEA, 2004). Assessment results should support that the disorder is having an adverse impact on performance in the general education classroom. As noted previously in Chapter 3, it is critical that the SLP and other professionals remember that if the EL has a communication problem it must be present across languages (Goldstein, 2004b; Kayser, 2002; Kohnert, 2008; Restrepo, 1997; Roseberry-McKibben, 2008).

Determining if a student has a disability is not the sole responsibility of the SLP. It is critical that *all* school professionals share information on the student with each other and that parents serve as active partners to help determine eligibility and appropriate educational services (Garcia, 2002). If the student is found to be eligible to receive services from the SLP then an Individual Education Plan (IEP) must be developed. The IEP should contain clear goals and objectives that will consider the student's strengths in L1 and L2. Information about each student's language proficiency should be clearly documented in the IEP so that SLPs can work with school professionals (e.g., ESOL professionals) and the parents to plan an appropriate and culturally responsive instructional program that addresses which language will be primary in instruction. It is important that SLPs know the eligibility criteria for their state.

Dismissal Decisions

Parents, teachers, SLPs, and professionals from other disciplines are encouraged to play a role in all aspects of decision making and problem solving related to the eligibility, placement, intervention, and dismissal of ELs with a communication disorder. Usually the decision to dismiss a student from speech-language services begins with the SLP. According to ASHA's best practices, students with communication disorders may be dismissed from receiving services only when they are no longer identified as having speech-language impairments and are no longer in need of special education services (ASHA, 2004). The SLP determines if the student met their IEP annual goals, conducts an assessment, and reviews all evaluation data to consider if the student no longer needs the services of the SLP. Dismissal from services may occur if the EL with a communication disorder meets the following criteria:

A. No longer has speech-language impairment;
B. Has a speech-language impairment, but it no longer affects his/her educational performance;
C. Has received speech-language services as special education and still has a speech-language impairment that affects his/her educational performance, but the child study team determines that he/she does not need special education; *or*
D. has received speech-language services as special education and still has a speech-language impairment that affects his/her educational performance, but the child study team determines that he/she does not need related services to benefit from special education.

When making decisions regarding dismissal, SLPs should follow the procedures established by their state and districts. Although all states adhere to IDEA requirements regarding dismissal, it is possible that various state laws and regulations may create additional requirements. For example, in Florida the dismissal policies and procedures are often found in the Special Programs and Procedures document of each respective school district as well as in technical assistance papers that provide guidance regarding state board rules (Florida Department of Education, 2010).

Steppling, Quattlebaum, and Brady (2007) have looked at the guidelines for dismissal as they are stated in IDEA and ASHA and identified several issues that the SLP needs to consider during the dismissal process. The IDEA guidelines for dismissal focus on measuring disabilities that affect educational performance, whereas the ASHA guidelines include educational goals and items that are linked to health status. The IDEA dismissal guidelines give the appearance that they are a broad outline that is connected with educational performance and that there are just a few questions that need to be answered in order for an EL with a communication disorder to be dismissed from SLP programs. On the other hand, the ASHA guidelines offer a more detailed list of considerations for dismissal. This important difference between the two set of guidelines might create a situation with important educational consequences for ELs with communication disorders if a child meets the criteria for dismissal under IDEA but still displays a disorder according to the ASHA criteria. For example, the IEP team might determine that the communication disorder of an EL with a communication disorder does not affect educational performance any longer, but still has a negative influence on social interaction. From an IDEA point of view, the student can be dismissed from the program, but from an ASHA perspective, the student needs to continue to be in the program.

Summary

In Chapters 6 and 7, we looked at a variety of procedures and instruments ESOL professionals and SLPs can use for assessing ELs and ELs with communication disorders. In the beginning of Chapter 6 we stressed the importance of collaboration between these two categories of professionals. Chapter 7 continues to highlight how critical the relationship between SLPs and ESOL professionals is in the assessment of ELs, and specifically ELs with communication disorders.

Collaboration is the recurring theme of this text. For this reason, we wanted to provide a comprehensive description of what each professional is doing at the identification stage, during the ongoing language proficiency assessment, and at the exiting/dismissal phase. When team members are familiar with the context in which their colleagues function, they can complement each other and collaborate to facilitate language and literacy development in ELs. These approaches and strategies are discussed in the following chapter.

References

Acevedo, M. A. (1993). Development of Spanish consonants in preschool children. *Journal of Childhood Communication Disorders, 15*(2), 9–15.

American Speech-Language-Hearing Association. (2004). *Admission/ discharge criteria in speech-language pathology* [Guidelines]. Available from www.asha.org/policy

American Speech-Language-Hearing Association. (n.d.). *Examples of state speech-language eligibility guidelines.* Retrieved from http:// www.asha.org/slp/schools/prof-consult/eligibility.htm

Anderson, R. (1995). Spanish morphological and syntactic development. In H. Kayser (Ed.), *Bilingual speech-language pathology: An Hispanic focus* (pp. 41–74). San Diego, CA: Singular.

Batsche, G., Elliott, J., Graden, J., Grimes, J., Kovaleski, & J., Prasse, D. (2005). *Response to intervention: Policy considerations and implementation.* Alexandria, VA: National Association of State Directors of Special Education.

Battle, D. (Ed.). (2002). *Communication disorders in multicultural populations* (3rd ed.). Woburn, MA: Butterworth-Heinemann.

Beck, A. R. (1995). Language assessment methods for three age groups of children. *Journal of Communication Development, 17*(2), 51–56.

Bedore, L. M., Pena, E. D., Garcia, M., & Cortez, C. (2005). Conceptual versus monolingual scoring: When does it make a difference? *Language, Speech, and Hearing Services in Schools, 36,* 188–200.

Bliss, L. S. (2002). *Discourse impairments: Assessment and intervention applications.* Boston, MA: Allyn & Bacon.

Bloome, D., Champion, T., Katz. L., Morton, M., & Muldrow, R. (2001). Spoken and written narrative development: African American preschoolers as storytellers and story makers. In J. Harris, A. Kamhi, & K. Pollock (Eds.), *Literacy in African American communities* (pp. 45–76). Mahwah, NJ: Erlbaum.

Brownell, R. (2000a). *Expressive One-Word Picture Vocabulary Test Spanish-Bilingual Edition manual.* San Antonio, TX: Pearson.

Brownell, R. (2000b). *Receptive One-Word Picture Vocabulary Test Spanish-Bilingual Edition manual.* San Antonio, TX: Pearson.

Brownell, R. (2010a). *Expressive One-Word Picture Vocabulary Test —Fourth Edition manual.* San Antonio, TX: Pearson

Brownell, R. (2010b). *Receptive One-Word Picture Vocabulary Test —Fourth Edition manual.* San Antonio, TX: Pearson.

Bruce, K. L., Lara-Alecio, R., Parker, R., Hasbrouck, J. E., Weaver, L., & Irby, B. (1997). Accurately describing the language. *Bilingual Research Journal, 21*(2&3), 123–145.

Burns, M. K., Griffiths, A. J., Parson, L. B., Tilly, W. D., & VanDerHeyden, A. (2007). *Response to intervention: Research to practice.* Alexandria, VA: National Association of State Directors of Special Education.

Burrus, E. A. & Haynes, W. (2009). *Professional communication in speech-language pathology. How to write, talk and act like a clinician.* San Diego, CA: Plural.

Butler, K. (1997). Dynamic assessment at the millennium: A transient tutorial for today! *Journal of Children's Communication Development, 19*, 43–54.

Caesar, L., & Kohler, P. (2007). The state of school-based bilingual assessment: Actual practice versus recommended guidelines. *Language, Speech, and Hearing Services in schools, 38*, 190–200.

CELF Technical Report. (2008). Retrieved from http://www.pearson assessments.com/NR/rdonlyres/F7DBBC32-B63E-4B8E-B1C4-59D 8358E5CA5/0/CELF_4_Tech_Report.pdf

Champion, T., & Mainess, K. (2003). Typical and disordered narration in African American children. In A. McCabe & L. S. Bliss, *Patterns of narrative discourse: A multicultural lifespan approach* (pp. 55–70). Boston, MA: Allyn & Bacon.

Champion, T., & Seymour, H. (1995). Narrative discourse among African American children. *Journal of Narrative and Life History, 5*, 333–352.

Collier, C. (2010). *RTI for diverse learners.* Thousand Oaks, CA: Sage.

Collier, c. (2011). Seven steps to separating difference from disability. Thousand Oaks, CA: Sage.

Cornejo, R. J., Weinstein, A., & C.Najar, C. (1983). *Eliciting spontaneous speech in bilingual students: Methods and techniques.* Las Cruces, N.M.: Educational Resources Information Center (ERIC), Clearinghouse on Rural Education and Small Schools (CRESS), New Mexico State University.

Crowley, C. J. (2003, October). Diagnosing communication disorders in culturally and linguistically diverse students. *ERIC Digest*, E650.

Dawson, J. I., Stout, C. E., & Elyer, J. A. (2003). *The Structured Photographic Expressive Language Test (SPELT-3)* (3rd ed.). DeKalb, IL: Janelle.

Echevarría, J. & Vogt, M.E. (2011). *Response to Intervention (RTI) and English learners.* Boston, MA: Pearson.

Ehren, B. J. (2005). Responsiveness to intervention and the speech-language pathologist [Special issue]. *Topics in Language Disorders, 25*(2).

Esparza-Brown, J. (2011). Personal communication.

Esparza-Brown, J., & Doolittle, J. (2008). A cultural, linguistic, and ecological framework for response to intervention with English language learners. *Teaching Exceptional Children, 40*(5), 67–72.

Esparza Brown, J., & Sanford, A. (March 2011). *RTI for English language learners: Appropriately using screening and progress monitoring tools to improve instructional outcomes.* Washington, DC: US Department of Education, Office of Special Education Programs, National Center on Response to Intervention.

Fantini, A. (1985). *Language acquisition of a bilingual child: A sociolinguistic perspective (to age 10).* San Diego, CA: College-Hill Press.

Florida Department of Education. (2010). *Exceptional student education eligibility for students with language impairments* [Technical assistance paper]. Retrieved from http://info.fldoe.org/docushare/dsweb/Get/Document-5952/dps-2010-179.pdf

Fuchs, D., & Deshler, D. D. (2007). What we need to know about responsiveness to intervention (and shouldn't be afraid to ask). *Learning Disabilities Research and Practice, 22,* 129–136.

Fuchs, D., Mock, D., Morgan, P. L., & Young, C. L. (2003). Responsiveness-to-intervention: Definitions, evidence, and implications for the learning disabilities construct. *Learning Disabilities Research and Practice, 18,* 157–171.

Garcia, S. (2002). Parent-professional collaboration in culturally sensitive assessment. In A. J. Artiles & A. A. Ortiz (Eds.), *English language learners with special education needs* (pp. 87–103). McHenry, IL: Center for Applied Linguistics and Delta Systems.

Goldfarb. R., & Serpanos, Y. (2009). *Professional writing in speech-language pathology and audiology workbook.* San Diego, CA: Plural.

Goldstein, B. (2000). *Cultural and linguistic diversity resource guide for speech-language pathologists.* San Diego, CA: Singular /Thompson Learning.

Goldstein, B. (2002). *Cultural and linguistic diversity resource guide for speech-language pathologist.* San Diego, CA: Singular /Thomson Learning.

Goldstein, B. (2004a). *Bilingual language development and disorders in Spanish-English speakers.* Baltimore, MD: Brookes.

Goldstein, B. A. (2004b). Bilingual language development and disorders: Introduction and overview. In B. A. Goldstein (Ed.), *Bilingual language development and disorders in Spanish-English speakers* (pp. 3–20). Baltimore, MD: Brookes.

Goldstein, B., & Iglesias, A. (1996). Phonological patterns in normally developing Spanish-speaking 3- and 4-year-olds of Puerto Rican descent. *Language, Speech, and Hearing Services in Schools, 27*(1), 82–90.

Greenfield, P. M. (1997). You can't take it with you. Why ability assessments don't cross cultures. *American Psychologist, 52*(10), 1115–1124.

Gutierrez-Clellen, V. F. (2000) Dynamic assessment: An approach to assessing children's language learning potential. *Seminars in Speech and Language, 21*(3), 215–222.

Gutiérrez-Clellen, V. F., Calderón, J., & Ellis Weismer, S. (2004). Verbal working memory in bilingual children. *Journal of Speech, Language, and Hearing Research, 47*, 863–877.

Gutiérrez-Clellen, V. F., & Pena, E. (2001). Dynamic assessment of diverse children: A tutorial. *Language, Speech, and Hearing Services in Schools, 32*, 212–224.

Gutiérrez-Clellen, V. F., & Quinn, R. (1993). Assessing narratives of children from diversecultural/linguistic groups. *Language, Speech, and Hearing Services in Schools, 24*(1), 2–9.

Gutiérrez-Clellen, V., Restrepo, M. A., & Bedore, L., Pena, E., & Anderson, R. (2000). Language sample analysis in Spanish-speaking children: Methodological considerations. *Language, Speech, and Hearing Services in the Schools, 31*, 88–98.

Hamayan, E., & Damico, J. (1991). *Limiting bias in the assessment of bilingual students.* Austin, TX: Pro-Ed.

Hammett Price, L., Hendricks, S., & Cook, C. (2010). Language sample analysis into clinical practice. *Language, Speech, and Hearing Services in the Schools, 41*, 206–222.

Hegde, M. N., & Maul, C. A. (2006). *Language disorders in children: An evidenced-based approach to assessment and treatment.* Boston, MA: Allyn & Bacon.

Hester, E. J. (2010). Narrative correlates of reading comprehension in African America children. *Contemporary Issues in Communication Science and Disorders, 37*, 73–85.

Hunt, K. W. (1964). *Grammatical structures written at three grade levels* (Research rep. no. 3). Champaign, IL: National Council of Teachers of English.

Hutchinson, T. (1996). What to look for in the technical manual: Twenty questions for users. *Language, Speech, and Hearing Services in Schools, 27*, 109–121.

Hux, K. (1993). Language sampling practices: A survey of nine states. *Language, Speech, and Hearing Services in Schools, 2*, 84–91.

Hux, K., Morris-Friehe, M., & Sanger, D. D. (1993). Language sampling practices: A survey of nine states. *Language, Speech, and Hearing Services in Schools, 24*, 84–91.

Individuals with Disabilities Education Act. (1997). 20 U.S.C. § 1400 et seq.

Individuals with Disabilities Education Act. (2004). Pub. L. No. 108-446, 118 Stat. 2647.

Jimenez, B. (1987). Acquisition of Spanish consonants in children aged 3–5 years, 7 months. *Language, Speech and Hearing Services in Schools, 18*, 357–363.

Juárez, M. (1983). Assessment and treatment of minority language-handicapped children: The role of the monolingual speech-language pathologist. *Topics in Language Disorders, 3*, 57–65.

Kayser, H. (1995). *Bilingual speech-language pathology. An Hispanic focus.* San Diego, CA: Singular.

Kayser, H. (1998). *Assessment and intervention resource for Hispanic children.* San Diego, CA: Singular.

Kayser, H. (2002). Bilingual language development and language disorders. In D. E. Battle (Ed.), *Communication disorders in multicultural populations* (2nd ed., pp. 157–196). Boston, MA: Butterworth-Heinemann.

Kayser, H. (2008). *Educating Latino preschool children.* San Diego, CA: Plural.

Kayser, H., & Restrepo, M. (1995). Language samples: Elicitation and analysis. In H. Kayser (Ed.), *Bilingual speech-language pathology: An Hispanic focus* (pp. 265–286). San Diego, CA: Singular.

Kemp, K., & Klee, T. (1997). Clinical language sampling practices: Results of a survey of speech-language pathologists in the United States. *Child Language Teaching and Therapy, 13*(2), 161–176.

Klecan-Aker, J., & Hedrick, D. (1985). A study of the syntactic language skills of normal school-age children. *Language, Speech, and Hearing Services in Schools, 16*, 187–198.

Klingner, J. K., & Edwards, P. A. (2006). Cultural considerations with response to intervention models. *Reading Research Quarterly, 41*, 108–117.

Klingner, J., & Harry, B. (2006). The special education referral and decision-making process for English language learners: Child study team meetings and placement conferences. *Teachers College Record, 108*(11), 2247–2281.

Kohnert, K. (2008). *Language disorders in bilingual children and adults.* San Diego, CA: Plural.

Kriticos, E. P. (2003). Speech-language pathologists' beliefs about language assessment of bilingual/bicultural individuals. *American Journal of Speech-Language Pathology, 12*, 73–91.

Laing, S. P., & Kamhi, A. (2003). Alternative assessment of language and literacy in culturally and linguistically diverse populations. *Language, Speech, and Hearing Services in Schools, 34*, 44–55.

Langdon, H. W. (1989). Language disorder or difference? Assessing the skills of Hispanic students. *Exceptional Children, 56*, 160–167.

Langdon, H. W. (1992). Language communication and sociocultural patterns in Latino families. In H. W. Langdon & L. L. Cheng (Eds.), *Hispanic children and adults with communication disorders: Assessment and intervention* (pp. 99–131). Gaithersburg, MD: Aspen.

Langdon, H. (2011). *Spanish Structured Photographic Expressive Language Test—3. II.* DeKalb, IL: Janelle.

Langdon, H. W., & Cheng, L. L. (2002). *Collaborating with interpreters and translators: A guide for communication disorders professionals.* Eau Claire, WI: Thinking.

Langdon, H., & Irvine Saenz, T. (1996). *Language assessment and intervention with multicultural students.* Oceanside, CA: Academic Communication Associates.

Leung, B. (1993). *Assessment considerations with culturally and linguistically diverse students.* Paper presented at National Association for Multicultural Education, Los Angeles, CA.

Lidz, C., & Pena, E. (1996). Dynamic assessment: The model, its relevance as a nonbiased approach, and its application to Latino American preschool children. *Language, Speech, and Hearing Services in the Schools, 27,* 367–372.

Linan-Thompson, S., & Ortiz, A. (2009). Response to intervention and English language learners: Instructional and assessment considerations. *Seminars in Speech and Language, 30,* 105–120.

Linares, N. (1981). Rules for calculating mean length of utterance in morphemes for Spanish. In J. Erickson & D. Omark (Eds.), *Communication assessment of the bilingual bicultural child* (pp. 291–295). Baltimore, MD: University Park Press.

Long, S. H., & Channell, R.W. (2001). Accuracy of four language analysis procedures performed automatically. *American Journal of Speech-Language Pathology, 10,* 180–188.

Long, S. H., Fey, M. E., & Channell, R. W. (2000). *Computerized Profiling (CP) (Version 9.2.7, MS-DOS)* [Computer software]. Cleveland, OH: Department of Communication Sciences, Case Western Reserve University.

MacWhinney, B. (1996). The CHILDES system. *American Journal of Speech-Language Pathology, 5,* 5–14.

MacWhinney, B. (2000a). *The CHILDES project: Tools for analyzing talk* (3rd ed.). Mahwah, NJ: Erlbaum.

MacWhinney, B. (2000b). *CLAN* [Computer software]. Pittsburgh, PA: Carnegie Mellon University.

Matsuda, M., & O'Connor L. (1993). *Creating an effective partnership: Training bilingual communication aides.* Paper presented at the annual conference of the California Speech-Language-Hearing Association, Palm Springs, CA.

Mattes, L.J., & and Saldana-Illingworth, C. (2008). *Bilingual communication assessment resource. Tools for assessing speech, language, and learning.* Oceanside, CA: Academic Communication Associates.

McCauley, R. J. (1996). Familiar strangers: Criterion-referenced measures in communication disorders. *Language, Speech, and Hearing Services in Schools, 27,* 122–131.

McCauley, R. J., & Swisher, L. (1984). Psychometric review of language and articulation tests for preschool children. *Journal of Speech and Hearing Disorders, 49,* 34–42.

Mellard, D. F., & Johnson, E. (2007). *RTI: A practitioner's guide to implementing Response to Intervention.* Thousand Oaks, CA: Corwin Press.

Merino, B. (1992). Acquisition of syntactic and phonological features in Spanish. In H. W. Langdon & L. Cheng (Eds.), *Hispanic children and adults with communication disorders: Assessment and intervention.* Gaithersburg, MD: Aspen.

Miller, J., & Iglesias, A. (2006). *Systematic Analysis of Language Transcripts (SALT), English & Spanish (Version 9)* [Computer software]. Madison, WI: Language Analysis Lab, University of Wisconsin–Madison.

Miller, J. F., & Chapman R. S. (2008). *Systematic Analysis of Language Transcripts (SALT)* [Computer software]. Madison, WI: University of Wisconsin–Madison, Waisman Center.

Miller, J. F., Freiberg, C., Rolland, M.-B., & Reeves, M. A. (1992). Implementing computerized language sample analysis in the public school. *Topics in Language Disorders, 12*(2), 69–82.

Moore, B. J., & Montgomery, J. K. (2008). *Making a difference for America's children — Speech-language pathologists in public schools* (2nd ed.). Greenville, SC: Thinking.

Murphy, B. C., & Dillon, C. (2008). *Interviewing in action in a multicultural world* (3rd ed.). Belmont, CA: Thomson Higher Education.

No Child Left Behind Act. (2001). 20 U.S.C. § 6301.

Ortiz, A. A. (1997). Learning disabilities occurring concomitantly with linguistic differences. *Journal of Learning Disabilities, 30,* 321–332.

Ortiz, A., & Yates, J. (2002). Considerations in the assessment of English language learners referred to special education. In A. J. Artiles & A. A. Ortiz (Eds.), *English language learners with special education needs* (pp. 65–86). McHenry, IL: Center for Applied Linguistics and Delta Systems.

Owens, R. E. (2004). *Language development: A functional approach to assessment and intervention* (4th ed.). Boston, MA: Allyn & Bacon.

Paradis, J. (2005). Grammatical morphology in children learning English as a second language: Implications of similarities with specific language impairment. *Language, Speech, and Hearing Services in Schools, 36*, 3, 172–187.

Pena, E. D., & Kester, E. S. (2004). Semantic development in Spanish-English bilinguals: Theory, assessment, and intervention. In B. A. Goldstein (Ed.), *Bilingual language development and disorders in Spanish-English speakers* (pp. 105–130). Baltimore, MD: Brookes.

Peña, E., Iglesias, A., & Lidz, C. S. (2001). Reducing test bias through assessment of children's word learning ability. *American Journal of Speech-Language Pathology, 10*, 138–151.

Pena, E., Quinn, R., & Iglesias, A. (1992). The application of dynamic methods to language assessment: A nonbiased procedure. *Journal of Special Education, 26*(3), 269–280.

Perona, K., Plante, E., & Vance, R. (2005). Diagnostic accuracy of the Structured Photographic Expressive Language Test: Third edition (SPELT-3). *Language, Speech, and Hearing Services in Schools, 36*, 103–115.

Plante, E., & Vance, B. (1994). Selection of preschool language tests: A data-based approach. *Language Speech and Hearing Services in Schools, 25*, 15–24.

Public Law 108-146. Retrieved from http://www2.ed.gov/legislation/FedRegister/finrule/2006-3/081406a.pdf

Pye, C. (1987). The Pye analysis of language. *Working Papers in Language Development, 3*, 1–37.

Restrepo, M. A. (1997). Guidelines for identifying primarily Spanish-speaking preschool children with language impairment. *Communication Disorders and Sciences in Culturally and Linguistically Diverse Populations, 3*(1), 11–13.

Restrepo, M. A., & Gutierrez-Clellen, V. (2004). Grammatical impairment in Spanish-English bilingual children. In B. Goldstein (Ed.), *Bilingual language development and disorders in Spanish-English speakers* (pp. 213–234). Baltimore, MD: Brookes.

Restrepo, M. A., & Silverman, S. W. (2001). Validity of the Spanish Preschool Language Scale-3 for use with bilingual children. *American Journal of Speech-Language Pathology, 10*, 382–393.

Retherford, K. (2000). *Guide to analysis of language transcripts* (3rd ed.). Eau Claire, WI: Thinking.

Rinaldi, C., & Samson, J. (2008). English language learners and response to intervention: Referral recommendations. *Teaching Exceptional Children, 40*(5), 6–14.

Rollins, P. R., McCabe, A., & Bliss, L. (2000). Culturally sensitive assessment of narrative in children. *Seminars in Speech and Language, 21*, 223–234.

Rosa-Lugo, L. I., Rivera, E., & Rierson, T. K. (October, 2010). The role of dynamic assessment within the response to intervention model in school-age English language learners. *Perspectives on School-Based Issues, ASHA Division 16, 11*(3), 91–106.

Roseberry-McKibben, C. (1993). *Bilingual classroom communication profile*. Oceanside, CA: Academic Communication Associates.

Roseberry-McKibbin, C. (2003). *Assessment of bilingual learners: Language difference or disorder? Video and workbook*. Rockbille Pike, MD: American Speech-Language-Hearing Association.

Roseberry-McKibbin, C. (2007). *Language disorders in children: A multicultural and case perspective*. Boston, MA: Allyn & Bacon.

Roseberry-McKibbin, C. (2008). *Multicultural students with special language needs* (3rd ed.). Oceanside, CA: Academic Communication Associates.

Saenz, T. I., & Huer, M. B. (2003). Testing strategies involving least biased assessment of bilingual children. *Communication Disorders Quarterly, 24*(4), 184–193.

Schnell de Acedo, B. (1994). Early morphological development: The acquisition of articles in Spanish. In J. Sokolov & C. Snow (Eds.), *Handbook of research in language development using CHILDES*. Hillsdale, NJ: Lawrence Erlbaum.

Schraeder, T. (2008). *A guide to school services in speech-language pathology*. San Diego, CA: Plural.

Schrank, F. A., Alvarado, C. G., & Wendling, B. J. (2010b). *Interpretive supplement: Instructional interventions for English language learners related to the Woodcock-Muñoz Language Survey—Revised Normative Update*. Rolling Meadows, IL: Riverside.

Schrank, F. A., Wendling, B., Alvarado, C., & Woodcock, R. (2010a). *Woodcock-Muñoz Language Survey—Revised Normative Update (WMLS-R NU)*. Itasca, IL: Riverside.

Semel, E., Wiig, E. H., & Secord, W. A. (2003). *The Clinical Evaluation of Language Fundamentals—Fourth Edition (CELF-4 English)*. San Antonio, TX: Pearson.

Semel, E., Wiig, E. H., & Secord, W. A. (2006). *The Clinical Evaluation of Language Fundamentals—Fourth Edition, Spanish Edition (CELF-4 Spanish)*. San Antonio, TX: Pearson.

Senaga, N., & Inglebret, E. (2003, November). *Assessment practices used by bilingual SLPs*. Paper presented at the meeting of the American Speech-Language-Hearing Association, Chicago, IL.

Seymour, H. N., Roeper, T. & de Villiers, J. G. (2005). *DELV-NR (Diagnostic Evaluation of Language Variation) Norm-Referenced Test*. San Antonio TX: Psychological Corporation.

Short, D. J., & Echevarria, J. (1999). *The Sheltered Instruction Observation Protocol: A tool for teacher-research collaboration and professional development* (Educational practice report no. 3). Santa Cruz, CA: Center for Research on Education, Diversity and Excellence.

Spaulding, T. J., Plante, E., & Farinella, K. A. (2006). Eligibility criteria for language impairment: Is the low end of normal always appropriate? *Language, Speech, and Hearing Services in Schools, 37*, 61–72.

Stallings, J. A., & Mohlman, G. G. (1988). Classroom observation techniques. In J. P. Keeves (Ed.), *Educational research, methodology, and measurement: An international handbook* (pp. 469–474). Oxford, UK: Pergamon.

Stein-Rubin, C., & Fabus, R. (2011). *A guide to clinical assessment and professional report writing in speech-language pathology*. Clifton Park, NY: Delmar.

Steppling, M., Quattlebaum, P., & Brady, D. E. (2007). Toward a discussion of issues associated with speech-language pathologists' dismissal practices in public school settings. *Communication Disorders Quarterly, 28*(3), 179–187.

Swisher, L. (1994). Learning and generalization components of morphological acquisition by children with specific language impairment: Is there a functional relation? *Journal of Speech and Hearing Research, 37*(6), 1406–1413.

Vygotsky, L. (1986). *Thought and language* (rev. ed.). Cambridge, MA: MIT Press.

Waxman, H. C., Padrón, Y., Franco-Feunmayor, S., & Huang, S.Y. (2009). Observing classroom instruction for ELLs from student, teacher, and classroom perspectives. *Texas Association for Bilingual Education, 11*(1), 63–95.

Webster, M. J., & Shelton, R. L. (1964). Estimation of mean length of response in children of normal and below average intellectual capacity. *Journal of Speech and Hearing Research, 7*, 98–100.

Werner, E. O., & Kresheck, J. D. (1983). *Structured Photographic Expressive Language Test—II*. DeKalb, IL: Janelle

Woodcock, R., Muñoz-Sandoval, A., Ruef, M., & Alvarado, C. (2005). *Woodcock-Muñoz Language Survey—Revised*. Itasca, IL: Riverside.

Zimmerman, I. L., Steiner, V. G., & Pond, R. E. (1992). *Preschool Language Scales* (3rd ed.). San Antonio, TX: Psychological Corporation.

Zimmerman, I. L., Steiner, V. G., & Pond, R. E. (2002a). *Preschool Language Scale-4*. San Antonio, TX: Psychological Corporation.

Zimmerman, I. L., Steiner, V. G., & Pond, R. E. (2002). *Preschool Language Scale-4 Spanish Edition*. San Antonio, TX: Psychological Corporation.

8

Approaches and Practical Strategies to Facilitate Language and Literacy Development in English Learners

Introduction

Promoting language and literacy development in ELs shares many commonalities with promoting language and literacy development in native speakers of English. However, depending on age and educational background, ELs also may have varying degrees of oral proficiency in English and literacy skills in their native language. There are a number of critical variables unique to ELs that affect the process and outcomes of literacy development. Understanding the needs of ELs can be difficult for literacy professionals because of these commonalities and differences. Although commonalities may seem to facilitate literacy development, they can be deceptively similar in appearance and possess different characteristics that may go unnoticed. Clear-cut differences may be more apparent, but their effects can be dissimilar to what might be expected.

In this chapter we summarize the findings of reading research from the National Early Reading Panel (NELP) (2008) and National Reading Panel (NRP) (2000). We examine how teaching reading may be affected by the second language acquisition process and the level of proficiency in ELs. Last, we highlight how the SLP and the ESOL professional can partner to implement and promote language and literacy development in ELs using some of the strategies that are discussed in this chapter.

Knowledge and Skills Necessary for Learning to Read

Learning to read for the first time involves developing the same knowledge and skills, regardless of whether the learner speaks one or two languages. According to the NELP (2008), research shows that preschool-age children must master six precursor skills in order to begin reading successfully.

The first skill, alphabet knowledge, pertains to knowing the names and sounds of printed letters. The second skill, phonological awareness, includes detecting, manipulating, or analyzing the sounds of spoken language. This involves separating or segmenting words, syllables, or phonemes, which are the smallest distinctions in sound that differentiate meaning (i.e., such as /p/ in pit; /b/ in bit versus [pʰ] in pat and [p'] in spat). Phonological awareness is independent of meaning. The third skill is rapid automatic naming of letters or digits. Similarly, the fourth skill involves the rapid automatic naming of common objects, such as a car or tree. The fifth skill is writing letters in isolation or writing one's name. Last, the sixth skill is phonological memory, which is the ability to remember what someone said for a brief time period. Table 8–1 summarizes the six skill areas.

In addition to these six necessary skills, the NELP (2008) found an additional five skills that are potentially important in developing the ability to read. These include: (1) concepts of print—print conventions such as left to right, front to back and print concepts such as book cover, author; (2) print knowledge—concepts of print, alphabet knowledge, and early decoding of sounds/symbols; (3) reading readiness—a combination of concepts of print, alphabet knowledge, vocabulary, memory, and phonological awareness; (4) oral language, including using vocabulary and grammar; and (5) visual processing, which involves matching or discriminating visual symbols.

Once the precursor reading skills are mastered, students in kindergarten through third grade develop more complex reading skills. The Center for the Improvement of Early Reading Achieve-

Table 8–1. Knowledge and Skills Necessary for Learning to Read

Language knowledge and skills learners must develop from birth to age 5	Alphabet knowledge
	Phonological awareness
	Rapid automatic naming of letters
	Rapid automatic naming of colors
	Writing name
	Phonological memory

Source: From *Developing Early Literacy: Report of the National Early Literacy Panel,* by National Early Literacy Panel, 2008, Washington, DC: National Institute for Literacy. Retrieved from http://www.nifl.gov/earlychildhood/NELP/NELPreport.html

ment (CIERA) reviewed more than 100,000 research studies on teaching reading in K–3 (Adler, 2001). From these studies, a clear picture of five necessary skills for successful reading emerged: (1) phonemic awareness; (2) phonics instruction; (3) fluency; (4) vocabulary; and (5) text comprehension.

The first necessary skill, *phonemic awareness*, is the ability to distinguish, identify, and manipulate phonemes. This is a skill that can be taught. Within the category of phonemic awareness, there are eight subskills, which we now examine in more detail.

The first subskill, isolating phonemes, is commonly taught by asking students to identify the first (or last) sound in a word. Phoneme identity involves asking learners to find the same sound in different words. Phoneme categorization requires learners to find the word that doesn't fit, such as in tip, cap, tap, and top. Blending phonemes requires learners to combine phonemes into a word, such as when a teacher pronounces the three phonemes /r/ /ə/ /g/ and asks children, "What words do those sounds make?" Segmentation of phonemes involves breaking words into separate phonemes. The teacher asks how many sounds are in the word "flat," and the students articulate each sound while clapping—/f/ clap /l/ clap /æ/ clap /t/ clap. In phoneme deletion, learners determine what remains when a phoneme is omitted, such as, "What is plate without the /p/?" The opposite of phoneme deletion, phoneme addition, involves adding a sound to an existing word, such as "What is the word if you add /s/ to the word "top"? Last, phoneme substitution switches one phoneme for another, as in the case of, "What happens if you change the /l/ in the word 'look' to /b/?" Although there are eight subskills, research shows that it is important for teachers to focus on only one or two different phonemic awareness activities.

Phonics instruction teaches how to use the relationships between letters and sounds to read and write. Explicit and systematic phonics instruction involves direct teaching of sound-letter correspondences in a determined sequence. Research shows that explicit, systematic phonics instruction leads to better reading outcomes. Systematic phonics instruction should begin in kindergarten and continue through first grade for the greatest impact on children's reading achievement. Other findings regarding phonics instruction indicate that it improves reading comprehension and is effective for children from different social and economic statuses. In addition, it is beneficial for struggling and at-risk readers, and is most effective when begun in kindergarten. It is important to note that phonics instruction is only one part of reading instruction during the K–3 continuum and is not sufficient for developing all the requisite skills.

Fluency is the rate and comprehension of reading. If a reader is fluent, then he/she can read text at his or her level accurately and quickly. When reading aloud, a fluent reader expresses the written text effortlessly and naturally. Fluent readers attend to meaning because they are capable of decoding the sounds of the letters with automaticity. Their main focus is on comprehension. Fluency is dependent on the subject and difficulty of the text, the reader's familiarity with the topic of the text, and the reader's amount of practice in reading the text. *The Nation's Report Card: Reading 2009* (National Center for Education Statistics, 2009) reported a close relationship between fluency and comprehension. Research shows that regular guided oral reading improves fluency and reading achievement. This can be accomplished by having students read a text multiple times (up to four times) until a particular fluency level is attained or by using instructional technology or peer tutoring. When selecting a text for building fluency, teachers should choose materials that are at the reader's independent reading level. The independent level text contains no more than 5% difficult words for the reader. Instructional level texts contain approximately 10% difficult words, and frustration level texts include more than 10% difficult words. Techniques such as taking turns reading a text with students (student-adult reading), choral reading, recorded reading, and peer reading help build fluency.

Vocabulary is one of the most important aspects of reading and involves both oral and print representation of words. Vocabulary comprehension consists of four modalities of language comprehension and expression: listening vocabulary (words comprehended by hearing others' speech), speaking vocabulary (words we use when speaking), reading vocabulary (words we understand when reading), and writing vocabulary (words we use in writing). Vocabulary is learned both informally and formally. Informal or indirect vocabulary learning comes from conversations with adults, listening to adults read, and independent reading.

Direct instruction of vocabulary is important and includes teaching specific words as well as strategies for learning new words. Specific word instruction techniques support learners' comprehension and use of new vocabulary and include: (1) pre-teaching words prior to encountering them in a reading passage; (2) multiple exposure to new terms; and (3) access to the same terms in different contexts. In selecting words to teach, three considerations can be helpful: the importance of the word, the usefulness of the word, and the difficulty of the word. Difficulty encompasses words with multiple meanings and idiomatic expressions. In learning new words, students move through becoming acquainted with the term to establishing meaning. There are four types of word learning: (1) learning a new meaning of a known word; (2) learning the meaning of a new word whose concept the learner knows; (3) learning the meaning of a new word whose concept the learner does not know; and (4) clarifying and enhancing the meaning of a word the learner knows. Developing strategies for learning new words include using dictionaries; learning about word parts, such as prefixes, word roots, and suffixes; and using context clues to understand word meaning.

The last skill, *text comprehension*, is the purpose of reading. According to the National Reading Panel Report (2000), good readers have a purpose for reading and think actively as they read. Research shows that specific comprehension strategy instruction improves text comprehension. The report identifies six strategies that improve text comprehension.

The first strategy, monitoring comprehension, indicates that readers are aware of what they understand and do not understand and use strategies to repair comprehension problems. Examples of monitoring comprehension strategies include identifying where and what the difficulty is, restating the difficult passage in the reader's own words, and reviewing previous and upcoming parts of the text.

The second strategy, using graphic and semantic organizers, enables learners to comprehend concepts and relationships among the concepts in a text. These tools help students see the text structure, examine relationships, and summarize the content of a text.

Answering questions, the third area, gives a purpose for reading, focuses attention on key elements, promotes active thought while reading, supports monitoring comprehension, and connects content of the reading to learners' background knowledge of the topic.

Similar to answering questions, the fourth area involves having students generate questions. This strategy promotes active processing of the text and monitoring of comprehension.

The fifth area, recognizing story structure, involves identifying the setting, events, reactions, and so forth, and how they are pulled together in a plot. Story maps are an effective means of depicting story structure.

Lastly, summarizing the important ideas in a text helps students identify and connect main ideas, omit unnecessary information, and remember what they read. Table 8–2 summarizes the National Reading Panel Report's (2000) findings.

Table 8–2. *The National Reading Panel Report's (2000) Findings*

Language knowledge and skills learners must develop, K–3	Phonemic awareness—Phoneme isolation, identity, categorization, blending, segmentation, deletion, addition, and substitution
	Phonics—Graphophonemic (combined letter and sound representation) relationships, letter-sound associations, letter-sound correspondences, sound-symbol correspondences, sound-spelling correspondences
	Fluency—Read a text accurately and quickly, focusing on comprehension
	Vocabulary—Listening, speaking, reading, and writing
	Text comprehension—Use strategies such as comprehension monitoring, graphic and semantic organizers, answering questions about the reading, generating questions about the reading, recognizing story structure, and summarizing.

Source: From *Teaching Children to Read: An Evidence-Based Assessment of the Scientific Research Literature on Reading and Its Implications for Reading Instruction—Reports of the Subgroups,* by National Reading Panel, April 2000. Retrieved from http://www .nationalreadingpanel.org/Publications/subgroups.htm

Adapting Literacy Activities for English Learners

As stated previously, developing ELs' reading skills has much in common with developing the reading skills of native speakers of English. Chapter 5 offered a detailed description of how teaching reading to ELs differs from native speakers. We will highlight a number of effective reading development activities that work for ELs as well as native speakers; however, we will first present simple guidelines developed and used with preservice and in-service general education teachers (Nutta, Mokhtari, & Strebel, 2012).

Teaching Reading

Unlike teaching subject matter content such as science or social studies to English learners, teaching language arts focuses primarily on language development. When teaching subject matter content, the point is for ELs to learn the concepts and skills of the discipline—language growth occurs as a collateral effect of comprehending those concepts and skills in the second language. However, when teaching language arts, including listening, speaking, reading, and writing in English, the point is to learn about the language and how to use it—in other words, the aim is language growth.

   Teachers of native speakers of English may assume that common techniques for teaching reading and writing are similarly appropriate for ELs and native speakers. This assumption is partly fueled by the use of the same terminology in both fields. For example, the emergent literacy development technique for native speakers known as the language experience approach (LEA) is also used for ELs in sheltered environments (i.e., classes with ELs only) (Dixon & Nessel, 2008). However, the *way* the technique is used differently with ELs than with native speakers who possess oral proficiency in English is the focus here.

   The goal of this approach is to use the students' own experiences and descriptions as reading material, ensuring that the content is familiar to all. During the initial phase of the LEA, the steps are the same for ELs and non-ELs: students participate in a shared experience and then recount their experience while the teacher transcribes their description. However, during the recounting of the experience, the teacher of ELs needs to scaffold their oral description of the experience by eliciting and elaborating on the input of the ELs and focusing attention on linguistic errors as appropriate. Although the outcome, having all students recite the finished product as the teacher leads them in choral reading of their class-generated text, is the same, the intermittent step of generating the oral description of the dictated text is very different. In addition, the complexity of the oral description that is transcribed will differ based on the students' level of English proficiency.

As a rule of thumb, Nutta, Mokhtari, and Strebel (2012) categorize the difference between the way a language arts (including reading) activity is used with ELs versus native speakers of English in four areas: *pitch*; *pace*; *portion*; and *perspective*.

Pitch refers to targeting the language used to the students' level of English proficiency. This is similar to using the appropriate reading materials for a particular grade level; however, age and grade do not determine English proficiency. An EL in first grade may be at a near-native level in English proficiency, and an EL in fifth grade may be at a beginning level of English proficiency. If the two students attempted to read a first grade text, everything else being equal, the first grader would perform better than the fifth grader. If the fifth-grade EL were in a sheltered reading class, the teacher would attempt to match the reading materials to the student's vocabulary and grammar knowledge and skills in English. In addition to the pitch of the reading text, the pitch of the teacher's oral language use (giving definitions, explanations, directions, etc.) needs to be adjusted to the level of the EL.

In addition to matching reading materials and instructional discourse to the EL's level of English proficiency, the content of the reading activity needs to be scaffolded to facilitate comprehension. Scaffolding takes place through controlling the pace of the lesson and the portion of the materials. The lower the EL's level of English proficiency, the slower the pace to unpack and scaffold the content. Providing ample time for frequent comprehension checks, repetition and rephrasing, giving definitions (which can often include acting out, drawing, etc.), and explaining new grammar is important. In a mixed classroom with ELs and native speakers, taking this extra time may not be practical, so coteaching or follow-up may be necessary.

Similar to the time constraints of pacing, the portion or amount of reading material in an activity must be adjusted for ELs. Native speakers may read four pages during a class and then answer comprehension questions, but ELs at low levels of proficiency may only be able to fully comprehend four sentences during the lesson. If the reading lesson focuses on understanding details, then the teacher may limit the material to four sentences from the text. If the reading lesson focuses on getting the main idea, then the teacher may choose to extract four key points and organize them in an outline. Because ELs need to understand new vocabulary, grammar, and often cultural references, they can be overwhelmed with too much content and will come away from the lesson without making gains.

Perspective pertains to the focus of the instruction. For a native speaker, a lesson using LEA may focus primarily on properly spelling and sounding out words the students dictate. For an EL a lesson using LEA may focus on syntactic errors, such as stating an adjective after a noun. Because ELs do not have the same oral proficiency and cultural background as the native English-speaking students, the issues that arise during reading instruction may be very different for ELs.

As we look at the following literacy development activities, we need to take into account the English proficiency of ELs and how this will affect the pitch, pace, portion, and perspective of the lesson.

Developing Reading Skills

The Center for Applied Linguistics (CAL) (n.d.) offers a variety of excellent activities for reading development. For example, some ideas for developing phonemic awareness (CAL, 2007, pp. 144–145) include:

◆ Rhyme hunt—Have students identify objects in the classroom and school that rhyme with words the teacher supplies. For example, students are told to find something that rhymes with "hat" and identify "mat." ELs may intersperse words from their native language or may mispronounce words in a way that makes them rhyme (spot and hat could rhyme if the EL pronounces /æ/ as /ɑ/).

◆ Find and say—Paste clip art or magazine pictures of at least two objects that begin with the same sound on card stock, putting together a set of different pictures depicting a variety of beginning sounds. Ask the student to pick a card, say the word and its beginning sound, and find another picture card of an object that begins with the same sound.

◆ Ball toss—Using a beach or NERF ball, state a word and toss the ball to a student, who then says another word that begins with the same sound. Keep tossing the ball until no one can think of another word for the sound. The game can be changed to say words that use the same vowel sound in a one-syllable word, such as hat and nap.

In the area of phonics, CAL (2007, p. 147) provides some examples of activities:

◆ Sorting alphabet cereal—Give each child a cup full of alphabet letter cereal and a paper plate. Each student (or pairs of students) should sort the letters and count the multiples. The teacher then makes a graph with each letter across the bottom and asks students to raise their fingers to show how many of the letters they have, plotting the total number of each letter on the graph.

◆ Letter formation—Have pairs or small groups use their bodies to form different letters and have the class state the letters.

To develop reading fluency, CAL (2007, p. 166) recommends Adler's (2001) activities. These include:

◆ Choral reading—Fluent reader reads the passage aloud while students listen, then class reads along in chorus with the fluent reader. Repeat the process four or five times to prepare students to read the passage independently.

◆ Reading in pairs—Pair students up, pairing one student who reads fairly well with another student who does not read as well. Have the better reader read the text while the other reader listens and follows the text silently. Switch readers and have the stronger reader assist the other with word recognition as needed. For ELs, the pairs can consist of an EL and a native speaker or an EL at one level of English proficiency and an EL at a higher level of English proficiency.

Vocabulary development, the fourth area of the National Reading Panel's research review, is especially critical for ELs. Peregoy and Boyle (2008, pp. 215–216, 219) offer several suggestions for EL vocabulary development:

◆ Word wheels—Make a circle in the center of a poster board and write a common word in the middle, for example, the word "good." Draw six lines like spokes outward from the circle, leaving enough space to write synonyms for good between each pair of lines.
◆ Teaching affixes—Show students a prefix in a common word and define it, for example, in "un-happy," "un" means "not." Ask students to think of other examples using this prefix. Make index cards with adjectives that can serve as base words with the prefix "un-" and have students work in pairs to match, define, and illustrate them.

The last area of the NRP (2000) findings focuses on text comprehension and teaching strategies for comprehension. CAL (2007, pp. 77–78) suggests Stauffer's (1975) sequence, the Directed Reading-Thinking Activity (DRTA). This sequence of five steps involves:

1. Previewing the content of the reading—vocabulary, structures, background knowledge—and introducing them to students;
2. Predicting: teacher preparing questions that guide students to scan passage headings and graphics;

3. Reading: students read alone, in pairs, or while someone else reads aloud and they note where predictions are confirmed or disproven;
4. Checking: students report prediction results and where the answers are found in the text; and,
5. Summarizing: students read the main points in the text and write them in his/her own words.

Developing Oral Proficiency in ELs

Depending on the learning context and age of the learner, specific activities for developing oral proficiency are helpful. These activities may take place in the mainstream classroom, in self-contained ESOL classes, or in consultation with the SLP. In general, ELs and English-speaking students in the lower grades are immersed in activities that build their oral proficiency, such as show and tell, picture books, and more. As they move to upper grades, students have fewer nonverbal cues to connect with new terms and phrases; therefore, working on specific speaking activities can help mitigate this shift. In addition, older students are more likely to have literacy skills in at least one language, so these can be used to foster oral proficiency as well (e.g., in a dialogue memorized for a skit). Last, some students in the upper grades may benefit from specific pronunciation exercises to help them distinguish phonemes that may not be the same in their native language.

Information Gap

An information gap is a second language learning activity intended to promote real communication in the language being acquired. In contrast with language learning approaches such as the audiolingual approach of the 1960s, which focused on learning contrived dialogues to facilitate conversational skills (Richards & Rodgers, 1986), information gap activities set up communication situations that are real.

For example, using a dialogue in an audiolingual approach, a person may ask where the library is and the other person responds that it is two blocks down the street on the right. Both speakers know that this is not a real dialogue; therefore, they do not use language spontaneously or for their own immediate communication needs. In contrast, an information gap activity creates a reason for one person to gather information from the other, thus prompting each person to use language purposefully. An example of an information gap activity follows:

> A teacher brings in a variety of clothing that she hangs up for the class to see. She calls upon two volunteers to role-play the information gap situation. Person one is given a card with a picture of a piece of clothing, such as a corduroy jacket with elbow patches. She must describe the jacket to person two, who takes the role of the salesperson, and ask if she has anything in the store that is similar. Person two finds the corresponding jacket from the clothes hung in the classroom, and offers to let person one try it on. They then improvise from there until completing the transaction.

Information gaps promote the use of vocabulary and phrases specific to a situation, and spontaneously emulates real communication. They are used to allow ELs to practice any type of vocabulary or discourse. Examples of information gap activities can be found at http://bogglesworldesl.com/information_gap.htm.

Jazz Chants

Invented by Carolyn Graham, an ESOL teacher with a jazz background, jazz chants (Graham, 1978) are similar to raps and choral activities. They focus on particular topics, vocabulary, and phrases to give ELs practice in pronouncing new words and sentences. Because they are chanted chorally, the intonation is exaggerated, which helps with prosody. There are a number of prepared jazz chant books with accompanying audio files; however, they are easy to create. Graham (1978; 2000) recommends identifying vocabulary and phrases for a topic of focus, then isolating a small sample for a jazz chant. She recommends selecting words that are one, two, or three syllables. For example, in a lesson on moon phases, some of the words might be: "moon," "full," "new," "phases," "waxing," "waning," "gibbous," "crescent," "quarter," and "full."

Full moon, waxing gibbous

New moon, waning crescent

First quarter, last quarter

Phases of the moon

Jazz chants can also be used to help students learn language functions and the proper intonation for expressing them. For example, in asking and giving permission:

Is this seat taken? May I sit here?

Is this seat taken? May I sit here?

Is this seat taken? May I sit here?

No, it's free. Have a seat! It's yours!

Each of the chants would be accompanied by rhythmic clapping and exaggerated intonation and stress on the stressed syllables and music can also be added.

Minimal Pairs

Minimal pairs focus on phonemes of contrast to help students whose native languages do not have the same distinctions. For example, the Arabic-speaking EL does not have a /p/ sound in their native language. This often leads to confusion, because the Arabic language does have the /b/, which is a similar sound. This can result in misunderstandings of both languages and often leads to errors stemming from not hearing the difference between the /p/ and /b/ sounds (e.g., pat and bat). If the EL were told, "Give him a pat," he or she may understand, "Give him a bat." Similarly, not having the phoneme /p/ in Arabic results in substituting the phoneme /b/ when attempting to pronounce a word in English, such as "Bark the car."

Minimal pair exercises often involve the selection of two words that differ in one phoneme. The first step is to have the learner identify which word has the targeted phoneme. For instance, the teacher would say, "park, bark" and would ask the learner to raise her hand when she heard the /p/ sound. After "park, bark" the teacher would say "bin, pin," and so forth. The /p/ phoneme could then be used in the medial position, such as "cable, maple," and also in the final position, "cap, cab." After the student develops a high success rate of identifying the /p/ phoneme, the teacher can then move to having the student pronounce each pair, ensuring that the /p/ sound is included in words that use it. It then becomes a type of pronunciation drill.

Although minimal pairs is primarily a listening and speaking activity, it has implications for reading and writing. An EL who could not distinguish the sounds would then have trouble spelling the word "park" in writing and might confuse the word "pole" for the word "bowl" in the sentence, "She was carrying a pole." Helping students to differentiate between sounds has far-reaching implications.

Cooperative Learning

The cooperative learning strategy is not specific to ELs, although it has many features that promote the development of oral language skills. Students work in teams and must interact to complete a given task. The interaction involves conversation and discussion, and often occurs between pairs or small groups of up to four people. This allows for multiple opportunities for negotiating meaning, which facilitates second language development.

According to Kagan (1994), a leading proponent of cooperative learning, a group activity must include four elements: positive interdependence, individual accountability, equal participation, and simultaneous interaction. In other words, everyone in the group is dependent on each other for the outcome; each member is evaluated for his/her contributions; everyone contributes and is on task; and everyone has a concurrent task.

An example of a cooperative learning activity for pairs is the think-pair-share strategy. The first step is for individuals in each pair to think about a question or problem that the teacher poses. Step two requires two students to share their thoughts with each other. The final step involves grouping the pairs with another pair to report their conclusions or share the pairs' conclusions with the entire class. The amount of time that each student spends speaking is greatly increased by participating in pair and small group activities rather than whole class instruction.

Developing Writing Skills

Writing skill development spans emergent writing stages — including letter formation, invented spelling, and approximated spelling — all the way to advanced composition skills, such as writing a research paper. In the following section, we highlight a sampling of writing activities. Peregoy and Boyle (2008) offer a wealth of resources that promote writing skill development at K–12 levels.

Language Experience Approach

The Language Experience Approach (Peregoy & Boyle, 2008, p. 297–300), described above as a reading skill development activity, can also be used as an early writing skill development activity. Using this approach, students participate in a shared experience that serves as the basis for subsequent storytelling. For example, the teacher and students may use a blender to grind peanuts into peanut butter. Following the experience, the teacher leads the students to retell what happened and then writes the students' dictation sentence-by-sentence on chart paper. The teacher then leads the class in a choral reading of the descriptive paragraph. Depending on the children's age, they may copy the paragraph or write and/or draw their own version of the story. If they have difficulty writing their own version, they can dictate the story to the teacher or an aide, who helps reinforce the narrative structure of a descriptive paragraph and grammar and usage conventions.

Dialogue Journals

Peregoy and Boyle (2008) point out that emergent writers need to develop fluency and automaticity in writing. The development of fluent writing skills requires practice in purposeful writing that is engaging and interesting to the student. Dialogue journals are like personal journals. Students share their personal thoughts and the teacher responds to the student by sharing their own personal thoughts. There is a regular exchange of journaling between the teacher and students. The role of the teacher is not to correct grammar or any other aspect of form, but to reply to the content of the entry. Students should be reminded that the teacher cannot necessarily respond to every issue raised in the dialogue journals, but if they would like a response on a specific point, they can underline it or write it in a different color. It's also important to set parameters for dialogue journals, as students may address inappropriate topics or reveal issues that the teacher must report.

Clustering and Mapping

Peregoy and Boyle (2008) suggest two types of graphic organizers to help plan for writing: clustering and mapping. Clustering helps writers identify vocabulary for their composition. The subject of the composition is placed at the center of the cluster. Students then begin to draw spokes from the center circle with words that relate to the topic. Words on the spokes can be added to the cluster as necessary (Figure 8–1).

Mapping is more detailed and organized than clustering, and can be used by writers at all levels. It uses more than single words in the graphic and moves the writer into the next stages of composition. If students were to take the composition of making peanut butter to the next step, they could first make a cluster and then categorize the content. Maps assist students to write about a topic in a logical and descriptive way (Figure 8–2).

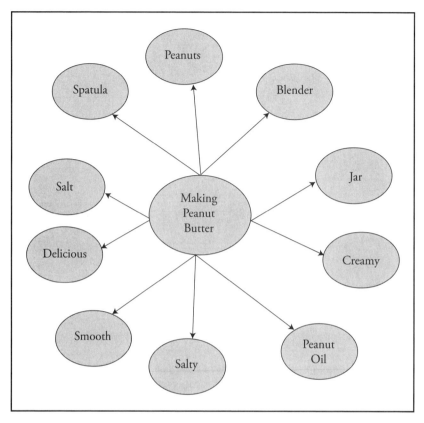

Figure 8-1. *Cluster about making peanut butter.*

Sentence Combining and Shortening

More advanced ELs, especially at the secondary level, can benefit from writing exercises that emphasize varied sentence construction. Peregoy and Boyle (2008) suggest sentence combining and sentence shortening as a way to help students write with more sophistication. In sentence combining, writers are given two or more sentences that present information on the same topic. Students are then required to find the best way to combine the sentences into one sentence, using relative phrases, subordinate clauses, etc. For example: (1) Mary ate her lunch; (2) Mary's lunch was delicious and nutritious; (3) Mary was in a hurry; and

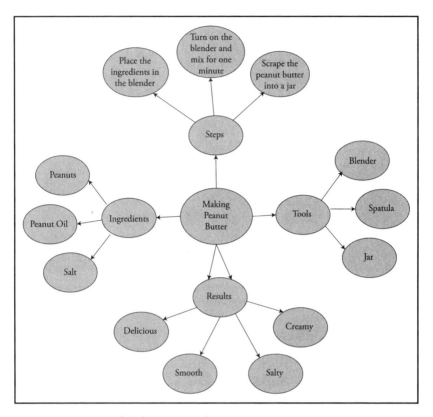

Figure 8–2. *Map of making peanut butter.*

(4) Mary only had a 15-minute lunch break. The combined sentence might look like this: Mary ate her delicious and nutritious lunch in a hurry because she only had a 15-minute lunch break.

   Sentence shortening addresses verbose sentences, challenging students to revise them into the shortest sentence possible without losing meaning. Sometimes this involves dividing a run-on sentence into two sentences, and sometimes it simply requires omitting extraneous words and phrases from the sentence. For example, in the sentence, "I had ice cream for dessert and it was chocolate chip, and I liked it a lot, and I ate every bite," the writer could revise it to two sentences, such as, "I had chocolate chip ice cream for dessert. I liked it so much that I ate every bite." The sentence, "Due to the fact that the economy is affected by the purchasing habits of the general population, people have an influence on the nation's financial health," can omit a number of superfluous words and rephrase the main concepts more simply, "People's purchasing habits affect the national economy."

SLPs and ESOL Professionals—Partners in Language and Literacy Development

The ASHA 2001 position statement *Roles and Responsibilities of SLPs with Respect to Reading and Writing in Children and Adolescents* set the stage for the involvement of the SLP in reading and writing. Specifically, SLPs were challenged to address reading and writing for struggling students and those with communication disorders. The established connections between spoken and written language and the reciprocal relationship between language and literacy competence makes the SLP a unique contributor in the implementation of evidence-based literacy strategies and interventions.

A requirement of IDEA (1997) is that intervention must be relevant to the expectations of the general education curriculum. Although SLPs traditionally have been trained in the language base of curriculum, including reading and writing, they have not always been familiar with or involved in incorporating the curriculum in their intervention (Ehren, 2006; Justice, 2006). With the increased emphasis on high performance standards brought on by educational reform and more emphasis in university training programs on the role of the SLP in language and literacy, many SLPs have become familiar with approaches and practical strategies that parallel the curriculum and facilitate language and literacy development. Specifically, SLPs work in partnership with other school-based professionals to help students meet the performance standards of a particular school district and state.

The No Child Left Behind Act of 2001 stressed that accountability for all students is the responsibility of all school-based professionals (e.g., mainstream, content-area, ESL, bilingual education teachers, and SLPs) who work with ELs. Specifically, several TESOL position papers (TESOL, 2003, 2005, 2007, 2010) have focused on the preparation and roles of the ESOL professional in the development of language and literacy in ELs. Similar to the SLP, they are charged with implementing evidenced-based instructional practices and making instruction comprehensible (Brisk, 2008; Menyuk & Brisk, 2005). However, unlike the SLP, the responsibilities of the ESOL professional primarily focuses on achievement in core subjects using standards-based instruction (TESOL, 2001, 2006, 2009). What makes this challenging is that ELs must achieve the standards in a language other than their native language, and often before the EL is literate in that language

A significant amount of research has been conducted during the past decades on literacy development in ELs. However, research on effective practices for ELs with a communication disorder is limited. In many instances, research that has been conducted on ELs has been generalized and applied to ELs with language disorders. For example, models to address literacy in ELs that involve native and second languages have been proposed (Gorman & Gillam, 2003; Gutierrez-Clellan, 1994; Klingner, Artiles, & Barletta, 2006; Lesaux & Siegel, 2003; Proctor, August, Carlo, & Snow, 2006; Restrepo & Towle-Harmon, 2008), as well as strategies for ELs in the beginning, intermediate, and advanced stages of literacy (Cloud, Genesee, & Hamayan, 2009). Systematic reviews have been conducted on ELs and literacy development. The goal of these reviews are to identify programs or interventions that can potentially have positive effects on reading achievement and English language development (Institute of Education Science, 2006, 2007a, 2007b; Thomason & Gorman, 2008).

This chapter does not provide an exhaustive list of strategies and approaches that have been used with ELs or ELs with communication disorders. Readers are directed to more specific sources for that purpose (i.e., Calderon, 2007; Diaz-Rico, 2004; Cloud, Genesee, & Hamayan, 2009; Peregoy & Boyle, 2008; Roseberry-Mckibben, 2007; Schatz, 2010). However, this chapter does serve as a starting point for the SLP and ESOL professional to consider *purposeful collaboration* in the planning and implementation of intervention services, specific treatment techniques, and programs for students exhibiting a communication disorder.

Summary

This chapter has provided several approaches and practical strategies to facilitate language and literacy development in ELs. Evidence-based approaches and strategies that will facilitate literacy skills in ELs continue to be needed. Research that informs practice suggests that ELs learn best when explicit instruction, modeling, and a multitude of effective strategies are used daily that involve students as active and engaged listeners. The involvement of all professionals in the development of language and literacy skills for ELs and ELs with communication disorders is necessary. The next chapter specifically discusses the collaboration of the SLP and ESOL professional and how this partnership is instrumental in promoting language and literacy in ELs with communication disorders.

References

Adler, C. R. (Ed). 2001). *Put reading first: The research building blocks for teaching children to read*, pp. 49–54. National Institute for Literacy. Retrieved from http://www.nifl.gov/partnershipforreading/publications/reading_first1text.html

American Speech-Language-Hearing Association. (2001). *Roles and responsibilities of speech-language pathologists with respect to reading and writing in children and adolescents* [Guidelines]. Available from www.asha.org/policy

Brisk, M. E. (Ed.). (2008). *Language, culture, and community in teacher education*. Mahwah, NJ: Lawrence Erlbaum.

Calderon, M. (2007). *Teaching reading to English language learners, grades 6–12*. Thousand Oaks, CA: Corwin Press.

Center for Applied Linguistics. (n.d.). Washington, DC. Retrieved from http://www.cal.org

Center for Applied Linguistics. (2007). *What's different about teaching reading to students learning English? Trainer's manual*. Washington, DC: Center for Applied Linguistics. Retrieved from http://www.cal.org/solutions/resources/index.html#1

Cloud, N., Genesee, F., & Hamayan, E. (2009). *Literacy instruction for English language learners*. Portsmouth, NH: Heinemann.

Diaz-Rico, L. T. (2004). *Teaching English learners. Strategies and methods*. Boston, MA: Pearson.

Dixon, C. N., & Nessel, D. (2008). *Using the language experience approach with English language learners: Strategies for engaging students and developing literacy*. Thousand Oaks, CA: Sage.

Ehren, B. J. (2006). Partnerships to support reading comprehension for students with language impairment. *Topics in Language Disorders*, *26*(1), 41–53.

Gorman, B. K., & Gillam, R. B. (2003). Phonological awareness in Spanish: A tutorial for speech-language pathologists. *Communication Disorders Quarterly*, *25*, 13–22.

Graham, C. (1978). *Jazz chants*. New York, NY: Oxford University Press.

Graham, C. (2000). *Jazz chants: Old and new*. New York, NY: Oxford University Press.

Gutierrez-Clellan, V. (1994). Syntactic complexity in Spanish narratives: A developmental study. *Journal of Speech and Hearing Research*, *37*, 645–654.

Individuals with Disabilities Education Act (IDEA). (1997). *Federal Register*, *62*(204). Part V, Department of Education, 34 CFR PARTSW 300, 303.

Institute of Education Science. (2006). Vocabulary improvement program for English language learners and their classmates. *IES What Works Clearinghouse Intervention Report*. Washington, DC: Author. Retrieved from http://www.asha.org/members/compendiumSearch Results.aspx?type=1&searchtext=Literacy

Institute of Education Science. (2007a). *Effective literacy and English language instruction for English learners in the elementary grades*. Washington, DC: Author. Retrieved from http://ies.ed.gov/ncee/ wwc/pdf/practiceguides/20074011.pdf

Institute of Education Science. (2007b). English language learners. *IES What Works Clearinghouse Intervention Report*. Washington, DC: Author. Retrieved from http://www.asha.org/members/compendium SearchResults.aspx?type=1&searchtext=Literacy

Justice, L. (2006). Evidence-based practice, response to intervention, and the prevention of reading difficulties. *Language, Speech, and Hearing Services in Schools*, *37*(4), 284–297.

Kagan, S. (1994). *Cooperative learning*. San Clemente, CA: Resources for Teachers.

Klingner, J. K., Artiles, A. J., & Barletta, L. M. (2006). English language learners who struggle with reading: Language acquisition or LD? *Journal of Learning Disabilities*, *39*, 108–128.

Lesaux, N. K., & Siegel, L. S. (2003). The development of reading in children who speak English as a second language. *Developmental Psychology*, *36*, 1005–1019.

Menyuk, P., & Brisk, M.E. (2005). *Language development and education: Children with varying language experience.* Hampshire, UK: Palgrave MacMillan.

National Center for Education Statistics. (2009). *The nation's report card: Reading 2009*(NCES 2010–458). Washington, DC: Institute of Education Sciences, US Department of Education.

National Early Literacy Panel. (2008). *Developing early literacy: Report of the National Early Literacy Panel.* Washington, DC: National Institute for Literacy. Retrieved from http://www.nifl.gov/earlychild hood/NELP/NELPreport.html

National Reading Panel. (2000, April). *Teaching children to read: An evidence-based assessment of the scientific research literature on reading and its implications for reading instruction — reports of the subgroups.* Retrieved from http://www.nationalreadingpanel.org/ Publications/subgroups.htm

No Child Left Behind (NCLB). (2001). 20 U.S.C (2001& Supp 2002). Washington, DC: US Department of Education.

Nutta, J. W., Mokhtari, K, & Strebel, C. (Eds.). (2012). *Preparing every teacher to reach English learners: A practical guide for teacher educators.* Cambridge, MA: Harvard Education Press.

Peregoy, S., & Boyle, O. (2008). *Reading, writing, and learning in ESL: A resource book for teaching K–12 English learners.* Boston, MA: Pearson.

Proctor, C. P., August, D., Carlo, M. S., & Snow, C. (2006). The intriguing role of Spanish language vocabulary knowledge in predicting English reading comprehension. *Journal of Educational Psychology, 98,* 159–169.

Restrepo, M. A., & Towle-Harmon, M. (2008, September 23). Addressing emergent literacy skills in English-language learners. *ASHA Leader.*

Richards, J. C., & Rodgers, T. S. (1986). *Approaches and methods in language teaching.* New York, NY: Cambridge Press.

Roseberry-McKibbin, C. (2007). *Language disorders in children: A multicultural and case perspective.* Boston, MA: Allyn & Bacon.

Schatz, M. (Ed.). (2010). *Education of English language learners (challenges in language and literacy).* New York, NY: Guildford.

Stauffer, R. (1975). *Directing the reading-thinking process.* New York, NY: Harper & Row.

TESOL. (2001). *ESL Standards into Classroom Practice: Grades Pre-K–2.* Alexandria, VA: Author.

TESOL. (2003). *Position statement on the preparation of pre-K–12 educators for cultural and linguistic diversity in the United States.* Alexandria, VA: Author. Retrieved from http://www.tesol.org/s_tesol/ seccss.asp?CID=32&DID=37

TESOL. (2005). *Position statement on highly qualified teachers under No Child Left Behind*. Alexandria, VA: Author. Retrieved from http://www.tesol.org/s_tesol/seccss.asp?CID=32&DID=37

TESOL. (2006). *PreK–12 English language proficiency standards*. Alexandria, VA: Author.

TESOL. (2007). *Position statement on the identification of English language learners with special educational needs*. Alexandria, VA: Author. Retrieved from http://www.tesol.org/s_tesol/seccss.asp?CID=32&DID=37

TESOL. (2009). *Integrating the paper to practice: Using the TESOL ELP standards in preK–12 classrooms*. Alexandria, VA: Author.

TESOL. (2010). *Position paper on language and literacy development for young English language learners (ages 3–8)*. Alexandria, VA: Author. Retrieved from http://www.tesol.org/s_tesol/seccss.asp?CID=32&DID=37

Thomason, K. M., Gorman, B. K., & Summers, C. (2008). English literacy development for English language learners: Does Spanish instruction promote or hinder? *EBP Briefs, 2*, 13–24. Retrieved from http://www.asha.org/members/compendiumSearchResults.aspx?type=1&searchtext=Literacy

9

The Power of Two: Directions for an Effective Collaboration Between SLPs and ESOL Professionals

Key Terms

EL—English Learner

ESOL—English for Speakers of Other Languages

IDEA—Individual Disabilities Education

SLP—Speech-Language Pathologist

Introduction

Collaboration and teamwork among various categories of education professionals are key elements in working with ELs with communication disorders. The team-based approach in identifying and educating students with special needs has been mandated since 1975, when Congress passed Public Law 94-142 (Education for All Handicapped Children Act), now known as IDEA (Individuals with Disabilities Education Act) (2004). One of the key provisions of IDEA was the creation of an individualized education program (IEP) for children with special needs, a concept that has at its core a group problem-solving approach to the identification and education of students with special needs. For this reason and many others, all categories of special education have strongly advocated collaboration with other professionals, parents, and school administrators.

Clearly, collaboration among SLPs and ESOL professionals can potentially affect the instruction of ELs with communication disorders in a very positive manner. However, in order to occur, collaboration needs to be systematic and constant. It is not enough for SLPs, educators, and other decision makers to meet once a year to review IEPs. Meetings should occur regularly and in a very well-defined context. These meetings should not be driven exclusively by compliance issues in an effort to avoid litigations. Instead, meetings should be a supportive group process where teachers, SLPs, related service professionals, parents, and administrators work collaboratively as valued team members and key decision makers in this process.

Do SLPs and ESOL professionals feel encouraged to collaborate when working with ELs with communication disorders? What are some of the perceptions, practices, and needs of educational professionals who work with ELs with special needs? A survey of 125 educational professionals working with ELs with special needs in the Washington, DC, area attempted to answer these significant questions (Roache, Shore, Gouleta, & Butkevich, 2003). The majority of the participants' responses indicated that they had the training and skills to work with EL students with special needs but were unclear about the roles, responsibilities, and practices of other school professionals who worked with ELs with special needs. Additionally, they noted that they had not received appropriate training on establishing effective frameworks for collaboration.

Notably, another finding revealed that administration often did not provide adequate support to foster collaboration with other school professionals in serving EL students with special needs. To achieve a successful collaboration, the roles and responsibilities of each professional needs to be well-defined. Then, collaboration needs to be structured and modeled after successful research-based examples of SLP-ESOL partnerships that generated tangible results for ELs with communication disorders. Last, it is important to have visible support from administration for a successful collaboration effort (Roache et al., 2003).

The Roles of SLPs and ESOL Professionals in Working with ELs with Communication Disorders

A first step to establish an effective collaborative environment between SLPs and ESOL professionals is to ensure that both disciplines know exactly what their respective roles and responsibilities are when working with ELs (Rosa-Lugo & Fradd, 2000). For this reason, let us first examine how the role of the ESOL professional is defined and how they perceive their role. Then, we will look at the role of the SLPs in working with ESOL instructors in school settings, from RtI or preassessment, assessment, and intervention stages.

ESOL Professionals: Roles and Perceptions

In accordance with state and federal laws, ESOL programs across the United States must make every effort to implement policies and procedures to meet the educational needs of students whose primary language is not English. A primary goal of all ESOL programs is to increase the proficiency levels of ELs in the areas of listening, speaking, reading, and writing. To achieve this goal, ESOL professionals assist in the identification of EL students, using appropriate and approved assessment tools. They create and maintain instructional classes that have a positive impact on students' learning the English language so that ELs can function independently and fully in general education classrooms upon passing English language proficiency assessments. To facilitate the academic success of ELs, the ESOL professional works with other instructional team members to: (a) plan culturally responsive instruction, (b) use appropriate accommodations and modifications, and (c) implement evidence-based strategies and techniques to make instruction comprehensible for ELs while promoting academic language development.

In addition to addressing the language needs of ELs, ESOL professionals have other roles. They are not simply teaching language; they are also assisting their students with the sometimes difficult transition to a new culture and set of expectations. As a resource teacher, they work with ELs to understand American culture and encourage students in regular education and work with school faculty and staff to understand other cultures. ESOL professionals also provide social and emotional support for ELs. While developing the language proficiency of their ELs, ESOL professionals promote academic achievement, social growth and acceptance, and self-confidence and self-worth. Many ELs arrive from countries and cultures that are different from the mainstream US. ESOL professionals are expected to provide support not only for their ELs, but also for students' families while they adjust to life in America. Providing opportunities for acculturation and socialization are important aspects of the ESOL professional's role.

ESOL professionals also act as student advocates in the school community. Many times, the parents of ELs do not have the language skills to participate in the decision-making processes involving their children. ESOL professionals often take on the roles and responsibilities of parents and act as a critical liaison between the student and other teachers and staff members As a consequence, ESOL professionals are an essential link between the school and the student's family. This connection can be vital when ELs or their families are isolated as a result of cultural differences or language barriers.

This description of ESOL professionals' roles is applicable to the expectations of ESOL professionals in many programs and schools across the US. However, it is important to know what

ESOL professionals think of their roles and how they view themselves in the educational context in which they function. Are these self-constructed roles congruent with the roles they are expected to perform in accordance with state and federal mandates?

DeGuerrero and Villamil (2000) explored ESL professionals' roles through metaphor analysis. In their study of 22 participants who were ESOL professionals in Puerto Rico, they looked at the metaphors ESOL professionals associated with their roles and identified no less than nine roles, listed in Table 9–1.

It is very important to note that most of the roles listed in Table 9–1 are exclusively addressing the language needs of ELs and do not focus on the other roles of ESOL professionals, such as advocating for their students or collaborating with other teachers and professionals who are teaching ELs. This reiterates the idea that collaboration occurs only when there is administrative commitment and solid and well-established mechanisms in schools and districts.

The Speech Language Pathologist's Role in ESOL Instruction

What is the role of SLPs in ESOL instruction? Because of SLPs' professional preparation, are they allowed to provide *direct instruction* to ELs? Briefly said, "no." The specialized competencies and the required education necessary to deliver ESOL instruction to ELs should not be assumed to be possessed by all SLPs. ESOL instruction requires academic preparation and experience in areas such as second language acquisition, linguistics, language teaching methodologies, assessment, and practicum, which may or may not be covered in SLPs' preparation programs. Therefore, SLPs without the mandatory training should not provide direct ESOL instruction to ELs. Instead, SLPs should collaborate and consult with ESOL instructors (ASHA, 1998).

SLPs providing services to school-age ELs with communication disorders should know the school district policy, state and federal laws, first and second language acquisition, culturally appropriate assessment methods and intervention techniques, and strategies for working with families and other professionals.

Table 9–1. *ESOL Professionals' Roles*

Role	Definition	Metaphor
Cooperative Leader	The ESOL professional guides and directs students, and establishes an atmosphere of trust in the classroom.	Coach
Challenger/Agent of Change	The ESOL professional creates challenges, brings about change, and procures opportunities for learning.	Gateway to the future
Knowledge Provider	The ESOL professional is the source of language.	Sun
Nurturer	The ESOL professional facilitates language growth and development and mediates language learning by giving constant feedback and support.	Gardener
Innovator	The ESOL professional keeps up with new methods and evidenced- based research in the field for classroom implementation	Explorer
Provider of Tools	The ESOL professional makes language available to students as a tool to construct meaning.	Tool carrier
Artist	The ESOL professional approaches teaching as an aesthetic experience and molds learners into works of art.	Potter
Repairer	The ESOL professional corrects students' language, strategies, and attitudes.	Mechanic of the mind
Gym Instructor	The ESOL professional treats students' minds as muscles that need to be trained and exercised.	Aerobics instructor

Source: Adapted from "Exploring ESL Teachers' Roles through Metaphor Analysis," by M. de Guerrero & O. Villamil, 2000, *TESOL Quarterly, 34*(2), 341–351.

SLPs should also know the process and procedures for identifying, placing, and serving ELs with special needs as well as the role of the SLP in the area of prevention (i.e., RtI). In providing services to ELs, SLPs should follow guidelines, competencies, and definitions outlined in various ASHA position papers and guidelines (i.e., *Clinical Management of Communicatively Handicapped Minority Language Populations*, ASHA, 1985; *Definitions of Communication Disorders and Variations*, ASHA, 1993; *Preferred Practice Patterns for the Professions of Speech-Language Pathology*, ASHA, 2004; *Scope of Practice, Speech-Language Pathology*, ASHA, 1996; *Social Dialects*, ASHA, 1983; *Roles and Responsibilities of Speech-Language Pathologists in School, 2010*). If the provider of speech and language services is a bilingual SLP, then the professional should meet the guidelines found in the *Bilingual Speech-Language Pathologists and Audiologists* position statement (ASHA, 1989), as well as federal and state requirements.

As stated before, ESOL instruction should be provided only by professionals with appropriate training and experience. The required knowledge, skills, and competencies for providing ESOL instruction may go beyond those provided in communication sciences and disorders preservice educational training programs. However, SLPs can play a key role by collaborating with providers of ESOL instruction, at any or all stages of service delivery. These ways of collaborating, suggested by ASHA (1998; 2010) are listed in Table 9–2. These roles are not mandatory but constitute possible avenues that SLPs and ESOL professionals may choose to foster collaboration.

Team-Building and Collaboration Models

In order to provide effective services to ELs with communication disorders, SLPs and classroom teachers should establish collaborative team relationships. Research suggests that a collaborative team approach is a very efficient way to promote positive outcomes for children with communication disorders (Moore-Brown & Montgomery, 2001). Collaboration can be defined as the

Table 9–2. *SLP-ESOL Collaboration at Preassessment, Assessment, and Intervention Stages for ELs with Communication Disorders*

Stage of Service Delivery	SLP-ESOL Collaboration

Preassessment	At this stage, the SLP may:
	1. collaborate with an ESOL professional on issues such as language development and code-switching in Els who are developing English proficiency; and
	2. provide information to and gather data from the ESOL professional including, but not limited to:
	  a. Els' socialization; and
	  b. patterns of first and second language development, and language use in the classroom and home.
	3. play a critical role in RtI efforts to include:
	  a. assisting general education classroom teachers and ESOL professionals to meet the needs of students in initial RTI tiers with an emphasis on the relevant language underpinnings of learning and literacy
	  b. collaborating with ESOL professional to provide their expertise in language, its disorders, and treatment

Assessment	At this stage, the SLP may: 1. Consult with ESOL professionals on issues such as the EL's performance on testing completed by the ESOL professional and the EL's performance on testing completed by the SLP; 2. Share evaluation results after the assessment regarding the EL's performance; and 3. Collaborate with the ESOL professional in developing an appropriate intervention plan, including: a. Adapting curricula to meet the EL's specific needs, such as modifying assignments, activities, and tests;

Table 9–2. *continued*

Stage of Service Delivery	SLP-ESOL Collaboration
Assessment *continued*	b. Considering the EL's individual needs and learning style; c. Selecting appropriate materials and instructional strategies; and d. Involving parents and caregivers in the EL's program of instruction.
Intervention	At this stage, the SLP-ESOL collaboration is an essential aspect of the educational and therapeutic process. This collaboration can occur in many ways, ranging from informal conversations to formal, planned activities. By collaborating, the SLP and ESOL professional should: 1. Share ideas and resources as well as plan and work together to coordinate goals and objectives; 2. Evaluate progress toward speech and/or language intervention goals and English language development goals; 3. Coordinate the instruction of English language development with the intervention for the communication disorder; 4. Consider cultural and linguistic factors that affect service delivery; and 5. Prepare for and participate in IEP reviews.

Source: Adapted from *Provision of Instruction in English as a Second Language by Speech-Language Pathologists in School Settings* [Technical Report], by American Speech-Language-Hearing Association, 1998. Retrieved from www.asha.org/policy; *Roles and Responsibilities of Speech-Language Pathologists in Schools* [Professional Issues Statement], by American Speech-Language-Hearing Association, 2010. Retrieved from www.asha.org/policy.

direct interaction between team members engaged in decision making as they work toward achieving a common goal (Friend & Cook, 2000). For example, collaboration between SLPs and ESOL professionals may involve working on a team for a short period of time, for example, when implementing specific instructional strategies and interventions for ELs who are struggling (RtI—Tier 1), making placement decisions for ELs with communication disorders, or for a more extended period of time, when team members develop and implement interventions for ELs with communication disorders.

Friend and Cook (2000) note that effective teams have a shared purpose, clearly defined roles, and shared leadership. However, effective teams do not occur without effort; they require time, commitment, and nurturing. According to McCartney (1999), successful collaboration can be threatened by several hurdles. First, team members might have individual assumptions concerning the model of collaboration to be used and different perceptions of their roles and responsibilities in participating and implementing a collaborative initiative. Additionally, members of the team may not be aware of the unique roles and responsibilities of each team member. When team members have overlapping responsibilities for only a subset of goals, collaboration may be limited to the shared tasks. Specifically, the ESOL professional may focus more on getting through the curriculum, whereas speech-language services are provided without considering the common core state standards (National Governor's Association, 2011). In spite of these difficulties, the outcomes of the collaborative team process can be highly beneficial for the team participants and, more important, for ELs with communication disorders and their families.

Team formation can be conceptualized as a developmental process that evolves through stages. Tuckman and Jensen (1977) described a five-stage model of team development: forming, storming, norming, performing, and adjourning. Based on the work of Lowe and Herranen (1978, 1982), Pena and Quinn (2003) looked at team development in speech-language pathology in the context of a school environment. The stages of team development they discussed are listed in Table 9–3.

Their observation and data analysis of the interactions between SLPs and ESOL professionals in classrooms generated several recommendations that SLPs and ESOL professionals should consider if they want to have effective teams. First, ESOL professionals need to be included in the preliminary sessions that are conducted at the onset of any SLP initiative; more spe-

Table 9–3. *Predictable Stages of Team Development*

Stage	Characteristics
Becoming Acquainted	Polite and impersonal, hierarchical interactions, autocratic leadership
Trial and Error	Intrateam alliances/factions, role conflict, attempts to coordinate and facilitate team function, ambiguity about role on team
Collective Indecision	False assumptions of shared responsibility, with little accomplished; avoidance of conflict and maintenance of equilibrium; decisions by default; general indecision and autocratic leadership
Crisis	Internal or external event forces team members to realize they are functioning ineffectively; crisis has function of either unifying or dissolving team; team members may react emotionally, express anger, concern, or uneasiness; productivity remains low
Tentative Purpose	Renegotiation of roles, realization that team members need to assume shared responsibility, consciousness of purpose, productivity remains low
Resolution	Concerted effort to work together as a team; development of effective communication strategies; genuinely shared leadership, decision making, and responsibility
Team Maintenance	Realization of the greater mission—meeting the client's needs, team functioning is effective, dependent on internal group process, conflicts are resolved quickly and with mutual respect

Source: From "Developing Effective Collaboration Teams in Speech-Language Pathology: A Case Study," by E. D. Pena & R. Quinn R, 2003, *Communications Disorders Quarterly, 24*(2), 53–63. Copyright 2003 by Sage. Adapted with permission.

cifically, they need to be included in the entry, orientation, and problem identification stages. The result of this inclusion is a shared understanding of the model and process of collaboration, on the one hand, and a set of common goals and purpose on the other hand. Many times, ESOL professionals believe that once the in-class screening, observations, and evaluations are completed, a more traditional pull-out model will be used and the SLPs will work one-on-one with ELs with communication disorders in a different setting. The presence of ESOL professionals at the initial stages of SLPs' program implementation will ensure that their presence in the classroom will be understood and accepted by teachers, thus making collaboration more effective and diffusing potential crises.

Additionally, collaboration needs to be voluntary. Teachers should be provided with rewards and incentive for participation and should be given sufficient time to participate in the collaboration process. Therefore, the administrators' support for the collaborative process is critical and must be demonstrated through meaningful incentives, including the allocation of time to dedicate to the process. Moreover, team members must see each other as peers. To ensure this aspect of collaboration and to foster collegiality, initial stages of any SLP project need to include teaching team members to plan collaboratively while being aware of the roles of different professionals in that process. Learning how to give constructive feedback and how to listen to such feedback may be important training in order to evaluate implementation of a given intervention. Finally, developing a shared definition of collaboration as it refers to the team is an important aspect of an effective collaborative effort.

Prelock, Miller, and Reed (1995) describe the key elements for establishing effective collaborative partnerships in the delivery of services to children with communication disorders. In terms of collaboratively planning and implementing lessons, they propose several transdisciplinary components that collaborative lesson plans need to include for effective delivery. The proposed framework establishes the roles during planned meetings and during lesson implementation, identifies concerns regarding student performance, selects educational goals, teaching techniques, and materials, as well as key vocabulary that needs to be covered during instruction. Special attention is given to data collection that focuses on student performance during class activities and other assessments. All these elements are outlined in Table 9–4.

Table 9–4. *Components of Collaborative Lesson Plans*

Component	Description
Roles during Planning Meetings	• Typically, a team meets once every 2 or 3 weeks and plans for a 2- to 3-week unit in 30 to 40 minutes. Initially, most teams should meet weekly for 30 minutes to plan single lessons. As teams became more time efficient, the need for weekly planning meetings will probably decrease. • The roles team members can take are as time managers/facilitators of the discussion during the meeting or as recorders responsible for writing the collaboratively planned lesson. • The time manager keeps the team on task and goal directed. • The facilitator ensures that all aspects of the lesson plan are covered and that all members of the team participate in the planning process. • The recorder writes the lesson plan.
Roles during Lesson Implementation	• There are three important roles in collaborative intervention: leader, helper, and data collector. • The leader is responsible for introducing the lesson, providing directions, and primarily teaching the lesson. • The helper keeps an eye on the lesson in progress to ensure the clarity of the message, to assist in student comprehension, and to make sure that the stated objectives are addressed. • The data collector verifies that the objectives are measurable and gathers the data during the presentation of the lesson.
Establishment of Collaborative Concerns	• Following role designation, the team identifies concerns regarding student performance for both identified students and total classroom needs. • By establishing collaborative concerns, a team can determine relevant curricular and speech-language goals.

continues

Table 9–4. *continued*

Component	Description
Selection of Goals	• Based on collaborative concerns, the team decides the number and content of lessons that are needed to be planned, emphasizing goals to address the student's performance.
Facilitating Techniques	• To support the communication needs of the identified student while in the classroom, facilitating techniques often are necessary. • Additionally, other students in the classroom have become familiar with these cues and use them in their interactions with the identified child.
Brainstorming	• Time is allotted for brainstorming the lesson activity (approximately 5–10 minutes). Once the brainstorming period has ended, a team decision for an activity can be made from the list of suggestions. • When making this decision, the team considers goals for the curriculum and for the identified student.
Outline of Procedures	• The procedures for a collaborative lesson are ordered and instructions and/or models to be used are listed.
Key Vocabulary	• In order to ensure student comprehension, it is critical to identify and teach key vocabulary within the collaborative lesson. Many students with communication disorders demonstrate deficits in learning, categorizing, and applying vocabulary within the classroom context. • The ESOL professional's knowledge of the vocabulary specific to the curriculum allows the SLP to predict breakdowns in understanding. Together, they can assist student learning.

Table 9–4. *continued*

Component	Description
Data Collection	• During lesson planning, a collaborative team decides what data are to be collected and in what manner. • Examples include tally data (a + / − system), narrative data useful for qualifying a process (e.g., noting how a student decodes unfamiliar words when reading a passage), videotapes of classroom interaction, journal entries, homework assignments, etc.
Material Preparation	• Preparing materials is divided equally among team members.
Follow-up Planning	• Follow-up can be implemented through homework, class work, or pull-out therapy.

Source: Adapted from "Collaborative Partnerships in a Language in the Classroom Program," by P. A. Prelock, B. E. Miller, & N. L. Reed, 1995, *Language, Speech, and Hearing Services in Schools, 26,* 286–292.

Based on these lesson plan components, an example of a collaborative lesson plan adapted from Prelock, Miller, and Reed (1995) is presented in Table 9–5. It is an SLP-ESOL team lesson plan designed for an EL with a communication disorder. The lesson plan contains the targeted curriculum, lists the targeted speech-language goals, as well as the facilitating techniques to address those goals. In addition, the lesson plan details the lesson procedures, targeted vocabulary, materials used, and indicates what types of data are to be collected.

The Power of Two + : Making Administrators Part of the Collaborative Process

It is true that the major players in an SLP-ESOL collaborative initiative are the SLPs and ESOL professionals, but administrators are important and powerful team members. Administrative

Table 9–5. *Example of Collaborative Lesson Plan*

<table>
<tr><td colspan="2" align="center">

Collaborative Classroom Lesson Plan

Grade: Kindergarten   Area: ESOL

PLANNING

Roles During Planning for EL with a Communication Disorder

Facilitator/Time Manager: SLP   Recorder: ESOL Professional

CLASSROOM INSTRUCTION/INTERVENTION

Roles During Classroom Instruction/Intervention

Leader: SLP

Partner: ESOL Professional

Data Collector: ESOL Professional

Establishing Current Collaborative Concerns:

need to get identified child involved; need strategies for turn taking and establishing eye contact

all children having difficulty understanding and applying letter-sound knowledge; need to develop metalinguistic skills

</td></tr>
<tr><td>

Targeted Curriculum Goals
</td><td>

• Students will identify and differentiate between symbols (e.g., letters, numbers).
</td></tr>
<tr><td>

Targeted Speech-Language Goals
</td><td>

• Students will recognize that symbols have meaning.

• Student will increase attention to the speaker and participation in class discussions.

• Student will increase use of intelligible speech when answering questions.
</td></tr>
<tr><td>

Facilitating Techniques
</td><td>

• ESOL professional will sit by student with a communication disorder to prompt attention.

• ESOL professional will correct production of back sounds using "hand to throat" cue.
</td></tr>
</table>

Table 9–5. continued

Brainstorming Activities	
Procedures	1. Discuss the meaning of symbols. 2. Have students identify the symbol or signs they see (e.g., restroom, street signs, fire drill, etc.). 3. Walk around school to find various symbols: take photographs or make drawings for inside vs. outside, restrooms, exit, wet floor, arrows for directions, traffic light, crosswalk, and poison. 4. Define symbols as signs that have meaning and can look like pictures, numbers, or letters.
Targeted Vocabulary	• symbol • letter • sign • sound
Materials	• photos/drawings of signs/symbols
Data Collection	1. Tally the number of times the student raises hand to volunteer and makes eye contact with leader. 2. Tally the number of times the student produces back sounds and is intelligible 3. Describe students' understanding of signs/symbols and the application to letters/sounds.
Follow-Up	1. Discuss the words and/or numbers on photos of signs that give the signs meaning. 2. Prepare a homework assignment that requires student to draw a sign found in their home/neighborhood. Student will provide the meaning of chosen sign.

Source: Adapted from "Collaborative Partnerships in a Language in the Classroom Program," by P. A. Prelock, B. E. Miller, & N. L. Reed, 1995, *Language, Speech, and Hearing Services in Schools, 26,* 286–292.

support is critical to the success of collaboration between SLPs and ESOL professionals. Administrators' engagement in and support of collaboration are constantly cited in research as factors that have a strong influence on the success of professional collaboration (Honigsfield & Dove, 2010). Many elements of effective collaboration, ranging from simple verbal encouragement to release time and money, are contingent on school administrators that are committed to supporting collaborative, inclusive learning environments for ELs. Given the importance of the role of the administrator in developing a school culture that promotes collaborative instructional practices, it is critical to consider how the SLP and ESOL team engage administrators to support professional collaboration.

Rea (2005) has several suggestions that the SLP-ESOL team should consider for the successful integration of administrators in the team's collaborative efforts. First, the SLP-ESOL team should involve administrators from the incipient stages of team building and goal setting. The SLP-ESOL team should share with administrators the team's long- and short-term implementation strategies, the research base that supports the instruction, and the anticipated need for resources. SLP and ESOL professionals should not assume that administrators know everything there is to know about collaboration, or the practices that the SLP and ESOL professional can engage in to collaboratively ensure the success of ELs and, specifically, ELs with communication disorders. Information about evidence-based practices and successful collaboration models should be shared.

Once the instruction process has started and the goals have been established, the SLP-ESOL team should schedule an observation. A preobservation conference is recommended so that administrators and the team can discuss the purpose of the observation and what the role and responsibility of each professional will be in the specific context. Setting specific times for observations increases the likelihood that the administrator will have an opportunity to see the team combine their competencies, knowledge, and skills to facilitate the success of ELs. The team will also have the opportunity to highlight specific aspects of their initiative. After observations, the teams should ask administrators for feedback on the team's performance, and incorporate their suggestions in future collaborative initiatives. If administrators cannot participate in class observations, the team can videotape their class and share particularly interesting segments with their administrator. It's important not only to choose positive instances but also to share problematic examples. This will provide administrators with the opportunity to provide feedback and constructive criticism.

The SLP-ESOL team should also make a special effort to involve parents as collaborators and contributors. To improve participation, collaboration, and service delivery with families from diverse backgrounds, professionals must understand and respect their culturally specific beliefs and values (Garcia, Mendez-Perez, & Ortiz, 2000; Kummerer, Lopez-Reyna, & Hughes, 2007; Lian & Fantanez-Phelan, 2001; Rodriguez & Olswang, 2003; Salas-Provance, Erickson, & Reed, 2002). Barriers to successful parental collaboration have been categorized as logistical or attitudinal (Nathenson-Mejia, 1994; Navarette, 1996; Violand-Sanchez, Sutton, & Ware, 1991). When working with diverse parents it is critical that professionals identify these potential barriers (i.e., language, time, money, safety, child care concerns, and investing in strategies to foster parent decision making.

Professional development is an area where the SLP-ESOL team can involve administrators quite extensively. Numerous professional development opportunities are available at the local, state, or national level. The SLP-ESOL-administrator team can share their initiatives on successful collaborations with other professionals in the field and obtain feedback from their colleagues with similar challenges and initiatives.

Creating collaborative environments is not an easy task. It requires effort, dedication, and action on everyone's part to include administrators. SLP and ESOL professionals should encourage administrators to be a leader in collaborative efforts. Without the explicit support of administrators, the success of the SLP-ESOL team is questionable, and can be a barrier in creating a supportive learning environment for ELs with a communication disorder.

Summary and Final Thoughts

In Chapter 1, we introduced the case of Rey, the 7-year-old EL in a second grade English-only classroom. We noted that he had behavior problems and did not always participate in class tasks.

Rey's oral language proficiency test results showed that he was limited in both English and Spanish. A bilingual general language performance test indicated that his Spanish performance was normal but his English performance was below average. The various professionals working with Rey needed to determine if he had a communication disorder; a disability; or if his school performance was related to his limited English proficiency and perhaps other factors. Rey's dilemma was offered as an example of circumstances that require professionals to have the valuable information presented in this book. Given the information presented in the subsequent chapters, Rey's situation is best addressed through the collaboration of the SLPs and ESOL professionals at his school. Collaborative partnerships between SLPs and ESOL professionals have very important implications for how school SLPs and ESOL professionals might approach assessment and classroom interventions for ELs and, specifically, ELs with communication disorders in the school setting.

Chapter 2 presented some of the challenges faced by SLPs and ESOL professionals in working with ELs. The professional organizations of both disciplines, ASHA and TESOL, provide recommended competencies and preferred practices used within each discipline to guide each professional. Well-prepared professionals in both fields would be familiar with the content of Chapter 3, which described the general EL population in the United States and offered definitions of the categories of ELs, as well as ELs with communication disorders.

Chapter 4 laid the foundational knowledge for analyzing whether Rey's English language development shows tendencies of a disorder or if it follows a normal process, offering an in-depth explanation of second language acquisition. In order for SLPs to conduct an accurate assessment of a communication disorder, they must be able to distinguish normal progression in a second language from those aspects of language that are characteristic of a communication disorder. When professionals are familiar with the natural variation in the language acquisition process and the different contexts of acquiring the language, they can begin to identify any traits that fall outside the expected range. Making a decision about a language disorder is a process that should take place over time, with multiple opportunities for observing and analyzing the student's language use. Knowing what to look for and documenting students' strengths and weaknesses is an important step in the identification of potential disorders.

Building on the information learned about general second language acquisition, Chapter 5 offered a definition of literacy and provided an overview of literacy development in ELs. Although there are many commonalities between first and second language reading and writing, a number of distinctions exist that could affect Rey's literacy skills. SLPs and ESOL professionals learned in Chapter 5 that they should pay attention to Rey's literacy in Spanish, oral language proficiency in English, age of arrival to the US mainland, expectations of the school experience, and his parents' educational levels. In addition, the first language issues that affect his literacy development in English include the contrasts between the English and Spanish languages, Rey's vocabulary knowledge in both languages, and his awareness of language in both English and Spanish, among other factors (Anderson, 2008). All these variables must be considered to determine if his performance is a result of a communication disorder or related to his stage of second language acquisition.

Understanding the definition of language proficiency and the importance of identification practices and protocols used by SLPs and ESOL professionals to determine language proficiency were the focus of Chapters 6 and 7. Rey's SLPs and ESOL professionals learned about specific standardized tests, alternative assessment protocols and procedures, and types of accommodations used to assess ELs and ELs with communication disorders. Chapter 7 concluded with a discussion on the importance of using multiple data sources to determine if Rey has a communication disorder or is demonstrating characteristics of a second language learner.

Because one focus of this text is literacy, in Chapter 8 we explored the various approaches and practical strategies in literacy instruction. By combining theory, research, and practice, we have explored several instructional strategies used in the instruction of ELs and adapted for use with ELs with communication disorders. Classroom practices and practical strategies to facilitate and support Rey's literacy development are offered as ways that can be used to improve his phonemic awareness, knowledge of phonics, fluency, vocabulary, and text comprehension.

In addition, suggestions were provided to Rey's professional team on how they can work together to facilitate his oral language and writing development.

To understand the basis of educational decisions made during the literacy instruction of ELs with communication disorders, we focused on the critical role of the SLP and ESOL professional in working with ELs in Chapter 9. Specifically, we highlighted the advantages and importance of collaboration in the four key components of literacy development for ELs with communication disorders (Figure 9–1). For example, one result of SLP-ESOL teamwork is that SLPs know what the literacy curriculum goals and classroom expectations are and ESOL professionals are more aware of how communication disorders affect the classroom performance of ELs. SLPs provide techniques to facilitate

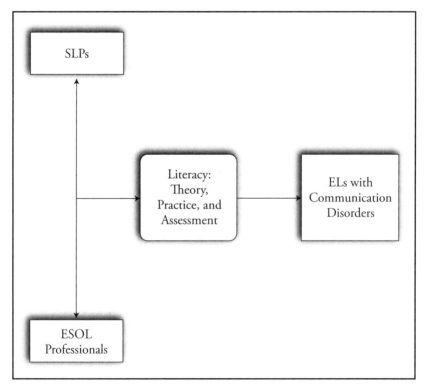

Figure 9–1. *Four key components of literacy development for ELs with communication disorders.*

language and literacy development in ELs with communication disorders. By building on these techniques, ESOL professionals can continue to address the communication needs of ELs with communication disorders through the provision of modified instruction and feedback.

The collaborative power of two professionals, the SLP and the ESOL professional, ensures continuity in practice and across settings, with the goal of ensuring that ELs with communication disorders succeed in the classroom. By collecting data on effective language and literacy interventions for ELs and collaboration situations, we can base our instructional decisions on evidence-based research. The benefits of this type of research effort are enormous and can only contribute in a positive manner to the success of literacy acquisition for ELs with communication disorders.

References

American Speech-Language-Hearing Association. (1983). Position paper: Social dialects and implications of the position on social dialects. *ASHA, 25*(9), 23–27.

American Speech-Language-Hearing Association. (1985). Clinical management of communicatively handicapped minority language populations. *ASHA, 27*(6), 29–32.

American Speech-Language-Hearing Association. (1989). Bilingual speech-language pathologists and audiologists. *ASHA, 31*, 93.

American Speech-Language-Hearing Association. (1993, March). Definitions of communication disorders and variations. *ASHA, 35*(Suppl. 10), 40–41.

American Speech-Language-Hearing Association. (1996, Spring). Scope of practice in speech-language pathology. *ASHA, 38*(Suppl. 16), 16–20.

American Speech-Language-Hearing Association. (1998). *Provision of instruction in English as a Second language by speech-language pathologists in school settings* [Position statement]. Retrieved from www.asha.org/policy

American Speech-Language-Hearing Association. (2004). *Preferred practice patterns for the profession of speech-language pathology.* Retrieved from www.asha.org/policy

American Speech-Language-Hearing Association. (2010). *Roles and responsibilities of speech-language pathologists in schools* [Professional issues statement]. Retrieved from www.asha.org/policy

American Speech-Language-Hearing Association. (2011). *Cultural competence in professional service delivery* [Professional issues statement]. Retrieved from www.asha.org/policy

Anderson, N. (2008). *Active skills for reading, book 3* (2nd ed.). Boston, MA: Heinle Cengage.

DeGuerrero, M. C., & Villamil, O. S. (2000). Exploring ESL teachers' roles through metaphoranalysis. *TESOL Quarterly*, *34*, 341–351.

Friend, M., & Cook, L. (2000). *Interactions: Collaboration skills for school professionals* (3rd ed.). New York, NY: Addison Wesley Longman.

Garcia, S. B., Mendez-Perez, A. M., & Ortiz, A. A. (2000). Mexican American mothers' beliefs about disabilities: Implications for early childhood intervention. *Remedial and Special Education*, *21*, 90–100.

Honigsfeld, A., & Dove, M. (2010). *Collaboration and co-teaching strategies for English learners*. Thousand Oaks, CA: Sage.

Individuals with Disabilities Education Act. (2004). Pub. L. No. 108-446, 118 Stat. 2647.

Kummerer, S. E., Lopez-Reyna, N. A., & Hughes, M. T. (2007). Mexican immigrant mothers' perceptions of their children's communication disabilities, emergent literacy development, and speech-language therapy program. *American Journal of Speech-Language Pathology*, *16*(3), 271–282.

Lian, M., & Fantanez-Phelan, S. (2001). Perceptions of Latino parents regarding cultural and linguistic issues and advocacy for children with disabilities. *Journal of the Association for Persons with Severe Handicaps*, *26*, 189–194.

Lowe, J., & Herranen, M. (1978). Conflict in teamwork: Understanding roles and relationship. *Social Work in Health Care*, *3*, 323–331.

Lowe, J., & Herranen, M. (1982). Understanding teamwork: Another look at the concepts. *Social Work in Health Care*, *7*, 1–11.

McCartney, E. (1999). Barriers to collaboration: An analysis of systemic barriers to collaboration between teachers and speech and language therapists. *International Journal of Language and Communication Disorders*, *34*, 431–440.

Moore-Brown, B., & Montgomery, J. K. (2001). *Making a difference for America's children: Speech-language pathologists in public schools*. Eau Claire, WI: Thinking.

National Governor's Association. (2011). *Realizing the potential: How governors can lead effective implementation of the Common Core State Standards*. Washington, D.C. Retrieved from http://www.nga.org/cms/home/nga-center-for-best-practices/center-publications/

page-edu-publications/col2-content/main-content-list/realizing-the-potential-how-gove.html

Nathenson-Mejia, S. (1994). Bridges between home and school: Literacy building activities for non-native English speaking homes. *Journal of Educational Issues of Language Minority Students, 14,* 149–164.

Navarette, Y. G. (1996). Family involvement in a bilingual school. *Journal of Educational Issues of Language Minority Students, 6,* 77–84.

Pena, E. D., & Quinn R. (2003). Developing effective collaboration teams in speech-language pathology: A case study. *Communications Disorders Quarterly, 24*(2), 53–63.

Prelock, P. A., Miller, B. E., & Reed, N. L. (1995). Collaborative partnerships in a language in the classroom program. *Language, Speech, and Hearing Services in Schools, 26,* 286–292.

Rea, P. J. (2005). Engage your administrator in your collaboration initiative. *Intervention in School and Clinic, 40*(5), 312–316.

Roache, M., Shore, J., Gouleta, E., & Butkevich, E. (2003). An investigation of collaboration among school professionals in serving culturally and linguistically diverse students with exceptionalities. *Bilingual Research Journal, 27*(1), 117–136.

Rodriguez, B. L., & Olswang, L. B. (2003). Mexican-American and Anglo-American mothers' beliefs and values about child rearing, education, and language impairment. *American Journal of Speech-Language Pathology, 12*(4), 452–462.

Rosa-Lugo, L. I., & Fradd, S. (2000). Preparing professionals to serve English-language learners with communication disorders. *Communication Disorders Quarterly, 22*(1), 29–42.

Salas-Provance, M., Erickson, J., & Reed, J. (2002). Disabilities as viewed by four generations of one Hispanic family. *American Journal of Speech-Language Patholo*gy, *11,* 151–162.

Tuckman, B., & Jensen, M. (1977). Stages of small group development revisited. *Group and Organizational Studies, 2,* 419–427.

Violand-Sanchez, E., Sutton, C. P., & Ware, H. W. (1991, Summer). *Fostering home-school cooperation: Involving language minority families as partners in education.* Washington, DC: National Clearinghouse on Bilingual Education.

A

ASHA and TESOL
Position Statements

- ◆ Appendix A1: ASHA Position Statements, Guidelines, and Technical Reports

- ◆ Appendix A2: TESOL Position Statements and Guidelines in Multicultural Populations

Purposeful collaboration by SLPs and ESOL professionals *in the identification, assessment, and management of* ELs and ELs with communication disorders requires competencies, knowledge, and skills to implement research-based practices. The American Speech-Language-Hearing Association (ASHA) and Teachers of English to Speakers of Other Languages (TESOL), professional associations, take official positions on a broad range of issues. Specifically, each discipline provides official documents that outline the guidelines and parameters of each profession in working with ELs.

Appendix A1 provides the links to ASHA position statements, guidelines, and technical reports. Appendix A2 provides the links to TESOL position statements and guidelines.

A 1
ASHA Position Statements, Guidelines, and Technical Reports

Communication Development and Disorders in Multicultural Populations

American Speech-Language-Hearing Association. (1983). *Social dialects* [Position statement]. Retrieved from www.asha.org/policy

American Speech-Language-Hearing Association. (1985). *Clinical management of communicatively handicapped minority language populations* [Position statement]. Retrieved from www.asha.org/policy

American Speech-Language-Hearing Association. (1989). *Bilingual speech-language pathologists and audiologists: Definition* [Relevant paper]. Retrieved from www.asha.org/policy

American Speech-Language-Hearing Association. (1993). *Definitions of communication disorders and variations* [Relevant paper]. Retrieved from www.asha.org/policy

American Speech-Language-Hearing Association. (1998a). *Provision of instruction in English as a second language by speech-language pathologists in school settings* [Position statement]. Retrieved from www.asha.org/policy

American Speech-Language-Hearing Association. (1998b). *Provision of instruction in English as a second language by speech-language pathologists in school settings* [Position statement]. Retrieved from www.asha.org/policy

American Speech-Language-Hearing Association. (1998c). *Students and professionals who speak English with accents and nonstandard dialects: Issues and recommendations* [Position statement]. Retrieved from www.asha.org/policy

American Speech-Language-Hearing Association. (1998d). *Students and professionals who speak English with accents and nonstandard dialects: Issues and recommendations* [Technical report]. Retrieved from www. asha.org/policy

American Speech-Language-Hearing Association. (2000). *Guidelines for the roles and responsibilities of the school-based speech-language pathologist* [Guidelines]. Retrieved from www.asha.org/policy

American Speech-Language-Hearing Association. (2001a). *Roles and responsibilities of speech-language pathologists with respect to reading and writing in children and adolescents* [Position statement]. Retrieved from www.asha.org/policy

American Speech-Language-Hearing Association. (2001b). *Roles and responsibilities of speech-language pathologists with respect to reading and writing in children and adolescents* [Technical report]. Retrieved from www.asha.org/policy

American Speech-Language-Hearing Association. (2002). *Knowledge and skills needed by speech-language pathologists with respect to reading and writing in children and adolescents* [Knowledge and skills]. Retrieved from www.asha.org/policy

American Speech-Language-Hearing Association. (2003). *American English dialects* [Technical report]. Retrieved from www.asha.org/policy

American Speech-Language-Hearing Association. (2004a). *Knowledge and skills needed by speech-language pathologists and audiologists to provide culturally and linguistically appropriate services* [Knowledge and skills]. Retrieved from www.asha.org/policy

American Speech-Language-Hearing Association. (2004b). *Preferred practice patterns for the profession of speech-language pathology* [Preferred practice patterns]. Retrieved from www.asha.org/policy

American Speech-Language-Hearing Association. (2005). *Cultural competence* [Issues in ethics]. Retrieved from www.asha.org/policy

American Speech-Language-Hearing Association. (2010a). *Roles and responsibilities of speech-language pathologists in schools* [Position statement]. Retrieved from www.asha.org/policy.

American Speech-Language-Hearing Association. (2010b). *Roles and responsibilities of speech-language pathologists in schools* [Professional issues statement]. Retrieved from www.asha.org/policy

American Speech-Language-Hearing Association. (2011a). *Cultural competence in professional service delivery* [Position statement]. Retrieved from www.asha.org/policy

American Speech-Language-Hearing Association. (2011b). *Cultural competence in professional service delivery* [Professional issues statement]. Retrieved from www.asha.org/policy

American Speech-Language-Hearing Association. (2011c). *The clinical education of students with accents* [Professional issues statement]. Retrieved from www.asha.org/policy

Code of Fair Testing Practices in Education. (2004). Washington, DC: Joint Committee on Testing Practices. Retrieved from http://www.asha.org/docs/html/RP2004-00195.html

A2

TESOL Position Statements and Guidelines in Multicultural Populations

Teachers of English to Speakers of Other Languages (TESOL). (1996). *Position statement of the TESOL board on language varieties*. Retrieved from http://www.tesol.org/s_tesol/sec_document.asp?CID=32&DID=381

Teachers of English to Speakers of Other Languages (TESOL). (1997). *Position statement of the TESOL board on African American vernacular English*. Retrieved from http://www.tesol.org/s_tesol/sec_document.asp?CID=32&DID=379

Teachers of English to Speakers of Other Languages (TESOL). (1999a). *Position statement on native language support in the acquisition of English as a second language (ESL)*. Retrieved from http://www.tesol.org/s_tesol/sec_document.asp?CID=32&DID=382

Teachers of English to Speakers of Other Languages (TESOL). (1999b). *Position statement on the acquisition of academic proficiency in English*. Retrieved from http://www.tesol.org/s_tesol/bin.asp?CID=32&DID=378&DOC=FILE.PDF

Teachers of English to Speakers of Other Languages (TESOL). (2000a). *Assessment and accountability of English for speakers of other languages (ESOL) students*. Retrieved from http://www.tesol.org/s_tesol/sec_document.asp?CID=32&DID=369

Teachers of English to Speakers of Other Languages (TESOL). (2000b). *Position paper on family involvement in the education of English for speakers of other languages (ESOL) students*. Retrieved from http://www.tesol.org/s_tesol/sec_document.asp?CID=32&DID=370

Teachers of English to Speakers of Other Languages (TESOL). (2003a). *Position statement on the preparation of pre-K–12 educators for cultural and linguistic diversity in the United States*. Retrieved from http://www.tesol.org/s_tesol/bin.asp?CID=32&DID=1301&DOC=FILE.PDF

Teachers of English to Speakers of Other Languages (TESOL). (2003b). *Position statement on teacher quality in the field of teaching English to speakers of other languages*. Retrieved from http://www.tesol.org/s_tesol/bin.asp?CID=32&DID=374&DOC=FILE.PDF

Teachers of English to Speakers of Other Languages (TESOL). (2003c). *Position paper on high-stakes testing for K–12 English language learners in the United States of America.* Retrieved from http://www. tesol.org/s_tesol/bin.asp?CID=32&DID=375&DOC=FILE.PDF

Teachers of English to Speakers of Other Languages (TESOL). (2004). *Position statement on multilingualism.* Retrieved from http://www. tesol.org/s_tesol/bin.asp?CID=32&DID=2933&DOC=FILE.PDF

Teachers of English to Speakers of Other Languages (TESOL). (2005a). *Position paper on assessment and accountability under NCLB.* Retrieved from http://www.tesol.org/s_tesol/bin.asp?CID=32&DID =4720&DOC=FILE.PDF

Teachers of English to Speakers of Other Languages (TESOL). (2005b). *Position statement on research and policy.* Retrieved from http:// www.tesol.org/s_tesol/bin.asp?CID=32&DID=3401&DOC=FILE.PDF

Teachers of English to Speakers of Other Languages (TESOL). (2005c). *Position statement on highly qualified teachers under No Child Left Behind.* Retrieved from http://www.tesol.org/s_tesol/bin.asp?CID=32 &DID=3400&DOC=FILE.PDF

Teachers of English to Speakers of Other Languages (TESOL). (2006a). *Position statement on the diversity of English language learners in the United States.* Retrieved from http://www.tesol.org/s_tesol/bin. asp?CID=32&DID=7212&DOC=FILE.PDF

Teachers of English to Speakers of Other Languages (TESOL). (October 2006b, amended October 2007). *Statement of principles and preliminary recommendations for the reauthorization of the elementary and secondary education act.* Retrieved from http://www.tesol. org/s_tesol/bin.asp?CID=32&DID=7211&DOC=FILE.PDF

Teachers of English to Speakers of Other Languages (TESOL). (2007a). *Position statement on teacher credentialing for teachers of English to speakers of other languages in primary and secondary schools.* Retrieved from http://www.tesol.org/s_tesol/bin.asp?CID=32&DID =8863&DOC=FILE.PDF

Teachers of English to Speakers of Other Languages (TESOL). (2007b). *Position statement on the identification of English language learners with special educational needs.* Retrieved from http://www.tesol .org/s_tesol/bin.asp?CID=32&DID=8283&DOC=FILE.PDF

Teachers of English to Speakers of Other Languages (TESOL). (2008). *Position statement on teacher preparation for content-based instruction.* Retrieved from http://www.tesol.org/s_tesol/bin.asp?CID=32 &DID=10882&DOC=FILE.PDF

Teachers of English to Speakers of Other Languages (TESOL). (2010a). *Position statement on the acquisition of academic proficiency in English at the postsecondary level.* Retrieved from http://www.tesol. org/s_tesol/bin.asp?CID=32&DID=13489&DOC=FILE.PDF

Teachers of English to Speakers of Other Languages (TESOL). (2010b). *Position paper on language and literacy development for young English language learners (ages 3–8)*. Retrieved from http://www.tesol.org/s_tesol/bin.asp?CID=32&DID=371&DOC=FILE.PDF

Teachers of English to Speakers of Other Languages (TESOL). (2011). *Increasing academic achievement and enhancing capacity for English language learners: Principles and recommendations for the reauthorization of the Elementary and Secondary Education Act.* Retrieved from http://www.tesol.org/s_tesol/bin.asp?CID=32&DID=13611&DOC=FILE.PDF

B
Professional Standards

◆ Appendix B1: ASHA Standards for the Certificate of Clinical Competence

◆ Appendix B2: TESOL/NCATE Standards for P–12 Teacher Education Programs

B1
ASHA Standards for the Certificate of Clinical Competence

The American Speech-Language-Hearing Association (ASHA) has defined a list of standards that must be acquired by graduate students in the course of their education and training. These standards ensure that new professionals to the field have the required experience, skills, and knowledge to effectively enter the workforce and to serve as innovators in the field.

ASHA Standard	Description
Standard III-B:	Knowledge of basic human communication and swallowing processes, including their biological, neurological, acoustic, psychological, developmental, and linguistic and cultural bases.
Standard III-C:	Knowledge of the nature of speech, language, hearing, and communication disorders and differences and swallowing disorders, including the etiologies, characteristics, anatomical/physiological, acoustic, psychological, developmental, and linguistic and cultural correlates.
Standard III-D:	Knowledge of the principles and methods of prevention, assessment, and intervention for people with communication and swallowing disorders, including consideration of anatomical/physiological, psychological, developmental, and linguistic and cultural correlates of the disorders.
Standard III-F:	Knowledge of processes used in research and the integration of research principles into evidence-based clinical practice.
Standard III-G:	Knowledge of contemporary professional issues.

ASHA Standard	Description
Standard IV-G:	Inclusion of supervised clinical experiences sufficient in breadth and depth to achieve the following skills outcomes: evaluation, intervention, and interaction and personal qualities.

For a complete list of Knowledge and Skills (KASA) requirements and objectives to prepare speech-language pathologists to meet competencies to work with English language learners, please see:

American Speech-Language-Hearing Association. (n.d.). *2005 standards and implementation procedures for the Certificate of Clinical Competence in speech-language pathology. Revised 2009.* Retrieved from http://www.asha.org/Certification/slp_standards/

B2
TESOL/NCATE Standards for P–12 Teacher Education Programs

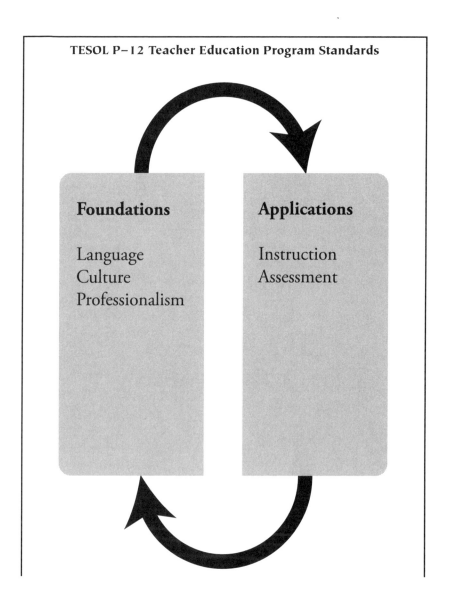

TESOL P–12 Teacher Education Program Standards

Foundations

Language
Culture
Professionalism

Applications

Instruction
Assessment

Language	Language as a system
	Language acquisition and development
Culture	Culture as it affects learning
Professionalism	Research and history
	Professional development, collaboration and advocacy
Instruction	Planning, implementing, and managing standards-based instruction for ELs in ESOL and content area classes
	Using resources and technology
Assessment	Language proficiency assessment for ELs
	Classroom-based assessment for ELs
	EL-specific assessment issues (accommodations, standardized tests, etc.)

For more information, see *TESOL/NCATE Standards for the Recognition of Initial TESOL Programs in P–12 ESL Teacher Education,* by Teachers of English to Speakers of Other Languages (TESOL) (http://www.tesol.org/s_tesol/seccss.asp?CID=219&DID=1689).

Index